Unsupervised Learning

Computational Neuroscience

Terrence J. Sejnowski and Tomaso A. Poggio, editors

Unsupervised Learning: Foundations of Neural Computation

edited by Geoffrey Hinton and Terrence J. Sejnowski

A Bradford Book
The MIT Press
Cambridge, Massachusetts
London, England

Library of Congress Cataloging-in-Publication Data

Unsupervised learning : foundations of neural computation / edited
 by Geoffrey Hinton and Terrence J. Sejnowski.
    p.   cm.—(Computational neuroscience)
 "A Bradford book."
 Includes bibliographical references and index.
 ISBN 978-0-262-58168-4 (pb.)
 1. Learning—Physiological aspects. 2. Neural networks.
3. Learning—Computer simulation. 4. Neural computers. I. Hinton,
Geoffrey E. II. Sejnowski, Terrence J. (Terrence Joseph) III. Series.
QP408.U57   1998
612.8'2—dc21   98-14784
                                                                     CIP
The MIT Press is pleased to keep this title available in print by manufacturing single copies, on demand, via digital printing technology.

CONTENTS

Introduction

Consider the problem of getting a neural network to associate an appropriate response with an image sequence. The obvious approach is to use supervised training. If the network has around 10^{14} parameters and only lives for around 10^9 seconds, the supervision signal had better contain at least 10^5 bits per second to make use of the capacity of the synapses. It is not immediately obvious where such a rich supervision signal could come from.

A more promising approach depends on the observation that images are not random but are generated by physical processes of limited complexity and that the appropriate response to an image nearly always depends on the physical causes of the image rather than the pixel intensities. This suggests that an unsupervised learning process should be used to solve the difficult problem of extracting the underlying causes, and decisions about responses can be left to a separate learning algorithm that takes the underlying causes rather than the saw sensory data as its inputs. Unsupervised learning can usually be viewed as a method of modeling the probability density of the inputs, so the rich sensory input itself can provide the 10^5 bits per second of constraint that is required to amke use of the capacity of the synapses.

The papers in this collection provide a sample of research on unsupervised learning. Some areas and important contributions are not represented either because an appropriate paper did not appear in *Neural Computation* or because of the limited space that was available. One entire area of research in unsupervised learning, self-organizing map formation, will appear as a separate volume in this series. Despite these limitations, the wide range of approaches that is included here serves as a guide to the development of the field of unsupervised learning.

Redundancy Reduction

One of the earliest formulations of unsupervised learning in the context of vision was the concept of redundancy reduction (Attneave 1954; Barlow 59; Barlow 1989). The goal was to find ways to compress the information contained in images, a goal that was also pursued in the commercial reduce the bandwidth needed to transmit images. In the case of visual system, information in the array of photoreceptors in the h number around 100 million, is compressed and represented s in around 1 million ganglion cells whose axons form the k and Redlich (1993) used an entropy reduction measure to er-surround receptive fields found in ganglion cells are optimal when the mapping is linear and the redundant information in the second-order correlations is removed. This was achieved by having lateral inhibition between neighboring cells.

Linsker (1986) had earlier shown that the same center-surround geometry for the receptive fields could be obtained in the context of a feedforward neural network that used a Hebbian form of synaptic plasticity. This approach, which he called "infomax," used a simple unsupervised Hebbian learning algorithm in the presence of noise on the inputs of the network and converged to the connection strengths needed for the center-surround geometry. It is unlikely that this learning mechanism is actually used in the retina, but it demonstrates that the response properties of neurons can be achieved with local learning rules and transmit visual images in an optimal way, in the sense defined by Atick and Redlich (1993).

Hebbian learning at a synapse depends jointly on the activity of the presynaptic neuron and the postsynaptic neuron. It is a biologically plausible leaning rule because it depends only on signals that are locally available at the synapse. Forms of Hebbian plasticity have been found in the hippocampus (Brown, Kairiss, and Keenan 1990) and the neocortex (Markram, Lubke, Frotscher, and Sakmann 1997).

Hebbian synapses are sensitive to information contained in the second-order correlations of the inputs. Zhang et al. (1993) demonstrate that properties of motion selective cells in the visual cortex, far removed from the retina, can also be understood using Hebbian synaptic plasticity in a feedforward network. The development of the visual cortex can also be modeled by a network with Hebbian plasticity (Miller, Keller and Stryker 1989; Obermayer and Sejnowski 1998).

Maximizing Mutual Information _____

There are many possible objective functions for unsupervised learning, each of which can be optimized to produce a representation that is particularly good at achieving some goal. In the case of reducing redundancy this means eliminating correlations and producing a compact code for the input. Linsker (1992) showed that a form of Hebbian learning was able to maximize the mutual information between the inputs and the outputs of a feedforward network in the presence of noise. The learning algorithm has two phases for learning, with the inputs present during the first phase of Hebbian learning and absent during the second, anti-Hebbian phase in which the sign of earning is reversed. The second phase is needed to calibrate the correlations that are induced in the output units by the intrinsic noise on the inputs. Sphased leraning algorithms were introduced by Crick and Mitchison (1983) and Hopfield, Feinstein, and Palmer (1983) for recurrent attractor networks that stored memories as stable states of the network, and for Boltzmann machines, which have hidden units to learn the higher-order structure of the inputs (Hinton and Sejnowski 1986).

Another way to detect higher-order structure of the inputs is to have a multilayer network and to introduce an objective function that measures coherence between different output units. Becker and Hinton (1993) introduced an objective function for maximizing the information that parameters extracted from different parts of an extended sensory input convey about some common underlying cause. The model used columns of feedforward networks and was able to detect disparity as an underlying cause from sterograms presented on the inputs. The learning algorithm, however, was quite complex and required the propagation of global information in the network to optimize the objective function.

In a movie, the temporal sequence of images is correlated and additional information can be extracted by lookking for temporal as well as spatial structure. For example, a movie of a rigidly moving object contains highly redundant information because the image of the object will appear in slightly different spatial locations on successive frames of the movie. Földiák (1991) showed how this translation invariance can be captured in simple feedforward network that used Hebbian synapses and an output layer of units with a short-term memory of previous inputs. The network was trained with moving lines and the response properties of neurons in the network were similar to those found in the visual cortex. This principle was generalized by Stone (1996), who applied it to learning stereo disparity from dynamic stereograms.

Independent Component Analysis _____

Neurons in the visual cortex have receptive fields that are compact and elongated, so that the best stimulus is often a thin bar or edge of light (Hubel and Wiesel 1968). The simple cells have separate excitatory and inhibitory subregions. Barlow conjectured that these neurons formed feature detectors that were maximally independent over the ensemble of natural images. Independence is a much stronger property than second-order decorrelation since independence entails that all higher-order correlations between pixels in the ensemble of images must also be zero. Field (1994) recognized that the output values of the feature detectors ought to have a sparse distribution with high kurtosis (many values near zero and a few quite high values). Field and Olshausen (1994) showed that an unsupervised learning algorithm that maximized sparseness produced visual feature detectors that resembled those found in the visual cortex.

Unsupervised learning algorithms have recently been found developed for finding independent components in linear mixtures and blind signal separation (Comon 1994). An efficient algorithm for Independent Component Analysis (ICA) of super-Gaussian signals was derived by Bell and Sejnowski (1995) from Linsker's infomax principle. When applied to natural images, ICA developed localized edge and and bar detectors similar to the simple cells that are found in the visual cortex (Bell and Sejnowski 1997). Amari

(1997) provided an improvement for speeding up this learning algorithm, and Lee, Girolami, and Sejnowski (1999) have extended it to sub-Gaussian sources. Other fast ICA algorithms have also been developed (Hyrarinen and Oja 1997). One of the advantages of these algorithms is that they are able to separate non-Gaussian sources, which are common in auditory and visual signal processing. One of the limitations is that the source model is linear and is not capable of adequately representing visual images with occlusion and other structured properties.

Clustering and Dimensionality Reduction

The goal of clustering is to group together similar inputs. Many algorithms exist for clustering in low-dimensional spaces, but the problem becomes more difficult as the dimensionality increases. Platt (1991) introduced an on-line clustering method that progressively adjusts the prototypes for each new input and adds a new prototype when none of the existing ones is sufficiently close by. This is an example of a constructive learning algorithm that adds resources sequentially as needed during the learning (Fahlman and Lebiere 1990). This approach has the advantage of starting out with relatively few parameters at the outset and avoids overfitting by increasing the number of parameters only when justified by additional inputs.

The distance measures used in most clustering algorithms are typically simple ones such as the Euclidean distance. However, two objects may be similar despite differences in position, orientation, and scale. Clustering with a graph-matching distance measure that incorporates these invariances, and which is also insensitive to permutation and missing data, was introduced by Gold, Rangarajan, and Mjolsness (1996). Their method is computationally efficient and scales well with the dimensionality of the problem.

A standard engineering technique for reducing the dimensionality of the input is to use Principal Component Analysis (PCA). This is computationally efficient, but it suffers from the limitation that the representation in the principal components is linearly related to the original input. A number of different research groups realized that this limitation of PCA can be overcome by combining it with clustering. The idea is to divide the data into clusters in such a way that the points in each cluster lie close to a plane. This can be done by using a simplified version of the expectation-maximization (EM) algorithm (Dempster, Laird, and Rubin, 1977), which alternates between an "E-step" that assigns each datapoint to the closest plane and an "M-step" that refits each plane to all the datapoints that have been assigned to it. Kambhatla and Leen (1997) demonstrate that this piecewise linear approach can be quite effective in modeling nonlinear manifolds. If high-dimensional data is projected onto a randomly oriented line it nearly always has an approximately Gaussian distribution. This suggests that directions in the input space that yield non-Gaussian distributions are interesting and that projections onto these directions would constitute interesting features. Intrator (1992) shows how neurons can discover such directions using a biologically plausible local algorithm called the BCM rule (Bienenstock, Cooper, and Munro, 1982).

Learning Probability Distributions

During supervised learning, each input vector comes with an associated desired output that is supplied by the teacher. Unsupervised learning is often characterized as supervised lerning with an unknown output. This makes it very hard to decide what counts as success and suggests that the central problem is to find a suitable objective function that can replace the goal of agreeing with the teacher. Many apparently different objectives have been proposed:

> Discover clusters in the data.
>
> Discover a mapping from the observed data to a set of pairwise decorrelated or statistically independent features.
>
> Discover temporal or spatial invariances in the data by getting modules to agree with each other.
>
> Discover unlikely coincidences of events whose joint probability far exceeds the product of their individual probabilities.
>
> Discover highly non-Gaussian projections of the data (projection pursuit).

It is less natural, but much more revealing, to view unsupervised learning as supervised learning in which the observed data is the *output* and for which there is no input. This makes it obvious that the model that generates the output must either be stochastic or must have an unknown and varying input in order to avoid producing the same output every time. Given this view, the obvious aim of unsupervised learning is to fit a generative model that gives high likelihood to the observed data.[1] This objective is often accompanied by the hope that the natural causes of the data will come to be represented by the activities of the hidden units.

The introduction of hidden processing units allows a network to represent a larger class of nonlinear functions using latent variables and to extract more complex nonlinear structure from the inputs with unsupervised learning. The Boltzmann machine is a recurrent network of stochastic units

---

[1] The generative model approach is closely related to the idea of finding an efficient code from which the data can be reconstructed, because any model that assigns high probability density to the data can be used for efficient data-compression in which the number of bits required to communicate a data vector approaches the negative log probability of the vector under the generative model.

with symmetric connections between them (Hinton and Sejnowski 1986) for which there is a Hebbian learning algorithm that reduces the Kullback-Liebler distance between the probability distribution of the inputs and that generated by the free-running network. The Boltzmann machine is a generative model in the sense that after learning is complete, the free-running network generates patterns on the input units with the same probability distribution that occurred during the training phase.

A major advantage of the generative approach is that it cleanly separates inference and learning. The inference process is given an observed data vector and a generative model, and assuming that the data came from the model, it computes the posterior probability distribution across the hidden states of the model, or an approximation to the posterior such as a random sample from it or a local peak. The learning process uses the inferred posterior distribution across hidden states to update the parameters of the generative model so that it is more likely to produce the observed data. In some popular and statistically improper generative models, such as principle components or vector quantization, the inference process is simple and can be performed by projection or by a winner-take-all competition. These degenerate cases have tended to conceal the true nature of unsupervised learning.

It is interesting to see how the five objectives above all make sense from the perspective of generative models. Clustering is just fitting a two-stage generative model in which we first make a discrete choice of a mixture component and then generate from a density determined by this component. The distance measure used for clustering corresponds to the negative log probability of the data under a component of the model. The usual hard assignment of a data vector to the closest cluster corresponds to approximating the posterior distribution over the hidden choices by the single most likely choice.

Discovering independent hidden features can be achieved by fitting a generative movel in which the activities of the hidden units are chosen independently. Some particularly tractable special cases arise when the observed data is modeled as a linear combination of the hidden unit activities plus additive Gaussian noise. If the hidden units have Gaussian priors, then this is factor analysis (Neal and Dayan 1997). If the hidden units have improper uniform priors, then it is principal components analysis. If the priors for the hidden units are independent but non-Gaussian, then it is ICA. The inference process for ICA becomes straightforward as the additive Gaussian observation noise goes to zero. For nonzero noise the posterior distribution over hidden states must be approximated, typically by finding its peak.

Discovering temporal invariances is just fitting a dynamical system (without driving inputs) in which the state-transition matrix for the hidden state space is the identity matrix. This makes it obvious that temporal invariance is naturally subsumed by linear dependence over time. If the observed data is modeled as a linear function of the hidden state space then temporal invariants can be learning by fitting a linear dynamical system.

Hidden units that represent unlikely coincidences arise naturally when fitting a generative model to data because they allow common conjunctions to have much higher density than they would get if their constituents were generated separately. The same applies to redundancies in general. An advantage of extracting redundancies by fitting a generative model is that it naturally makes differenet units within a layer do different things. No special decorrelating mechanism is required to make different units grab different redundancies. Also, in a multilayer generative model the lower layers can maximize the probability density of the observed data by extracting redundancies among which there are easily extracted redundancies. There is no necessity for the lower hidden layers to extract features that are fully decorrelated or statistically independent. All that is required is that the features should be statistically independent *given* the features in the layer above. So it makes sense to extract natural causes of images like noses and mouths because they are approximately statistically independent *given the face* even though they are very highly correlated.

Discovering very non-Gaussian projections is just what a linear generative model containing a single hidden unit will do if it is given (or allowed to empirically construct) a non-Gaussian prior for the activity of a hidden unit. Assume that the generative model treats the observed data as the output of the model plus Gaussian noise. To maximize the log likelihood of the data the model needs to account for as much of the variance in the data as possible without using improbable states of the hidden unit and without using large generative weights that dilute the probability density of the hidden activities. So the hidden unit needs to have a lot of variance in its activity but as little entropy as possible. This is a natural definition of what it means to be far from Gaussian, since the Gaussian distribution maximizes entropy for a given variance.

Much of the progress in the last few years has come from fitting linear generative models with a single layer of hidden units. In the longer term it seems likely that these simple models will have to be replaced by nonlinear generative models with multiple hidden layers. Consider, for example, the problem of extracting from an intensity image the three position and three orientation parameters of a rigid three-dimensional object. Suppose we want the activities of hidden units to represent these "instantiation" parameters explicitly or to represent posterior distributions in the space of instantiation parameters. The instantiation parameters are nonlinearly related to pixel intensities, so even if we ignore the formidable problems of image segmentation, no linear generative model will suffice. One approach (Gold, Rangarajan, and Mjolsness 1996) is to transform pixel intensities into the image coordinates of identified fragments. The alternative is to have a multilayer, nonlinear model in which units in higher layers somehow represent the instantiation parameters of progressively larger and more complex fragments of objects. To achieve economy and generalization it seems essential for each fragment to potentially be generated by many different larger fragments in the layer above so the connectivity cannot be restricted to a tree structure. This is precisely the sort of architecture that is found in the cerebral cortex.

A major challenge for unsupervised learning is to get a system of this general type to learn appropriate representations for images. The major difficulty is that it is intractable to compute the full posterior distribution across hidden states in such a complex generative model.[2] One ray of hope is that the standard EM method of fitting models to data can be generalized so that learning can proceed effectively even if the posterior distribution is only approximated. Neal and Hinton (1998) show that a quantity equivalent to free energy is minimized by alternating between a partial M-step that improves the log likelihood of the data given the assumed distribution over hidden states and a partial E-step that improves the approximation to the true posterior distribution. The free energy is equivalent to the description length used by Zemel and Hinton (1995) and it can also be viewed (with a sign reversal) as the log likelihood of the data under the model penalized by a measure of the difficulty of performing inference with the model. The penalty is just the Kullback-Liebler divergence between the approximating distribution and the true posterior distribution. Retrospectively, it is easy to see that a biological organism would much rather have a model in which correct inference can be approximated easily than a model which gives slightly higher likelihood to the data but in which the posterior distribution is hard to approximate. So we arrive at a new objective function for unsupervised learning that recognizes the difficulty of performing inferencein sophisticated generative models and builds in a measure of the tractability of inference. Helmholtz machines (Dayan, Hinton, Neal, and Zemel 1996) are an attempt to optimize such an objective function using top-down connections for the generative model and feedforward, bottom-up connections for the approximate inference process.

References _____

Amari, S.-I. (1998) Natural gradient works efficiently in learning. *Neural Computation* 10(2):252–276. Reprinted in this volume.

Atick, J. J. and Redlich, A. N. (1993) Convergence algorithm for sensory receptive field development. *Neural Computation* 5(1):45–60. Reprinted in this volume.

Attneave, F. (1954) Informational aspects of visual perception. *Psychological Review* 61:183–193.

_____

[2] For one-dimensional strings of n symbols produced by a stochastic context-free grammar it is possible to consider all $O(n^2)$ possible connected substrings and so the posterior distribution over parses can be computed exactly. This is not possible for two-dimensional images because there are exponentially many connected subregions.

Barlow, H. B. (1959) Sensory mechanisms, the reduction of redundancy, and intelligence. In National Physical Laboratory Symposium No. 10, *The Mechanisation of Thought Processes*, pp. 535–559. London: Her Majesty's Stationary Office.

Barlow, H. B. (1989) Unsupervised learning. *Neural Computation* 1(3):295–311. Reprinted in this volume.

Becker, S. and Hinton, G. E. (1993) Learning mixture models of spatial coherence. *Neural Computation* 5(2):267–277. Reprinted in this volume.

Bell, A. J. and Sejnowski, T. J. (1995) An information-maximization approach to blind separation and blind deconvolution. *Neural Computation* 7(6):1129–1159. Reprinted in this volume.

Bell, A. J. and Sejnowski, T. J. (1997) The "independent components" of natural scenes are edge filters. *Vision Research*, 37:3327–3338.

Bienenstock, E. L., Cooper, L. N., and Munro, P. W. (1982) Theory for the development of neuron selectivity: orientation specificity and binocular interaction in visual cortex. *Journal of Neuroscience* 2:32–48.

Brown, T., Kairiss, E., and Keenan, C., (1990). Hebbian synapses: biophysical mechanisms and algorithms, *Ann. Rev. Neurosci.* 13:475–511.

Comon, P. (1994) Independent component analysis: a new concept? *Signal Processing* 36:287–314.

Crick, F. and Mitchison, G. (1983) The function of dream sleep. *Nature* 304:111–114.

Dayan, P., Hinton, G. E., Neal, R. M., and Zemel, R. S. (1995) The Helmholtz machine. *Neural Computation* 7(5):889–904. Reprinted in this volume.

Dempster, A. P., Laird, N. M., and Rubin, D. B. (1977) Maximum likelihood from incomplete data via the EM algorithm. *Journal of the Royal Statistical Society* 39:1–38.

Fahlman, S., and Lebiere, C. (1990). The cascade-correlation learning architecture. In Touretzky, D. (ed.), *Advances in Neural Information Processing Systems* 2, pp. 524–532, San Mateo, CA: Morgan Kaufmann.

Field, D. J. (1994) What is the goal of sensory coding? *Neural Computation* 6(4):559–601. Reprinted in this volume.

Foldiak, P. (1991) Learning invariance from transformation sequences. *Neural Computation* 3(2):194–200. Reprinted in this volume.

Gold, S., Rangarajan, A. and Mjolness, E. (1996) Learning with preknowledge: clustering with point and graph matching distance measures. *Neural Computation* 8(4):787–804. Reprinted in this volume.

Hinton, G. and Sejnowski, T. (1986) Learning and relearning in Boltzmann machines. In Rumelhart, D. and McClelland, J. (eds.), *Parallel Distributed Processing*, volume 1, chapter 7, pp. 282–317. Cambridge, MA: MIT Press.

Hopfield, J. J., Feinstein, D. I., and Palmer, R. G. (1983) "Unlearning" has a stabilizing effect in collective memories. *Nature* 304(5922):158–159.

Hubel, D. H. and Wiesel, T. N. (1968) Receptive fields and functional architecture of monkey striate cortex. *J. Physiol.* 195:215–244.

Hyvarinen, A. and Oja, E. (1977) A fast fixed-point algorithm for independent component analysis. *Neural Computation* 9(7):1483–1492. Reprinted in this volume.

Intrator, N. (1992) Feature extraction using an unsupervised neural network. *Neural Computation* 4(1):98–107. Reprinted in this volume.

Kambhatla, N. and Leen, T. K. (1997) Dimenison reduction by local principal component analysis. *Neural Computation* 9(7):1493–1516. Reprinted in this volume.

Lee, T.-W., Girolam, M., and Sejnowski, T. J. (in press) Independent component analysis using an extended infomax algorithm for mixed sub-Gaussian and super-Gaussian sources. *Neural Computation* 11(2).

Linsker, R. (1986) From basic network principles to neural architecture: emergence of spatial-opponent cells. *Proceedings of the National Academy of Sciences of the United States of America* 83:7508–7512.

Linsker, R. (1992) Local synaptic learning rules suffice to maximize mutual information in a linear network. *Neural Computation* 4(5):691–702. Reprinted in this volume.

Markram, H., Lubke, J., Frotscher, M., and Sakmann, B. (1977) Regulation of synaptic efficacy by coincidence of postsynaptic APs and EPSPs. *Science* 275:213–215.

Miller, K. D., Keller, J. B., and Stryker, M. P. (1989) Ocular dominance column development: analysis and simulation. *Science* 245:605–615.

Neal, R. M. and Dayan, P. (1997) Factor analysis using delta-rule wake-sleep learning. *Neural Computation* 9(8):1781–1803. Reprinted in this volume.

Neal, R. and Hinton, G. E. (1998) A new view of the EM algorithm that justifies incremental and other variants. In M. I. Jordan (ed.), *Learning in Graphical Models*. Dordrecht: Kluwer Academic Press.

Obermayer, K. and Sejnowski, T. J. (1998) *Self-Organizing Map Formation: Foundations of Neural Computation*. Cambridge, MA: MIT Press.

Olshausen, B. A. and Field, D. J. (1996) Emergence of simple-cell receptive field properties by learning a sparse code for natural images. *Nature* 1381:607–609.

Platt, J. (1991) A resource-allocating network for function interpolation. *Neural Computation* 3(2):213–225. Reprinted in this volume.

Stone, J. V. (1996) Learning perpetually salient visual parameters using spatiotemporal smoothness constraints. *Neural Computation* 8(7):1463–1492. Reprinted in this volume.

Zemel, R. S. and Hinton, G. E. (1995) Learning population codes by minimizing description length. *Neural Computation* 7(3):549–564. Reprinted in this volume.

Zhang, K., Sereno, M. I., and Sereno, M. E. (1993) Emergence of position-independent detectors of sense of rotation and dilation with Hebbian learning: an analysis. *Neural Computation* 5(4):597–612. Reprinted in this volume.

1

Unsupervised Learning

H.B. Barlow
Kenneth Craik Laboratory, Physiological Laboratory,
Downing Street, Cambridge, CB2 3EG, England

What use can the brain make of the massive flow of sensory information that occurs without any associated rewards or punishments? This question is reviewed in the light of connectionist models of unsupervised learning and some older ideas, namely the *cognitive maps* and *working models* of Tolman and Craik, and the idea that redundancy is important for understanding perception (Attneave 1954), the physiology of sensory pathways (Barlow 1959), and pattern recognition (Watanabe 1960). It is argued that (1) The redundancy of sensory messages provides the knowledge incorporated in the maps or models. (2) Some of this knowledge can be obtained by observations of mean, variance, and covariance of sensory messages, and perhaps also by a method called "minimum entropy coding." (3) Such knowledge may be incorporated in a model of "what usually happens" with which incoming messages are automatically compared, enabling unexpected discrepancies to be immediately identified. (4) Knowledge of the sort incorporated into such a filter is a necessary prerequisite of ordinary learning, and a representation whose elements are independent makes it possible to form associations with logical functions of the elements, not just with the elements themselves.

1 Introduction

Much of the information that pours into our brains throughout the waking day arrives without any obvious relationship to reinforcement, and is unaccompanied by any other form of deliberate instruction. What use can be made of this impressive flow of information? In this article I hope, first, to show that it is the redundancy contained in these messages that enables the brain to build up its "cognitive maps" or "working models" of the world around it; second, to suggest initial steps by which these might be formed; and third, to propose a structure for the maps or models that automatically ensures their access and use in everyday perception, and represents percepts in a form suitable for detecting the new associations involved in ordinary learning and conditioning.

Self-organization has been a major preoccupation of those interested in neural networks since the early days, and the volume edited by Yovits *et al.* (1962) gives an overview of some of this work; it is interesting to compare this with the systematic and much more developed treatment in the book on the subject by Kohonen (1984). One goal has been to explain topographic projections of sensory pathways and the occurrence of feature-selective neurons without depending completely on genetic specification (see especially von der Malsburg 1973; Nass and Cooper 1975; Cooper *et al.* 1979; Perez *et al.* 1975; Fukushima 1975, 1980; Swindale 1980, 1982; Barrow 1987). Another goal has been to explain the automatic separation and classification of clustered sensory stimuli (Rosenblatt 1959, 1962; Uttley 1958, 1979). The *informon* (Uttley 1970), for example, separated frequently occurring patterns from among a background of randomly associated elements, and it mimicked many aspects of the model of Rescorla and Wagner (1972) for conditioning and learning (Uttley 1975). Grossberg (1980) mainly emphasized the interactions between supervised and unsupervised learning. The *adaptive critic* in the pole-balancing scheme described by Barto *et al.* (1983) improved learning performance by observing the pattern of recurring correction-movements and their outcomes. Self-organization may be mediated by the *competitive learning* analyzed by Rummelhart and Zipser (1985), which has been applied to the generation of feature specificity by Barrow (1987) and to a hippocampal model by Rolls (1989). The hierarchical mapping scheme of Linsker (1986, 1988) shows spontaneous self-organization, and his *infomax* principle develops further some ideas related to those Uttley (1979) proposed. Linsker's networks can produce an organization reminiscent of the cortex both spontaneously, and in response to regularities of the incoming signals. From an informational viewpoint the recent exploration by Pearlmutter and Hinton (1986) of unsupervised procedures for discovering regularities in the input is especially relevant.

Much of this paper has antecedents in the above work as well as in theories about the importance of redundancy in perception (Attneave 1954; Barlow 1959) and pattern recognition (Watanabe 1960, 1985). However, I have also tried to relate unsupervised learning to ideas about cognitive processes developed by Tolman (1932) and Craik (1943). Since these ideas provide a link with traditional psychology they will be briefly described.

1.1 Cognitive Maps and Working Models. Tolman (1932) worked within the behaviorists' tradition, but he disagreed with the rigidity of their explanations, feeling that these did not adequately convey the richness of the knowledge about their environment that maze-running rats clearly possessed and freely utilized. As he said, "behavior reeks of purpose and of cognition," and the structured knowledge of the environment that he argued for was subsequently called a *cognitive map*. Craik (1943), in his shorter, more philosophically oriented, book proposed that "thought models, or parallels, reality." These *working models* embodied the essential features and interactions in the world that fed the senses, so that the outcomes of various possible actions could be correctly predicted; this is very similar to the way Tolman thought of cognitive maps being used by his rats.

What is the source of the extensive and well-organized knowledge of the environment implied by the possession of a cognitive map or working model? Though their structure may be genetically determined, the specific evidence they incorporate can be obtained only from the sensory messages received by the brain, and it is argued below that it is the statistical regularities in these messages that must be used for this purpose. This is an extraordinarily complex and difficult task, for it requires something like a major program of scientific research to be conducted at a precognitive level. There is plenty of room for genetic help in doing this, but once the nature of the task has been defined the statistical aspects can be approached systematically. In the next sections this is attempted for the first few steps, and a new method of finding these regularities — minimum entropy coding — is proposed.

2 Redundancy Provides Knowledge

There are genuine conceptual difficulties in applying information theory to the nervous system. These start with the paradox that although redundancy is claimed to be terribly important, sensory pathways are said to eliminate or reduce it rather than preserve it. Some of these difficulties (such as that one) disappear upon better understanding of information theory, but others do not: it is, for instance, difficult to apply the concepts when one is uncertain about the information-bearing features of the messages in nerve fibres, and about the overall plan used to represent information in the brain. In the next section these difficulties are avoided by talking about the sensory stimuli applied to the animal rather than the messages these arouse, and by doing this the definitions can be made precise.

In principle, the maximum rate of presentation of usable information to the senses can be specified if one knows the psychophysical facts about their discriminatory capacities; call this C bits/sec. Now look at the actual rate at which information is delivered, and call this H bits/sec; then the redundancy is simply $C - H$ bits/sec, or $100 \times (C - H)/C\%$. There remains a problem about measuring H, for the lower limit to its value can be calculated only if one knows all there is to know about the constraints operating in the world that gives rise to our sensations, and this point can obviously never be reached. Fortunately the concept of redundancy remains useful even if H is calculated using incomplete knowledge of the constraints, for this defines an upper limit to H and a lower limit to the redundancy.

It is confusing to refer to these $C - H$ bits/sec as information, but the technically correct term, redundancy, is almost equally misleading, for it suggests that this part of the sensory inflow is useless or irrelevant, whereas it is the potential source of all the available knowledge about the constant or semiconstant patterns and regularities in an animal's environment. *Knowledge* is perhaps the best term for it, though it may seem paradoxical that this knowledge of the world around us can be derived only from the redundancy of the messages. The point can be illustrated by briefly considering what nonredundant sensory stimuli would be like.

Completely nonredundant stimuli are indistinguishable from random noise. Thus, such a visual stimulus would look like a television set tuned between stations, and an auditory stimulus would sound like the hiss on an unconnected telephone line. Though meaningless to the recipient, technically such signals convey information at the maximum rate because they cannot be predicted at all from other parts of the message; $H = C$ and there is no redundancy. Thus, redundancy is the part of our sensory experience that distinguishes it from noise; the knowledge it gives us about the patterns and regularities in sensory stimuli must be what drives unsupervised learning. With this in mind one can begin to classify the forms the redundancy takes and the methods of handling it.

3 Finding and Using Sensory Redundancy

Some features of sensory stimuli are almost universal. For instance, the upper part of the visual field is imaged on the lower part of the retina in an erect animal, and it is almost always more brightly illuminated. In animals such as cats that have a reflecting tapetum one usually finds that it is confined to the part receiving the image of the lower, dimmer, part of the visual field while the reflecting tapetum is replaced by a densely absorbing pigment in the part receiving the bright image; the result is to greatly reduce the amount of scattered light obscuring the image in its dimmer parts.

The many ways that redundant aspects of sensory stimuli are reflected in permanent features of the sensory system are themselves interesting, but here we are concerned with learning-like responses. To exploit redundant features the brain must determine characteristics of the stimuli that behave in a nonrandom manner, so one can consider methodically the various measures that could be made on the messages in order to characterize these regularities statistically.

3.1 Mean. One starts with the mean, taken over the recent past. In vision, this can assume any value from a few thousandths up to many thousands of cd/m^2, but it behaves in a very nonrandom manner because it tends to stay rather constant for quite long periods. I have been sitting at my desk for the past hour, and during this time the mean luminance has always been close to $10 \text{ cd}/m^2$; the constancy of this mean is a highly nonrandom feature and the visual system takes advantage of it to adjust the sensitivity of the pathways to suit the limited range of retinal illuminations it will receive. Much is understood about these adaptational mechanisms, but the principles are well understood by communication engineers and I shall go ahead to consider more interesting types of redundancy. However the way in which coding by the retina changes with the mean luminance of the images is a simple paradigm of unsupervised learning, and the one we are closest to understanding physiologically.

3.2 Variance. The variance of sensory signals probably does not show the constancy over short periods combined with very large changes over long periods that is characteristic of the mean, though a walker in mist or a fish in murky water would certainly be exposed to signals with an exceptionally low range of image contrasts and hence low variance. After the transformations in the retina, taking account of changes in the variance of the input signals is actually very nearly equivalent to adjusting for the mean values of the signals in the "on" and "off" systems, and it has been suggested that such *contrast gain control* occurs in primary visual cortex (Ohzawa *et al.* 1982, 1985).

One might perhaps consider next the higher moments of the distributions of input stimuli on the many input channels, but it is hard to imagine that adapting to these would have any great advantages and I know of no evidence that natural systems respond in any way to them. Hence the next step is the large one of considering the patterns of *correlation* between the inputs on different channels.

3.3 Covariance. The simplest measure of the correlated activity of sensory pathways would be the covariance between pairs of them. Just as adaptational mechanisms take advantage of the mean by using it as an expected value and expressing values relative to it, so one might take advantage of covariance by devising a code in which the measured correlations are "expected" in the input, but removed from the output by forming a suitable set of linear combinations of the input signals. It is possible to form an uncorrelated set of signals in a neural network with a rather simple scheme of connection and rule of synaptic modification (Barlow 1989; Barlow and Földiák 1989; see also Kohonen 1984). The essential idea is that each neuron's output feeds back to the other inputs through anti-Hebbian synapses, so that correlated activity among the outputs is discouraged. Such a network would account for many perceptual phenomena hitherto explained in terms of fatigue of pattern selective elements in sensory pathways, and it also offers a mechanism for some forms of the "unconscious inference" described by von Helmholtz (1925) and modern psychologists of perception (Rock 1983). These aspects are discussed in the references cited above, and here some of the possible extensions of the principle will be mentioned.

So far it has been supposed that the covariance is worked out from paired values occurring at the same moment, but this need not be the case. Sutton and Barto (1981) have discussed temporal relationships in conditioning, and there are several synaptic mechanisms that might depend on the correlation between synaptic input at one moment and post-synaptic depolarization at a later moment; a transmitter might cause lingering "eligibility" for subsequent reinforcement, or a synaptic rewarding factor or reverse transmitter released by a depolarized neuron might be optimally picked up by presynaptic terminals some moments after they had themselves been active. Decorrelating networks based on such principles would "expect" events that occurred in often-repeated sequences, and would tend to respond less strongly to frequently occurring sequences and more strongly to abnormal ones. It is easy to see how such a mechanism might explain aftereffects of motion.

A consequence of using covariances is that, since the inputs are taken in pairs, the number of computations increases in proportion to the square of the number of inputs. This means that it would be impossible to decorrelate the whole sensory input; the best that could be done would be to decorrelate local sets of sensory fibers. However, the process could then be repeated, possibly organizing the decorrelated outputs of the first stage according to principles other than their topographical proximity, such as proximity in color space or similarity of direction of motion (Barlow 1981; Ballard 1984). Such hierarchical decorrelation processes may have considerable potential, but there is no denying that the methods so far considered only begin the task of finding regularities in the sensory input.

3.4 Rules for Combination or Agglomeration. Decorrelation separates variables that are correlated, but if the correlation between two variables is very strong they might be conveying the same message, and then one should combine them. For instance, taste information is carried by a large number of nerve fibers each of which has its characteristic mixture of sensitivities to the four primary qualities, salt, sweet, sour, and bitter. We have shown (Barlow and Földiák 1989) how these can be decorrelated in groups of four to yield the four primary qualities, but one might expect all the outputs for one quality then to be combined on to a much smaller number of elements, for without doing this they just seem to replicate the information needlessly.

There is need for an operation of this sort in many situations: for instance, to exploit the fact that there are only two dimensions of color (in addition to luminance), to exploit the prevalence of edges in ordinary images, to combine in one entity the host of sensory experiences for which we use a single word or name, and to do the same for a commonly repeated phrase or cliché. Pearlmutter and Hinton (1986) consider a related problem, that of finding input patterns that occur more often than would be expected if the constituent features occurred independently.

Finding that some combinations occur more often than expected is the converse of finding that some combinations do not occur at all, as is the case when the number of degrees of freedom or dimensions in a set of messages is less than would appear from the form of the messages. The set of N features spans less than an N-dimensional space because certain combinations do not occur, and exploiting this is just the kind of simplification that would enable one to make useful cognitive maps and working models. Principle component analysis will do what is required, and it is believed that the method described in the next section will also, but it is natural to look for network methods, especially as these have already achieved some success (for example, Oja 1982; Rumelhart and Zipser 1985; Pearlmutter and Hinton 1986; Földiák 1989).

3.5 Minimum Entropy Coding. As with decorrelation the idea is to find a set of symbols to represent sensory messages such that, in the normal environment, each symbol is as nearly as possible independent of the others, but there are two differences: first, it is applicable to discretely coded, logically distinct variables rather than continuous ones, and second it takes into account all possible nonrandom relations between the outputs, not just the pairwise relationships of the covariance matrix. To make the principle clear the simple example of coding keyboard characters in 7 binary digits to find alternatives to the familiar 7-bit ASCII code will be considered. The advantages of examining this are its familiarity, its simplicity, and the fact that samples of normal English text are readily available from which the nonrandom character frequencies can be determined.

If a sample of ordinary text is regarded simply as a string of independent characters randomly selected from the alphabet with the probabilities given by their frequency of occurrence in ordinary text, the average entropy of the characters H_c is given by the familiar expression:

$$H_c = -\sum P_c \log P_c \tag{3.1}$$

where P_c are the probabilities of the mutually exclusive set of characters.

Each of the characters is represented by a 7-bit word, and the entropies for each bit can be obtained by measuring their frequencies in a sample of text. The entropy expression for the bits takes the form:

$$H_i = -(P_i \log P_i + Q_i \log Q_i) \tag{3.2}$$

where H_i is the average entropy of the ith bit, P_i is its probability, and Q_i is $1 - P_i$.

An estimate of the average character entropy can be obtained by adding the 7-bit entropies, but it is important to realize that this can never be less, and will usually be greater, than the character entropy given by the original expression (3.1). The reason for this is the lack of independence between the values of the bits; if it were true for all the 7 bits that their values were completely independent of the other bits occurring in any combination, then the two estimates would be equal. The object is to find a code for which this is true, or as nearly true as possible, and the method of doing this is to find a code that minimizes the sum of the bit entropies — hence the name. If the minimum is reached and the bits are truly independent we call it a *factorial* code, since each bit probability or its complement is then a factor of the probability of each of the input states.

The maneuver can be looked at another way. The seven binary digits of the ASCII code can carry a maximum of 7 bits, but actually carry less when used to transmit normal text, for two reasons. First, the bit probabilities are a long way from 1/2, which would yield the maximum bit entropy; this form of redundancy is explicit and causes no trouble, for the probability of each of the 7 bits is available wherever they are transmitted and easily measured. Second, there are complicated interdependencies among the bits, so the conditional bit probabilities are not the same as the unconditional ones; this form of redundancy is troublesome, for it is not available wherever the bits are transmitted and to describe it completely one needs to know the conditional probabilities of each bit for all combinations of other bits. If both of these forms of redundancy were taken into account the information conveyed per ASCII word would of course be the same as H_c of expression (1), i.e., about 4.3 bits, and no change of the code would alter this. However, changing the code does change the relative amounts of the two forms of redundancy, and by finding one that minimizes the sum of the bit entropies one maximizes the redundancy that results from bit probabilities deviating from 1/2. This leaves less room for redundancy from interdependencies between the bits; the troublesome form of redundancy is squeezed out by maximizing the other less troublesome form.

The minimum entropy principle should be generally applicable and clearly goes further than decorrelation, which considers only the outputs in pairs. It can also be used to compare and select from codes that change the number of channels or dimensionality of the messages. The entropy is a locally computable quantity, and by minimizing it one can increase the independence of the outputs without actually measuring the frequencies of all the possible output states, which would often be an impossible task. An accompanying article (Barlow *et al.* 1989) goes into some of the practical and theoretical problems in finding minimum entropy codes.

In this section it has been suggested that the statistical regularities of the incoming sensory messages might be measured and used to change the way they are coded or represented. It is easy to see that this would have advantages, analogous to those conferred by automatic gain control, in ensuring a compact representation within the dynamic range of the representative elements, but there may be more profound benefits attached to a representation in which the variables are independent in the environment to which the representation has been adapted. To understand these one must consider the main task for which our perceptions are used, namely the detection of new associations and their utilization in ordinary learning and conditioning.

4 Ordinary Learning Requires Previous Knowledge _____

Over the past 20 years the work of Kamin (1969), Rescorla and Wagner (1972), Mackintosh (1974, 1983), Dickinson (1980), and others has brought about a very big change in the way theorists approach the learning problem. Whereas previously they tended to think in terms of mechanistic links whose strengths were increased or decreased according to definable laws, attention has now shifted to the computational problem that an animal solves when it learns. This started with the realization and experimental demonstration of the fact that the detection of new associations is strongly dependent on other previously and concurrently learned associations, many of which may be "silent" in that they do not themselves produce overt and obvious effects on outward behavior. As a result of this change it is at last appreciated that the brain studied in the learning laboratory is doing a profoundly difficult job: it is deducing causal links from which it can benefit in the world around it, and it does this by detecting suspicious coincidences; that is, it picks up associations that are surprising, new, or different among those that the experimenter offers it.

To detect new associations one must detect changes in the probabilities of certain events, and once this is realized an important role for unreinforced experience becomes clear: it is to find out and record the a priori probabilities, that is, the normal state of affairs, or what usually happens. Though this elementary fact does not seem to have been much emphasized by learning theorists it is obviously crucial, for how can something be recognized as new and surprising if there is no preexisting knowledge about what is old and expected?

4.1 Detecting New Associations. The basic step in learning is to detect that event C predicts U; C might be the conditional, U the unconditional stimulus of Pavlovian conditioning, or C might be a motor action and U a reinforcement in operant conditioning, or they might be successive elements in a learned sequence. Unsupervised learning can help with at least two aspects of this process: first, the separate representation of a wide range of alternative Cs, and second, the acquisition of knowledge of the normal probabilities of occurrence of these possible conditional stimuli.

It is often tacitly assumed that all alternative conditioning stimuli can be separated by the brain and their occurrences independently registered in some way, but one should not blandly ignore the whole problem of pattern recognition, and the massive interconnections we know exist between the neurons of the brain means that the host of alternative Cs are unlikely to be completely separable unless there are specific mechanisms for ensuring that they are. The tacit assumption that the probabilities of occurrence of these stimuli, or of their cooccurrence with U, are known is equally unjustified, though it is evident that if they were not there would be no sound basis for judging that a particular C had become a good predictor of U. The logical steps necessary to detect an association between C and U will be considered in more detail to show the importance both of knowledge of their normal probabilities and of the separability of alternative conditional stimuli.

The only way to establish that C usefully predicts U is to disprove the null hypothesis that the number of occasions U follows C is no more than would be expected from chance coincidences of the two events; it is easy to see that if this null hypothesis is correct, no benefit can possibly result from using C as a predictor of U. To know the expected rate of chance coincidences one must either have measured the normal rate of the compound event (U following C) directly, or have knowledge of the normal probabilities of occurrence, P(C) and P(U); further if these probabilities are to be used it must be reasonable to assume they are independent. This prior knowledge is clearly necessary before new predictive associations can be detected reliably. Now consider the difficulties that arise if a particular C cannot be fully resolved or separated from the alternative Cs.

Failure of resolution or separation means that the registration of the occurrence of an event is contaminated by occurrences of other events. Estimates of the probabilities of occurrence of C both with and without U would be misleading if based on these contaminated counts, and their use would cause failures to detect associations that were present and the detection of spurious associations that did not exist. Thus, if counts of alternative events like C are to be used to detect causal factors, they must be adequately resolved or separated if learning is to be efficient and reliable.

4.2 Independence Is Needed for Versatile Learning. Now reconsider the two ways, measurement and calculation, of estimating the compound event probability P(U following C). Directly measuring it is adequate and plausible when one has prior expectations about the possible conditional stimuli C, especially as in either scheme one must somehow be able to detect the occurrence of this sequence when it occurs. But calculating P(U following C) from P(C) and P(U) is much more versatile, for the following reason. Measuring the rates of N coincidences such as "U following C" just gives these rates and no more, whereas knowledge of the probabilities of N independent events enables one to calculate the probability of all possible logical functions of those events, at least in principle. This gigantic increase in the number of null hypotheses whose predictions can be specified and tested gives an enormous advantage to the method of calculating, rather than measuring, the expected coincidence rates. However, calculating P(U following C) from the probabilities of its constituents depends on the formation of a representation in which the constituent events can be relied on to be independent until the association that is to be detected occurs.

To summarize: to detect a suspicious coincidence that signals a new causal factor in the environment one should have access to prior knowledge of the probabilities of simpler constituent events, and these simpler events should be separately registered and independent on the null hypothesis from which one wishes to advance. It is obviously an enormously difficult and complicated task to generate such a representation, and the types of coding discussed above are only first steps; however, the versatility of subsequent learning must depend critically on how well the task has been done.

4.3 Some Other Issues. The approach taken here might be criticized on the grounds that the problem facing the brain in learning is considered in too abstract a manner, the actual mechanisms being ignored. For example, the logic of the situation requires that the numbers of occurrences and joint occurrences be somehow stored, and one might point to this as the major problem, rather than the way the numbers are used. It certainly is a major problem, but the attitude adopted here is that one is not going to get far in understanding learning without recognizing the logic of inductive inference, since this dictates what quantities actually need to be stored; it seems obvious that this problem should be looked at first.

There must be many ways in which the brain fails to perform the idealized operations required to detect new causal factors. It performs approximations and estimates, not exact calculations, but one cannot appreciate the mistakes an approximation will lead to without knowing what the exact calculation is. It is likely that many of the features of learning stem from the nature of the problem being tackled, not from the specific details of the mechanisms, and it is foolish to confuse the one with the other through failing to attend to the complexity of the task the brain appears to perform so effectively.

There is another somewhat irrelevant issue. If it was known with certainty that a predictive relation between C and U existed it would still have to be decided whether it should be acted on. This theoretically depends on whether P(U following C) is high enough for the reward obtained when U does follow C to outweigh the penalty attached to the behavior needed to reap the reward when U fails to materialize; that is a different matter from deciding whether the relation exists, and for the present it can be ignored.

4.4 Storing and Accessing the Model. So far no means has been proposed for performing the computations suggested above, nor for storing and accessing the knowledge of the environment that the model contains. One possibility is to form a massive memory for the usual rates of occurrence of various combinations of sensory inputs. Something like this may underlie our ability to say "the almond is blossoming unusually early this year" and to make similar cognitive judgments, but the comparative judgments of everyday perception are certainly made in quite a different way. When we see white walls in a dimly lit room we do not observe their luminance, then refer to a memorized look-up table that tells us what luminances are to be called white when the mean luminance is such and such; instead we have mechanisms (admittedly not yet fully understood) that automatically compare the signals generated by the image of the wall with signals from other regions, and then attach the label "white" wherever this comparison yields a high value.

This automatic comparison was regarded above as a way of eliminating the redundancy involved in signaling the mean luminance on every channel, and it should now be clear how the various other suggested forms of recoding do much the same operation for other "expected" statistical regularities in the sensory messages. One can regard the model or map as something automatically held up for comparison with the current input; it is like a negative filter through which incoming messages are automatically passed, so that what emerges is the difference between what is actually happening and what one would expect to happen, based on past experience. In this way past experience can be made continuously and automatically available.

5 Discussion

Since the early days of information theory it has been suggested that the redundancy of sensory stimuli is particularly important for understanding perception. Attneave (1954) was the first to point this out, and I have periodically argued for its importance in understanding both the physiological mechanisms of sensory coding, and higher level functions including intelligence (Barlow 1959, 1961, 1987). One can actually trace the line of thought back to von Helmholtz (1877, 1925), and particularly to the writings of Ernst Mach (1886) and Karl Pearson (1892) about "The Economy of Thought." To what extent is this line of thought the same as that of Tolman and Craik on cognitive maps and working models?

They are certainly closely related, for they both say that the regularities in the sensory messages must be recorded by the brain for it to know what usually happens. However, redundancy reduction is the more specific form of the hypothesis, for I think it also implies that the knowledge contained in the map or model is stored in such a form that the current sensory scene is automatically compared with it and the discrepancies passed on for further consideration — the idea of the model as a negative filter.

There is perhaps something contradictory and intuitively hard to accept in this notion, especially when applied to the cognitive knowledge of our environments to which we have conscious access. When we become aware that the almond is blossoming unusually early, we think this is an absolute judgment based on comparisons with past, positive experiences, and not the result of a discrepancy between present experience and unconscious rememberings of past blossomings. Perhaps the negative filter idea applies only to the unconscious knowledge that our perceptions use so effectively, with quite different mechanisms employed at the higher levels to which we have conscious access. On the other hand redundancy reduction may be the deeper view of how our brains handle sensory input, for it may describe the goal of the whole process, dictating the form of representation as well as what is represented; we should not be too surprised if our introspections turn out to be misleading on such a matter, for they may be concerned with guiding us how to tell others about our experiences, not with informing us how the brain goes about its business.

The discussion should have demonstrated that there is a close relationship between the properties of the elements that represent the current scene, the model that tells one "what usually happens," and the ease with which new associations can be detected and learned. But the recoding methods suggested above are unlikely to be complete, and it is worth listing other factors that must be important in determining the utility of representations.

5.1 Other Factors Affecting the Utility of Representations.

1. The best method of detecting a target in a noisy background is to derive a signal that picks up all the energy available from the signal with the minimum contamination by energy from its background — the principle of the matched detector. This principle must be very important when detecting events in the environment that are associated with rewards or punishments, but there is no guarantee that the code elements of a minimum entropy code (or any other code that is unguided by reinforcement) will be well matched to these classes of events. Though a priori probabilities can be calculated for any logical function of the inputs if the representative elements are independent, this calculation is not necessarily as accurate as that obtained from a matched filter.

2. It is also important that a coding scheme should lead to appropriate generalization. Probably representative elements should start by responding to a wider class of events than that to which, under the influence of "shaping," they ultimately respond. To meet this

requirement mechanisms additional to minimum entropy coding
are required.

3. Items such as the markings of prey, predators, or mates may have a
biological significance that is arbitrary from an informational viewpoint.

4. Sensory scenes and stimuli that have been reinforced obviously
have special importance, and they should therefore have a key role
in classifying sensory stimuli.

It is clear that the minimum entropy principle is not the only one
on which the representation of sensory information should be based.
Nonetheless a code selected on this principle stores a wealth of knowledge about the statistical structure of the normal environment, and the
independence of the representative elements gives such a representation
enormous versatility. It is relatively easy to devise learning schemes capable of detecting specific associations, but higher mammals appear to
be able to make associations with entities of the order of complexity that
we would use a word to describe. As George Boole (1854) pointed out,
words are to the elements of our sensations like logical functions to the
variables that compose them. We cannot of course suppose that an animal
can form an association with any arbitrary logical function of its sensory
messages, but they have capacities that tend in that direction, and it is
these capacities that the kind of representative schemes considered here
might be able to mimic.

References

Attneave, F. 1954. Informational aspects of visual perception. *Psychol. Rev.* **61**,
183–193.
Ballard, D.H. 1984. Parameter networks. *Artificial Intell.* **22**, 235–267.
Barlow, H.B. 1959. Sensory mechanisms, the reduction of redundancy, and
intelligence. In National Physical Laboratory Symposium No. 10, *The Mech-
anisation of Thought Processes.* Her Majesty's Stationery Office, London.
Barlow, H.B. 1961. Possible principles underlying the transformations of sensory
messages. In *Sensory Communication*, W. Rosenblith, ed., pp. 217–234. MIT
Press, Cambridge, MA.
Barlow, H.B. 1981. Critical limiting factors in the design of the eye and visual
cortex. The Ferrier lecture, 1980. *Proc. Roy. Soc. London, B* **212**, 1–34.
Barlow, H.B. 1987. Intelligence: The art of good guesswork. In *The Oxford
Companion to the Mind*, R.L. Gregory, ed., pp. 381–383. Oxford University
Press, Oxford.
Barlow, H.B. 1989. A theory about the functional role and synaptic mechanism
of visual after-effects. In *Vision: Coding and Efficiency*, C. Blakemore, ed.
Cambridge University Press, Cambridge.

Barlow, H.B., and Földiák, P. 1989. Adaptation and decorrelation in the cortex. In *The Computing Neuron*, R. Durbin, C. Miall, and G. Mitchison, eds. New York: Addison-Wesley.

Barlow, H.B., Kaushal, T.P., and Mitchison, G.J. 1989. Finding minimum entropy codes. *Neural Comp.* **1**, 412-423.

Barrow, H.G. 1987. Learning receptive fields. *Proc. IEEE First Int. Conf. Neural Networks, Cat.* # 87TH0191-7, pp. IV-115–IV-121.

Barto, A.G., Sutton, R.S., and Anderson, C.W. 1983. Neuronlike adaptive elements that can solve difficult learning control problems. *IEEE Transact. Systems, Man, Cybernet.* **SMC-13**(5), 835–846.

Boole, G. 1854. *An Investigation of the Laws of Thought*. Dover Publications Reprint, New York.

Cooper, L.N., Liberman, F., and Oja, E. 1979. A theory for the acquisition and loss of neuron specificity in visual cortex. *Biol. Cybernet.* **33**, 9–28.

Craik, K.J.W. 1943. *The Nature of Explanation*. Cambridge University Press, Cambridge.

Dickinson, A. 1980. *Contemporary Animal Learning Theory*. Cambridge University Press, Cambridge.

Földiák, P. 1989. Adaptive network for optimal linear feature extraction. In *Proc. IEEE INNS Int. Joint Conf. Neural Networks*, Washington DC.

Fukushima, K. 1975. Cognitron: A self-organising multi-layered neural network. *Biol. Cybernet.* **20**, 121–136.

Fukushima, K. 1980. Neocognitron: A self-organising neural network model for a mechanism of pattern recognition unaffected by shift of position. *Biol. Cybernet.* **36**, 193–202.

Grossberg, S. 1980. How does a brain build a cognitive code? *Psychol. Rev.* **87**, 1–51.

Kamin, L.J. 1969. Predictability, surprise, attention and conditioning. In *Punishment and Aversive Behavior*, B.A. Campbell and R.M. Church, eds., pp. 279–296. Appleton-Century-Crofts, New York.

Kohonen, T. 1984. *Self-Organisation and Associative Memory*. Springer-Verlag, Berlin.

Linsker, R. 1986. From basic network principles to neural architecture (series). *Proc. Natl. Acad. Sci. U.S.A.* **83**, 7508–7512, 8390–8394, 8779–8783.

Linsker, R. 1988. Self-organisation in a perceptual network. *Computer* (March 1988), 105–117.

Mach, E. 1886. *The Analysis of Sensations, and the Relation of the Physical to the Psychical*. Translation of the 1st, revised from the 5th, German Edition by S. Waterlow. Open Court, Chicago and London. (Also Dover reprint, New York, 1959.)

Mackintosh, N.J. 1974. *The Psychology of Animal Learning*. Academic Press, London.

Mackintosh, N.J. 1983. *Conditioning and Associative Learning*. Oxford University Press, Oxford.

Nass, M.M., and Cooper, L.N. 1975. A theory for the development of feature detecting cells in visual cortex. *Biol. Cybernet.* **19**, 1–18.

Ohzawa, I. Sclar, G., and Freeman, R.D. 1982. Contrast gain control in the cat visual cortex. *Nature (London)* **298**, 266–278.

Ohzawa, I. Sclar, G., and Freeman, R.D. 1985. Contrast gain control in the cat's visual system. *J. Neurophysiol.* **54**, 651–667.

Oja, E. 1982. A simplified neuron as a principal component analyser. *J. Math. Biol.* **15**, 267–273.

Pearlmutter, B.A., and Hinton, G.E. 1986. G-maximization: an unsupervised learning procedure for discovering regularities. In *Proc. Conf. Neural Networks Comp.* American Institute of Physics.

Pearson, K. 1892. *The Grammar of Science*. Walter Scott, London.

Perez, R., Glass, L., and Shlaer, R. 1975. Development of specificities in the cat visual cortex. *J. Math. Biol.* **1**, 275-288.

Rescorla, R.A., and Wagner, A.R. 1972. A theory of Pavlovian conditioning: Variations in effectiveness of reinforcement and non-reinforcement. In *Classical conditioning II: Current Research and Theory*, A.H. Black and W.F. Prokasy, eds., pp. 64–99. Appleton-Century-Crofts, New York.

Rock, I. 1983. *The Logic of Perception*. MIT Press, Cambridge, MA.

Rolls, E.T. 1989. The representation and storage of information in neuronal networks in the Primate cerebral cortex and hippocampus. In *The Computing Neuron*, R. Durbin, C. Miall, and G. Mitchison, eds. Addison-Wesley, New York.

Rosenblatt, F. 1959. Two theorems of statistical separability in the Perceptron. In National Physical Laboratory Symposium No. 10, *Mechanisation of Thought Processes*, 419–456. Her Majesty's Stationery Office, London.

Rosenblatt, F. 1962. *Principles of Neurodynamics*. Spartan Books, Washington, DC.

Rumelhart, D.E., and Zipser, D. 1985. Feature discovery by competitive learning. *Cog. Sci.* **9**, 75-112. (Also in *Parallel Distributed Processing, Vol 1*, pp. 151–193, MIT Press, Cambridge, MA, 1986).

Sutton, R.S., and Barto, A.G. 1981. Towards a modern theory of adaptive networks: Expectation and prediction. *Psychol. Rev.* **88**, 135–170.

Swindale, N.V. 1980. A model for the formation of ocular dominance stripes. *Proc. Roy. Soc. London B* **208**, 243–264.

Swindale, N.V. 1982. A model for the formation of orientation columns. *Proc. Roy. Soc. London B* **215**, 211–230.

Tolman, E.C. 1932. *Purposive Behavior in Animals and Men*. The Century Company, New York.

Uttley, A.M. 1958. Conditional probability as a principle in learning. *Actes 1re Congrés Cybernetiques. Namur, 1956.* J. Lemaire, ed. Gauthier-Villars, Paris.

Uttley, A.M. 1970. The Informon: A network for adaptive pattern recognition. *J. Theoret. Biol.* **27**, 31–67.

Uttley, A.M. 1975. The Informon in classical conditioning. *J. Theoret. Biol.* **49**, 355–376.

Uttley, A.M. 1979. *Information Transmission in the Nervous System*. Academic Press, London.

von der Malsburg, C. 1973. Self-organisation of orientation sensitive cells in the striate cortex. *Kybernetik* **14**, 85–100.

von Helmholtz, H. 1877. *The Sensations of Tone.* (by A.J. Ellis 1885). Reprinted Dover, New York, 1954.

von Helmholtz, H. 1925. *Physiological Optics Volume 3: The Theory of the Perceptions of Vision.* Translated from 3rd German Edition (1910). Optical Society of America, Washington, DC.

Watanabe, S. 1960. Information-theoretical aspects of Inductive and Deductive Inference. *I.B.M. J. Res. Dev.* **4**, 208–231.

Watanabe, S. 1985. *Pattern Recognition: Human and Mechanical.* Wiley, New York.

Yovits, M.C., Jacobi, G.T., and Goldstein, G.D. 1962. *Self-organizing Systems.* Spartan Books, Washington, DC.

2

Local Synaptic Learning Rules Suffice to Maximize Mutual Information in a Linear Network

Ralph Linsker
IBM Research Division, T. J. Watson Research Center,
P. O. Box 218, Yorktown Heights, NY 10598 USA

A network that develops to maximize the mutual information between its output and the signal portion of its input (which is admixed with noise) is useful for extracting salient input features, and may provide a model for aspects of biological neural network function. I describe a local synaptic learning rule that performs stochastic gradient ascent in this information-theoretic quantity, for the case in which the input–output mapping is linear and the input signal and noise are multivariate gaussian. Feedforward connection strengths are modified by a Hebbian rule during a "learning" phase in which examples of input signal plus noise are presented to the network, and by an anti-Hebbian rule during an "unlearning" phase in which examples of noise alone are presented. Each recurrent lateral connection has two values of connection strength, one for each phase; these values are updated by an anti-Hebbian rule.

1 Introduction

The idea of designing a processing stage so as to maximize the mutual information (MI) between its output and the signal portion of its input (which is admixed with noise) is attractive as a way to use sensory input optimally, and to extract statistically salient input features (Linsker 1988; Atick and Redlich 1990). For the idea to be practical for use by biological systems or in large synthetic networks, it is important that the required optimization be implemented by a local algorithm—one that uses only information currently available at the node or connection that is to be modified. This paper presents such an algorithm for the case in which the input–output transformation is linear and the signal and noise distributions are multivariate gaussian. The algorithm performs stochastic gradient ascent in the MI.

Local network algorithms have been described for several tasks that differ from the present one but are related to it: (1) principal component analysis (PCA) (Földiák 1989; Leen 1991; Sanger 1989), which identifies high-variance linear combinations of inputs, but does not take account of noise; (2) smoothing and predictive filtering (Atick and Redlich 1991),

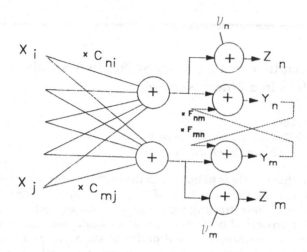

Figure 1: Linear network, showing feedforward paths (solid lines) and lateral recurrent connections (dashed lines).

which approximate MI maximization in certain limiting cases; and (3) MI maximization in a probabilistic winner-take-all network (Linsker 1989b), a nonlinear case in which only one output node "fires" at any given time, simplifying the computation of the MI.

The paper is organized as follows: Section 2 states the optimization problem. The algorithm is presented in Section 3, illustrated by a numerical example in Section 4, and discussed in a broader context in Section 5. Mathematical details are given in the Appendix.

2 The Optimization Problem

A linear feedforward network (indicated by the solid-line paths in Fig. 1) is presented with a sequence of input vectors X. Each vector is the sum of an input signal S and input noise N, where S and N are independently drawn from multivariate gaussian distributions whose means are zero. The network's output is $Z \equiv CX + \nu$, where the noise ν_n added at each output is an independent gaussian random variable of zero mean and nonzero variance.

The ensemble-averaged mutual information $R(Z, S)$ between Z and S, also called the Shannon information rate for the $S \rightarrow Z$ mapping, is the information that the output Z "conveys about" the input signal S. It equals $H(Z) - H(Z \mid S)$, where $H(Z)$ denotes the entropy of Z, and $H(Z \mid S)$

denotes the average over S of the conditional entropy of Z given S. [Note that $H(Z \mid S)$ equals the entropy of the noise contribution to Z, which is $CN + \nu$.] The entropy of a gaussian distribution having covariance Q is (Shannon and Weaver 1949), apart from an irrelevant constant term,

$$H = (1/2) \ln \det Q \qquad (2.1)$$

Therefore

$$R(Z, S) \equiv H(Z) - H(Z \mid S) = (1/2)[\ln \det Q^L - \ln \det Q^U] \qquad (2.2)$$

where

$$\begin{aligned} Q^L &\equiv \langle [C(S+N) + \nu][C(S+N) + \nu]^T \rangle = C q^L C^T + r \qquad (2.3) \\ Q^U &\equiv \langle (CN + \nu)(CN + \nu)^T \rangle = C q^U C^T + r \qquad (2.4) \end{aligned}$$

$q^L \equiv \langle (S+N)(S+N)^T \rangle = \langle SS^T \rangle + \langle NN^T \rangle$, $q^U \equiv \langle NN^T \rangle$, and $r \equiv \langle \nu \nu^T \rangle$.

Both S and N may have statistical correlations. Correlations in the input noise N may arise because of sensor design, or because correlations were induced at earlier stages of a multistage processing network, or because N represents environmental features that we do not want the network to respond to (e.g., "semantic noise").

In any case, if the network is to learn to maximize $R(Z, S)$, it must learn to distinguish input signal from noise. We will do this using a training process that consists of two phases. In "learning" or L phase, the network is shown examples of $X \equiv S+N$. In "unlearning" or U phase, the network is shown examples $X \equiv N$ of input noise alone. Performing gradient ascent on $R(Z, S)$ then consists of alternately performing gradient ascent on $H(Z)$ during L phase, and gradient descent on $H(Z \mid S)$ during U phase. Each of these tasks is performed, during its respective phase, by the local algorithm described in the next section.[1]

3 Local Synaptic Modification Rule _____

3.1 Performing Gradient Ascent in the Entropy of the Output Activity.
We show first how to perform gradient ascent in the entropy H of the output of a linear mapping. (Derivations are relegated to the Appendix.)

Let X be an input vector, $Y \equiv CX$, and $Z \equiv Y + \nu$ be the output. X has covariance matrix $q \equiv \langle XX^T \rangle$, and the output Z has covariance

---

[1]Throughout the paper, the covariance matrix of the input X is denoted by $q \equiv \langle XX^T \rangle$, and that of the output $Z = CX + \nu$ by $Q \equiv \langle ZZ^T \rangle$. When used, the superscript L or U specifies whether the covariance matrix refers to the "learning" or "unlearning" phase. Since $X = S+N$ during L phase and $X = N$ during U phase, the expressions for $q^{L,U}$ and $Q^{L,U}$ used in equations 2.3 and 2.4 are obtained. Angle brackets denote an ensemble average, and superscript T denotes the transpose.

$Q \equiv \langle ZZ^T \rangle = CqC^T + r$. We assume for now that r is independent of C. Using equation 2.1 we obtain

$$\partial H / \partial C_{ni} = (Q^{-1}Cq)_{ni} \qquad (3.1)$$

If the Q^{-1} factor were absent, we would obtain the gradient ascent "batch update" learning rule: $\Delta C_{ni} = \gamma \partial H / \partial C_{ni} = \gamma (Cq)_{ni} = \gamma \langle Y_n X_i \rangle$. The local Hebbian rule $\Delta C_{ni} = \gamma Y_n X_i$ would perform stochastic gradient ascent in H. The Q^{-1} factor, however, introduces a complicated dependence on the activities at all other nodes.

To compute equation 3.1 using a local learning rule, we augment the feedforward network that maps $X \rightarrow Y \rightarrow Z$ (solid lines of Fig. 1) by adding lateral connections of strength F_{nm} (dashed lines) from each node m to each node n (including $m = n$). The lateral connections do not directly affect the network output Z; they are used only to compute the weight changes ΔC. We choose the strength matrix to be

$$F = I - \alpha Q \qquad (3.2)$$

($\alpha > 0$, and I is the identity matrix) and recursively define a sequence of activity vectors $y(t)$ by

$$y(0) = Y; \qquad y(t+1) = Y + Fy(t) \qquad (3.3)$$

If α is chosen so that $y(t)$ converges (see Appendix), then $\alpha y(\infty) = Q^{-1}Y$ and we obtain the batch update learning rule

$$\Delta C_{ni} = \gamma \partial H / \partial C_{ni} = \gamma \alpha \langle y_n(\infty) X_i \rangle \qquad (3.4)$$

The Hebbian rule $\Delta C_{ni} = \gamma \alpha y_n(\infty) X_i$, using the iterated activity $y(\infty)$ rather than Y, performs stochastic gradient ascent in H.

The lateral connection strengths F depend on C through Q. An estimate $\tilde{Q}$ of Q is computed as a running average, or trace, over recent input presentations. The initial $\tilde{Q}$ is chosen arbitrarily, and $\tilde{Q}_{nm}$ is updated at each presentation by

$$\Delta \tilde{Q}_{nm} = (1/M)(Y_n Y_m + r_{nm} - \tilde{Q}_{nm}) \qquad (3.5)$$

(If r is not explicitly known, $Z_n Z_m$ may be used in place of $Y_n Y_m + r_{nm}$.) We define the strength $F_{nm} \equiv \delta_{nm} - \alpha \tilde{Q}_{nm}$. Thus ΔF_{nm} contains the anti-Hebbian term $[-(\alpha/M)Y_n Y_m]$.

An empirically useful, although not theoretically guaranteed, way to keep α at a proper value for convergence of $y(t)$ is to monitor whether $y(t)$ has "settled down" by a specified time T. For example, define p as the sum over all nodes n (optionally averaged over a running window of recent presentations) of $[y_n(T+1) - y_n(T)] \times [y_n(T) - y_n(T-1)]$. If $y(T)$ has nearly converged to $y(\infty)$, $|p|$ will be smaller than a specified tolerance ϵ. (The converse is not guaranteed.) If $p > \epsilon$, $y(t)$ is converging too slowly and α should be increased. If $p < -\epsilon$, $y(t)$ is oscillating and α should be decreased. (An analytic condition for convergence is discussed in the Appendix. That condition cannot directly be used to choose α, since it makes use of the eigenvalues of Q, which are not available to the network.)

To summarize, the local algorithm for stochastic gradient ascent in H is: Choose initial C (e.g., randomly) and $\tilde{Q}$ (e.g., $= 0$). Then do repeatedly the following steps, which we will refer to as "Algorithm A":

1. Select X; compute $Y = CX$, $Z = Y + \nu$.

2. Update lateral connections: Change $\tilde{Q}$ using equation 3.5.

3. Recursive activation: Compute $\{y(t), t \leq T + 1\}$ using equation 3.3 with $F = I - \alpha\tilde{Q}$.

4. Convergence check (e.g., using p as above). If α needs to be modified, go back to step 3.

5. Update feedforward connections: Change C_{ni} by $\Delta C_{ni} = \gamma \alpha y_n(T)X_i$.

During a start-up period, train $\tilde{Q}$ until it converges, but leave C unchanged, by skipping steps 3–5.

3.2 Gradient Ascent in Mutual Information; "Learning" and "Unlearning" Phases. Combining the two training phases (see equations 2.2 and 3.4), we obtain for the batch update rule

$$\Delta C_{ni} = \gamma \partial R(Z, S)/\partial C_{ni} = \gamma[\alpha_L \langle y_n(\infty; L)X_i \rangle_L - \alpha_U \langle y_n(\infty; U)X_i \rangle_U] \quad (3.6)$$

Here $\langle \ldots \rangle_\phi$ denotes an average over a set of presentations appropriate to phase ϕ—that is, $X \equiv S + N$ for L phase, and $X \equiv N$ for U phase. Each iterated activity $y_n(\infty; \phi)$ is computed using the lateral connection matrix $F^\phi = I - \alpha_\phi \tilde{Q}^\phi$ appropriate to that phase.

Stochastic gradient ascent in $R(Z, S)$ is obtained by starting with arbitrary C, $\tilde{Q}^L$, and $\tilde{Q}^U$, and repeatedly performing Algorithm A alternately (1) for L phase, updating $\tilde{Q}^L$, α_L (if necessary), and C; and (2) for U phase, updating $\tilde{Q}^U$, α_U (if necessary), and C.

3.3 Constraints and "Resource Costs". In general, maximizing the above $R(Z, S)$ will cause elements $|C_{ni}|$ to increase without limit. Some "resource cost" penalty function P, or some explicit constraint on C, is therefore typically included as part of the optimization problem. Maximizing $[R(Z, S) - P]$ instead of $R(Z, S)$ poses no additional difficulty, provided $\partial P/\partial C_{ni}$ can be computed locally (at each node or connection) by the network. Two useful cases are $P \propto \Sigma_n (1 - g_n)^2$, where (1) $g_n = \Sigma_i C_{ni}^2$ or (2) $g_n = V_n$, and where

$$V_n \equiv \langle Y_n^2 \rangle_L = (Cq^L C^T)_{nn} \quad (3.7)$$

is the output variance at node n during L phase (before adding output noise ν_n).

3.4 A Constraint on the Number of Discriminable Output Values at Each Node. Realistic nonlinear processing elements typically have limited dynamic range. This limits the number of output values that can be discriminated in the presence of output noise. One way to introduce a similar limitation in our linear network is to penalize deviations from $V_n = 1$ as above.

In this subsection we explore a different way to limit the effective dynamic range of each node. We multiply the output noise at each node n by the factor $V_n^{1/2}$, so that increasing V_n does not change the number of discriminable output values. That is, $Z_n = Y_n + \nu_n$ with $\nu_n = V_n^{1/2} \nu_n'$ and $\langle \nu_n'^2 \rangle = \beta$ (= constant).[2] When this is done, the variance of each ν_n depends on C (through V_n) and contributes additional terms to the gradient of $R(Z, S)$. We obtain (see Appendix for derivation of equations 3.8 and 3.10)

$$\partial R(Z, S)/\partial C_{ni} = [(Q^L)^{-1}Cq^L]_{ni} - [(Q^U)^{-1}Cq^U]_{ni} \\ + \beta[(Q^L)^{-1} - (Q^U)^{-1}]_{nn}(Cq^L)_{ni} \tag{3.8}$$

(note the term in β is new).

To derive a learning rule for batch update, we must express $[(Q^\phi)^{-1}]_{nn}$ in terms of local quantities. To do this, we recursively compute (during each phase ϕ)

$$y'(0; \phi) = \nu'; \qquad y'(t + 1; \phi) = \nu' + F^\phi y'(t; \phi) \tag{3.9}$$

The prime on y' indicates that the input to the recursion is now ν', rather than CX as before. We find

$$\Delta C_{ni} = \gamma \partial R(Z, S)/\partial C_{ni} \tag{3.10} \\ = \gamma\{\alpha_L \langle y_n(\infty)X_i \rangle_L - \alpha_U \langle y_n(\infty)X_i \rangle_U + (W_n^L - W_n^U)\langle Y_n X_i \rangle_L\}$$

where

$$W_n^\phi = \alpha_\phi \langle y_n'(\infty; \phi)\nu_n' \rangle \tag{3.11}$$

To derive a learning rule for update after each presentation, we associate with each node n an estimate or trace $\tilde{W}_n^\phi$ of W_n^ϕ obtained by choosing an initial $\tilde{W}^\phi$, then updating $\tilde{W}_n^\phi$ by $\Delta \tilde{W}_n^\phi = (1/M)[\alpha_\phi y_n'(\infty; \phi)\nu_n' - \tilde{W}_n^\phi]$. The learning rule is then as stated following equation 3.6, with the addition that $y'(t; \phi)$ is recursively computed and equations 3.10 and 3.11 are used.

---

[2]We could instead have rescaled the output Y_n to unit variance before adding output noise of constant variance β, yielding $Z_n = V_n^{-1/2}Y_n + \nu_n'$. The resulting $R(Z, S)$ is the same in both cases.

4 Illustrative Example

The operation of the local learning rule for update after each presentation in the case of constrained dynamic range (previous subsection) is illustrated by a numerical example.

Each input signal vector S is a set of values at D uniformly spaced sites on a one-dimensional "retina" having periodic boundary conditions. S is obtained by convolving white noise with a gaussian filter, so that $\langle S_i S_j \rangle = \exp[-(s_{ij}/s_0)^2]$ (apart from a negligible deviation due to the boundary condition), where $s_{ij} \equiv \min(|i-j|, D - |i-j|)$. The input noise is white; each component N_i of noise vector N is an independent gaussian random variable of mean zero and variance η. Thus $\langle N_i N_j \rangle = \eta \delta_{ij}$.

There are D' output nodes n. The initial C_{ni} values are drawn independently from a uniform distribution with mean zero. Initial $\tilde{Q}(\phi)$ and $\tilde{W}_n(\phi)$ are set to zero. Parameter values used are $D = 16$; $D' = 8$; $s_0 = 3$; input noise variance $\eta = 0.25$; output noise variance $\beta = 0.5$; $\gamma = 5 \times 10^{-5}$; $\alpha_L = 0.445$ to 0.475 (automatically adjusted to keep the convergence measure $|p| < \epsilon = 10^{-4}$ for $T = 16$); $\alpha_U = 1$; $M = 400$. C is held fixed for the first 800 input presentations to allow $\tilde{Q}^\phi$ to converge. During the development of C, a running estimate (trace) of each output variance V_n is used to rescale C_{ni} (multiplying it by $V_n^{-1/2}$) so that each V_n remains close to unity. [This rescaling of C for each node n is done for convenience, and has no effect on the value of $R(Z, S)$, as discussed in the previous subsection.] Note that γ was conservatively chosen for slow but accurate convergence of C; no attempt was made to optimize the rate of C development.

The resulting weight vector $(C_{n1}, \ldots, C_{nD})$ for each output node n in general spans the entire "retina." [No penalty for long connections has been included; see Linsker (1989a) for discussion of a similar case.] Since the input covariance matrix is Toeplitz ($\langle SS^T \rangle_{ij}$ is a function of $i - j$), the eigenvectors of $\langle SS^T \rangle$ are states (in weight space) having definite spatial frequency k. It is therefore more revealing to show the development of the Fourier components $(\hat{C}_{n1}, \ldots, \hat{C}_{nk}, \ldots, \hat{C}_{nD})$ of C for various n, rather than exhibiting the C_{ni} themselves. Figure 2 shows the squared magnitude $|\hat{C}_{nk}|^2$ for two of the eight nodes n, and the sum of this quantity over all eight nodes, at several stages during training.

The summed squared magnitude develops a "bandpass filter" appearance for the following reasons. For each n, C_{ni} starts as white noise and loses its high spatial frequency components during development, since the input signal is spatially correlated over short distances. The Fourier components of the connection strength also tend to decrease at low spatial frequencies k, where the input signal-to-noise ratio is largest, since devoting a large connection strength to transmitting a high-SNR component would be wasteful of the limited available output variance. Bandpass filter solutions have also been found for similar MI maximiza-

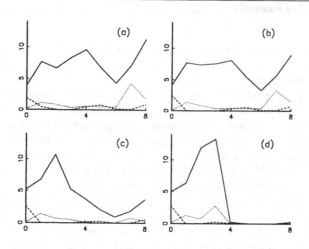

Figure 2: Example of development of Fourier transform $\hat{C}_{nk}$ of C_{ni} for output nodes n, input sites i, and spatial frequencies k. Plotted are $|\hat{C}_{nk}|^2$ (dotted and dashed curves) for two of the eight nodes n, and $\Sigma_n|\hat{C}_{nk}|^2$ (solid curve), vs. $|k|$, at (a) start of development (random C); (b,c) two intermediate times; (d) final state to which C has converged. Corresponding values of $R(Z, S)$ are (a) 2.00, (b) 2.33, (c) 2.87, (d) 3.04. See text for parameter values used.

tion problems, in special cases where the form of C has been restricted to a translationally invariant Ansatz (e.g., $C_{ni} \equiv C[(n/D') - i/D]$) [cf. Linsker (1989a) and Atick and Redlich (1990)].

5 Discussion

It is useful and perhaps striking that learning rules constructed from simple Hebbian and anti-Hebbian modification of feedforward and lateral connections can perform gradient ascent in the mutual information to any desired accuracy, with no need for additional network complexity or nonlocal rules.

The maximization of mutual information appears to have value for extracting statistical regularities, building "feature" analyzers, and generating fruitful comparisons with biological data. For synthetic networks, the existence of a local algorithm increases the likelihood of feasible and efficient hardware implementations. For biological networks, such an algorithm is crucial if the proposed optimality principle or some variant of it is to be seriously considered as a candidate for a general task that a neural processing stage may learn to perform (Linsker 1988).

5.1 Relation to PCA. The optimization principle is related to PCA in the special case that the input noise covariance $\langle NN^T \rangle \equiv \eta I$ and output noise variance $\beta \to 0$. Then the D' output nodes develop to span a D'-dimensional leading PCA subspace of the input space. Although the present MI-maximization algorithm is necessarily more complex, it resembles in some respects the PCA algorithm proposed by Földiák (1989).

An extension of PCA that is of practical interest for improving image SNR (Green *et al.* 1988) corresponds to the case in which the input noise N may have arbitrary correlations and one wants to select those components of the input that have maximum SNR in order to reconstruct a less-noisy version of the input. The present work provides a local network algorithm suitable for selecting the appropriate components.

5.2 More General Distributions and Mappings. In the case of gaussian-distributed inputs to a linear processing stage, treated here, MI maximization strikes a balance between (1) maximizing the fraction of each node's output variance that reflects variance in the input signal as opposed to the input noise; (2) removing correlations among different nodes' output signal values, thereby reducing redundancy (Barlow 1989), when the output noise variance β is small; and (3) *introducing* redundancy to mitigate the information-destroying effects of output noise when β is large.

The present algorithm can be applied to signal and noise distributions that are not multivariate gaussian, as well as to multistage processing systems in which a nonlinear transformation may be applied between stages. In these more general cases, the algorithm can be expected to strike a balance among the same three goals, although in general the MI will not be thereby maximized (since the MI reflects higher order correlations as well). The present learning algorithm, and extensions thereof, are likely to be well suited to nonlinear multistage networks in which one wishes to analyze low-order statistical correlations at each stage, with the goal of extracting higher-order featural information after a sequence of stages.

5.3 Lateral Connectivity and the Role of Selective "Unlearning". Two features of the lateral connectivity in the present work are of interest. First, the lateral connection strengths F_{nm} depend on the correlation between output activities. (They may in general also depend on the distance between output nodes; we have omitted this for simplicity.) Second, two phases—"learning" and "unlearning"—are used for distinguishing input signal from input noise, both of which may have correlational structure. The lateral connection strength depends on which phase the network is in at a given time. It would be of great interest to know to what extent biological learning rules and network architectures may exhibit qualitatively similar features.

Two-phase learning, with input signal present in one phase and absent in the other, has played a role in some earlier work directed toward other goals.

1. A Boltzmann machine learns to generate activation patterns over a subset of nodes whose probability distributions are as nearly as possible the same during two phases: (i) when the nodes' activities are clamped by the inputs, and (ii) when they are free-running (Hinton and Sejnowski 1983).

2. "G-maximization" produces a single node whose output is maximally different, in the presence of input correlations, from what it would be if its inputs were uncorrelated (Pearlmutter and Hinton 1986).

3. The A_{R-P} rule for reinforcement learning (Barto and Anandan 1985) uses a rule similar to Hebbian update when the output is "successful," and anti-Hebbian update otherwise. We may draw an analogy between reinforcement learning and the present work on unsupervised learning: "Success" may indicate that the network is responding to combinations of input that are relevant to the intended goal (hence to combinations that constitute input "signal"), while "failure" may indicate that the input combinations that evoked the response constitute "semantic noise." Extensions of the present algorithm along these lines may be applicable to reinforcement learning.

4. Finally, Crick and Mitchison (1983) have suggested that dream sleep may serve a selective "unlearning" role, by suppressing parasitic or otherwise undesired network interactions. The present algorithm offers a concrete example of the utility of such an "unlearning" process in a simple network.

6 Appendix

Derivation of equation 3.1: Since Q is a positive definite symmetric matrix, it can be shown that $\ln \det Q = \mathrm{Tr} \ln Q$, and that the differential quantity $dH = (1/2)d(\mathrm{Tr} \ln Q) = (1/2)\mathrm{Tr}(Q^{-1}dQ)$. Also, $\partial Q_{mp}/\partial C_{ni} = (Cq)_{mi}\delta_{pn} + (Cq)_{pi}\delta_{mn}$, where δ denotes the Dirac delta function. Therefore, $\partial H/\partial C_{ni} = (Q^{-1}Cq)_{ni}$.

Derivation of equation 3.4: The recursive method is due to Jacobi. Equations 3.2 and 3.3 yield $\alpha y(\infty) = \alpha \Sigma_{t=0}^{\infty} F^t Y = \alpha(I - F)^{-1}Y = Q^{-1}Y$. Combining this result with equation 3.1 yields the desired result.

Convergence condition for α (see text following equation 3.5): Let f denote the eigenvalues of F, and let $\lambda_{\pm}$ denote the maximum and minimum eigenvalues of Q ($0 < \lambda_- \le \lambda_+$). Iff $\alpha < 2/\lambda_+$, then $\max |f| < 1$ and the series $(I - F)^{-1} = \Sigma_{t=0}^{\infty} F^t$ converges.

For faster convergence, $\max |f|$ should be small. When $\alpha = 2/(\lambda_+ + \lambda_-)$, $\max |f|$ is minimized and equals $(\lambda_+ - \lambda_-)/(\lambda_+ + \lambda_-)$. The convergence rate is slow when $\max |f|$ is close to unity, i.e., when the condition number of Q, λ_+/λ_-, is large. Note that the variance of the output noise term ν_n can be used to control the condition number: increasing all output noise variances by a constant increases λ_+ and λ_- by the same amount, hence decreases the condition number and improves convergence.

Derivation of equations 3.8 and 3.10: $V_m = (Cq^L C^T)_{mm}$ yields $\partial V_m/\partial C_{ni} = 2(Cq^L)_{ni}\delta_{mn}$. We also have

$$Q^L_{mp} = (Cq^L C^T)_{mp} + \beta V_m \delta_{mp} \tag{A.1}$$

hence

$$\partial Q^L_{mp}/\partial C_{ni} = (Cq^L)_{mi}\delta_{pn} + (Cq^L)_{pi}\delta_{mn} + 2\beta(Cq^L)_{ni}\delta_{mn}\delta_{pn} \tag{A.2}$$

and

$$\partial[(1/2)\ln\det Q^L]/\partial C_{ni} = [(Q^L)^{-1}Cq^L]_{ni} + \beta[(Q^L)^{-1}]_{nn}(Cq^L)_{ni} \tag{A.3}$$

Subtracting the corresponding expression involving Q^U yields equation 3.8. Next, using equation 3.9 and $\langle \nu'_m \nu'_n \rangle = \beta\delta_{nm}$, we obtain

$$
\begin{aligned}
\alpha_\phi \langle y'_n(\infty;\phi)\nu'_n \rangle &= \alpha_\phi \langle [\Sigma_{l=0}^{\infty}(F^\phi)^l \nu']_n \nu'_n \rangle = \langle [(Q^\phi)^{-1}\nu']_n \nu'_n \rangle \\
&= \Sigma_m [(Q^\phi)^{-1}]_{nm}\langle \nu'_m \nu'_n \rangle = \beta[(Q^\phi)^{-1}]_{nn}
\end{aligned} \tag{A.4}
$$

Combining this result with $(Cq^L)_{ni} = \langle Y_n X_i \rangle_L$ yields equation 3.10.

References

Atick, J. J., and Redlich, A. N. 1990. Towards a theory of early visual processing. *Neural Comp.* **2**, 308–320.

Atick, J. J., and Redlich, A. N. 1991. Predicting ganglion and simple cell receptive field organizations. *Int. J. Neural Syst.* **1**, 305–315.

Barlow, H. B. 1989. Unsupervised learning. *Neural Comp.* **1**, 295–311.

Barto, A. G., and Anandan, P. 1985. Pattern-recognizing stochastic learning automata. *IEEE Trans. Sys. Man Cybern.* **15**, 360–375.

Crick, F. H. C., and Mitchison, G. 1983. The function of dream sleep. *Nature (London)* **304**, 111–114.

Földiák, P. 1989. Adaptive network for optimal linear feature extraction. In *Proc. IEEE/INNS Intern. Joint Conf. Neural Networks, Washington, DC*, Vol. 1, pp. 401–405. IEEE Press, New York.

Green, A. A., Berman, M., Switzer, P., and Craig, M. D. 1988. A transformation for ordering multispectral data in terms of image quality with implications for noise removal. *IEEE Trans. Geosci. Remote Sensing* **26**, 65–74.

Hinton, G. E., and Sejnowski, T. J. 1983. Optimal perceptual inference. *Proc. IEEE Conf. Computer Vision*, 448–453.

Leen, T. K. 1991. Dynamics of learning in linear feature-discovery networks. *Network* **2**, 85–105.

Linsker, R. 1988. Self-organization in a perceptual network. *Computer* **21**(March), 105–117.

Linsker, R. 1989a. An application of the principle of maximum information preservation to linear systems. In *Advances in Neural Information Processing Systems 1*, D. S. Touretzky, ed., pp. 186–194. Morgan Kaufmann, San Mateo, CA.

Linsker, R. 1989b. How to generate ordered maps by maximizing the mutual information between input and output signals. *Neural Comp.* **1**, 402–411.

Pearlmutter, B. A., and Hinton, G. E. 1986. G-maximization: An unsupervised learning procedure for discovering regularities. In *Neural Networks for Computing*, J. S. Denker, ed., pp. 333–338. American Institute Physics, New York.

Sanger, T. 1989. An optimality principle for unsupervised learning. In *Advances in Neural Information Processing Systems 1*, D. S. Touretzky, ed., pp. 11–19. Morgan Kaufmann, San Mateo, CA.

Shannon, C. E., and Weaver, W. 1949. *The Mathematical Theory of Communication.* Univ. of Illinois Press, Urbana.

3

Convergent Algorithm for Sensory Receptive Field Development

Joseph J. Atick
The Rockefeller University, 1230 York Avenue,
New York, NY 10021 USA

A. Norman Redlich
School of Natural Sciences, Institute for Advanced Study,
Princeton, NJ 08540 USA

An unsupervised developmental algorithm for linear maps is derived which reduces the pixel-entropy (using the measure introduced in previous work) at every update and thus removes pairwise correlations between pixels. Since the measure of pixel-entropy has only a global minimum the algorithm is guaranteed to converge to the minimum entropy map. Such optimal maps have recently been shown to possess cognitively desirable properties and are likely to be used by the nervous system to organize sensory information. The algorithm derived here turns out to be one proposed by Goodall for pairwise decorrelation. It is biologically plausible since in a neural network implementation it requires only data available locally to a neuron. In training over ensembles of two-dimensional input signals with the same spatial power spectrum as natural scenes, networks develop output neurons with center-surround receptive fields similar to those of ganglion cells in the retina. Some technical issues pertinent to developmental algorithms of this sort, such as "symmetry fixing," are also discussed.

1 Introduction

Recent theoretical results on neural processing support the idea that efficiency of information representation in the sensory pathways could have cognitive advantages [Barlow 1989 (+REFS); Linsker 1988; Atick and Redlich 1990]. This is a predictive idea since it leads to the hypothesis that much of the processing in the early stages is geared toward recoding incoming sensory signals into a more efficient form. Starting with natural signals one can assess the efficiency of the sampled representation formed by the array of sensory cells and mathematically derive recodings that would improve the efficiency. These recodings can then be compared with the multistages of neural processing observed.

One form of efficient representations that figures prominently in the recent literature is the so called "minimum entropy" one,[1] where the sum of the individual entropies for the elements of the representation (e.g., pixels) is minimal for the ensemble of natural signals (Field 1987; Barlow 1989; Barlow *et al.* 1989; Atick and Redlich 1990, 1992). This minimum is achieved when there is the least possible statistical dependence between elements. The idea that the nervous system could be engaged in trying to build such a minimum entropy representation of the environment has been tested in the limited context of retinal processing (Atick and Redlich 1992). There it was assumed that the retina, being the first stage in the visual pathway, could reduce pixel-entropy by eliminating no higher than two-point correlations (pairwise correlations). The linear transform on the photoreceptor activities needed to achieve pixel–pixel decorrelations was shown to agree with observed retinal filters—after being careful to take noise into account.

In general, the problem of finding entropy reducing maps is very difficult. It is also very unlikely that one will be able to analytically solve for the explicit form of these maps as was done for the pairwise decorrelating map in the retina. An alternate approach is to use neural networks to try to compute these maps. What one needs are developmental algorithms that iteratively reduce statistical dependence among the elements of the representation as a network is trained over more sensory inputs, and preferably algorithms that are guaranteed to converge to the optimal maps.

In this paper we derive a simple developmental algorithm, for the linear class of maps, which we prove lowers pixel-entropy at each learning stage. For this class of maps lowering pixel-entropy is equivalent to decreasing pairwise correlations at each step. The algorithm turns out to be identical to one originally introduced by Goodall (1960) who was interested in decorrelation in a different context. When introduced, Goodall's algorithm was proven—without reference to an entropy measure—to converge to the solution that pairwise decorrelates. For us this old proof is an independent check of convergence since our entropy measure has no local minima. Therefore our demonstration that the Goodall algorithm successively lowers the entropy is sufficient in itself to prove it converges to the global minimum. This minimum entropy solution is the one that we have previously shown predicts the linear processing observed in the retina—after incorporating noise filtering. One major purpose of this paper is to demonstrate that these ganglion cell receptive fields can also be developed by applying the Goodall algorithm to an ensemble with the same second-order statistical properties (same power spectrum) as natural scenes. Also we expect insight gained from this simple algorithm to be helpful in discovering more complex algorithms capable of produc-

---

[1]In previous papers we have referred to this as minimum redundancy representation, since it eliminates the part of redundancy that is due to statistical dependence among the elements.

ing minimum entropy representations for nonlinear maps that reduce statistical dependence beyond pairwise decorrelation.

We should point out that there are several other pairwise decorrelating algorithms in the literature (Kohonen and Oja 1976; Oja 1982; Linsker 1986; Barlow and Foldiak 1989; Foldiak 1989; Sanger 1989; Rubner and Schulten 1990). However, the algorithm that we are presenting here is of particular interest to us since it is proven to reduce our previously introduced entropy measure. Another nice property of this algorithm is its locality in the sense that all of the data needed by a synapse to modify its strength is available at the input to the neuron. This means that the algorithm is at least plausibly one that might be implemented biologically.

By actually attempting here to derive receptive fields based on a "natural" input ensemble we are also forced to face an important issue that also arises in implementing similar decorrelation algorithms, but has not to our knowledge been resolved. The problem is that decorrelation itself does not guarantee a unique solution for the receptive fields, and most of the solutions are not localized. This problem can be traced to a large symmetry under which any decorrelating solution remains decorrelating. Here we theoretically analyze the requirements for fixing this symmetry and we find a simple way to do so that leads to localized receptive fields.

2 Entropy Reduction and Convergence

We begin by assuming that the sensory input signal $\{S_i\}$, representing the set of photoreceptor responses, is recoded through a linear map K_{ij} to the set of outputs $\{O_i\}$, which in the retina are the ganglion cell responses:

$$O_i = \sum_j K_{ij} S_j \tag{2.1}$$

As in our previous work (Atick and Redlich 1990, 1992), we introduce an "entropy" measure $E\{K\}$, that grades different recodings K according to how well they minimize the sum of pixel entropies, without overall loss of information:

$$E\{K\} = \mathrm{Tr}(K \cdot R \cdot K^T) - \log \det(K^T \cdot K) \tag{2.2}$$

In 2.2 $R_{ij} \equiv \langle S_i S_j \rangle$ is the autocorrelator for the input ensemble, with brackets denoting ensemble average; boldface denotes matrices. Minimizing the first term was shown to be equivalent to minimizing the sum of the individual pixel entropies, while the second term acts to enforce reversibility of the map (no information loss). When the measure 2.2 is minimized, $\delta E/\delta K = 0$, one gets a decorrelating solution K satisfying

$$K \cdot R \cdot K^T = 1 \tag{2.3}$$

which when convoluted with a noise filter was shown to reproduce ganglion cell receptive fields (Atick and Redlich 1992).

Although mathematically it is straightforward to find a decorrelating
solution $\mathbf{K}$ satisfying 2.3, it is not clear how a network of neurons can
arrive at such a $\mathbf{K}$. What is needed is a biologically plausible developmental algorithm that can be proven to converge to a $\mathbf{K}$ satisfying 2.3.
One way to do this is to find a small update $\delta\mathbf{K}$ for the map $\mathbf{K}$ that is
guaranteed to lower $E\{\mathbf{K}\}$ at each step. This requires that the change in
$E\{\mathbf{K}\}$ due to $\delta\mathbf{K}$ must be negative:

$$\delta E\{\mathbf{K}\} = \mathrm{Tr}\left(\frac{\delta E}{\delta\mathbf{K}} \cdot \delta\mathbf{K}^T\right) < 0 \tag{2.4}$$

One obvious possibility is to use gradient descent $\delta\mathbf{K}^T = -(\delta E/\delta\mathbf{K})^T$.
However this leads to a nonlocal algorithm that at each update stage
requires the computation of an *inverse* matrix. We propose instead the
update

$$\delta\mathbf{K}^T = -\mathbf{K}^T \cdot \left[\frac{\delta E}{\delta\mathbf{K}}\right] \cdot \mathbf{K}^T \tag{2.5}$$

where from 2.2

$$\frac{\delta E}{\delta\mathbf{K}} = 2\left[\mathbf{K} \cdot \mathbf{R} - (\mathbf{K}^T)^{-1}\right] \tag{2.6}$$

Like gradient descent this update always reduces $E\{\mathbf{K}\}$ since by 2.4 and
2.5

$$\delta E\{\mathbf{K}\} = -\mathrm{Tr}\left([\mathbf{K} \cdot \mathbf{R} \cdot \mathbf{K}^T - \mathbf{1}][\mathbf{K} \cdot \mathbf{R} \cdot \mathbf{K}^T - \mathbf{1}]^T\right) \tag{2.7}$$

which is always negative (or zero upon convergence) since $\mathrm{Tr}(\mathbf{M}\cdot\mathbf{M}^T) > 0$
for any matrix $\mathbf{M} \neq 0$. (For the mathematically minded reader this shows
that E can be thought of as a Lyapunov functional.)

The next step is to show that the update 2.5 can be implemented as an
algorithm requiring no nonlocal calculations. For this we rewrite 2.5 as
an update for $\mathbf{K}^{-1}$ instead of $\mathbf{K}^T$, using the fact $\delta\mathbf{K}^{-1} = -\mathbf{K}^{-1}\cdot\delta\mathbf{K}\cdot\mathbf{K}^{-1}$. For
later convenience, we also change notation now and define $\mathbf{W} \equiv \mathbf{K}^{-1}$; the
variables W_{ij} will designate the actual synaptic strengths in the feedback
network introduced in the next section. Then in terms of $\mathbf{W}$ the algorithm
2.5 becomes

$$\tau\frac{d\mathbf{W}}{dt} = \mathbf{R} \cdot \left(\mathbf{W}^{-1}\right)^T - \mathbf{W} \tag{2.8}$$

where τ is a time constant setting the update rate. Although $\mathbf{W}^{-1}$ does
appear in 2.8, it appears in the combination $\mathbf{R} \cdot (\mathbf{W}^{-1})^T$, which as will be
discussed in the next section is equal to $\langle S_i O_j\rangle$, and thus in the network

implementation no nonlocal computations will be needed. The algorithm 2.8 can be recognized as the ensemble averaged form of the Goodall (1960) algorithm.

Since direct minimization of $E\{\mathbf{K}\}$ in 2.2 gives the global minimum 2.3 with no local minima, our demonstrating that 2.8 or 2.5 always reduces $E\{\mathbf{K}\}$ is sufficient to prove convergence. However, for completeness we shall also give the old proof of convergence (Goodall 1960) that does not require a minimization measure. One reason we give this proof here is that it leads us to rewrite the update algorithm 2.8 in yet another form that will be useful in our later discussion of symmetry fixing and locality. To start the proof we need, in addition to 2.8, the transpose equation

$$\frac{d\mathbf{W}^T}{dt} = \left(\mathbf{W}^{-1}\right) \cdot \mathbf{R} - \mathbf{W}^T \tag{2.9}$$

using $\mathbf{R} = \mathbf{R}^T$. By multiplying 2.8 from the right by $\mathbf{W}^T$ and 2.9 from the left by $\mathbf{W}$ and then adding the resulting equations, we arrive at the integrable differential equation

$$\tau\frac{d}{dt}\left(\mathbf{W}\cdot\mathbf{W}^T\right) = 2\left(\mathbf{R} - \mathbf{W}\cdot\mathbf{W}^T\right) \tag{2.10}$$

which has the solution

$$\mathbf{W}\cdot\mathbf{W}^T = \mathbf{R} - e^{-2t/\tau}\mathbf{C} \tag{2.11}$$

where $\mathbf{C}$ is a constant matrix determined by initial conditions. In the limit where t/τ becomes large $\mathbf{W}\cdot\mathbf{W}^T = \mathbf{R}$, which is just the minimum $E\{\mathbf{K}\}$ solution 2.3 since $\mathbf{W} \equiv \mathbf{K}^{-1}$.

3 Network Implementation

In this section we discuss a network implementation of the above algorithm. As shown in Figure 1 the network has one nontrivial layer, with feedforward connections directly from the input S_i and lateral feedback connections among the neurons. It is assumed that the input S_i is directly connected only to the ith neuron, with link strength unity. The plastic links in this network are the lateral feedback links that connect the output of the jth neuron back to the input of the ith neuron with link strength W_{ij}. The neurons are assumed to be linear, thus the dynamics of this network can be written as

$$T\frac{dO_i}{dt} = S_i - \sum_j W_{ij}O_j \tag{3.1}$$

where O_i is the output of the ith neuron, S_i is its feedforward input, and

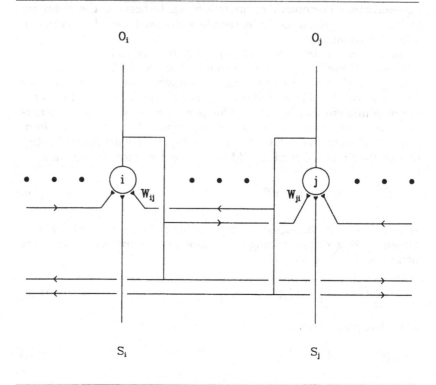

Figure 1: The architecture of the network used for decorrelation. It is assumed that the ith neuron receives direct input with synaptic weight unity from S_i and feedback input from the outputs of all neurons with weights W_{ij}. Only the feedback links W_{ij} are updated during learning.

T is a time constant. Below we shall assume that $T \ll \tau$ for the update algorithm 2.8 so we can safely approximate the system by its equilibrium solution, $dO_i/dt = 0$,

$$S_i = \sum_j W_{ij}O_j \qquad (3.2)$$

This shows that the matrix W_{ij} can be identified with the *inverse* of the retinal kernel K_{ij} introduced above, so W_{ij}^{-1} corresponds to the ith ganglion cell's receptive field.

In terms of the network variables S_i, O_j, W_{ij}, the algorithm 2.8 can be written as

$$\tau \frac{dW_{ij}}{dt} = \langle S_i O_j \rangle - W_{ij} \qquad (3.3)$$

where the brackets denote an ensemble average. To see that this is the same as 2.8 note that $\langle S_i O_j \rangle = \sum_k \langle S_i S_k \rangle W_{jk}^{-1}$ and $\langle S_i S_j \rangle = R_{ij}$. As long as τ is much greater than the characteristic time scale of the ensemble we can remove the averaging brackets in 3.3 and finally arrive at the algorithm that requires no a priori knowledge of any ensemble properties (no prior knowledge of **R**)

$$\tau \frac{dW_{ij}}{dt} = S_i O_j - W_{ij} \qquad (3.4)$$

Another significant fact about 3.4 is that it is biologically plausible in the sense that all of the data, S_i, O_j, W_{ij} needed for the ith neuron to update its synaptic links, W_{ij}, is available locally to that neuron (see Fig. 1).

In Section 6 we simulate 3.4 for an ensemble of inputs with the same autocorrelator as natural scenes. But before we can do that we need to discuss the important technical issue of the nonuniqueness of the decorrelating solutions, and the related problem of nonlocalized receptive fields.

4 Finding Localized Receptive Fields

We would like next to apply the learning algorithm 3.4 to generate linear receptive fields for an ensemble of "natural" input images. However, if one naively employs this learning algorithm, the receptive fields very often turn out to be nonlocalized, and thus do not resemble those of retinal ganglion cells. The problem is that the algorithm 3.4 or 2.8, though guaranteed to converge to a pairwise decorrelating solution, $\mathbf{W} \cdot \mathbf{W}^T = \mathbf{R}$, does not find a unique solution W, and most of the solutions are not localized. The source of the nonuniqueness is that $\mathbf{W} \cdot \mathbf{W}^T$ possesses a large symmetry, since any transform $\mathbf{W} \rightarrow \mathbf{W} \cdot \mathbf{U}$ of a solution $\mathbf{W}$ by any orthogonal matrix $\mathbf{U}$ ($\mathbf{U} \cdot \mathbf{U}^T = 1$) is also a solution. This means that there is a whole class of acceptable solutions parameterized by $\mathbf{U}$. However, from a biological point of view, most of these solutions are unacceptable since they correspond to nonlocalized receptive fields.

So the problem is to eliminate the extra symmetry $\mathbf{U}$ in a way that guarantees localization. In other words, we wish to remove the extra degrees of freedom in $\mathbf{W}$ due to this symmetry by constraining the form of $\mathbf{W}$, while preserving its decorrelating property: $\mathbf{W} \cdot \mathbf{W}^T = \mathbf{R}$. One type of constraint that does this is

$$\mathbf{W} = \mathbf{W}^T \qquad (4.1)$$

since there is no longer any freedom to multiply $\mathbf{W}$ by $\mathbf{U}$ without violating this condition. That this condition removes all the extra freedom follows from the fact that the number of independent components of the matrix

W that are eliminated is $N(N-1)/2$, which is precisely the number of independent components in **U**.

The reason for our choice of constraint 4.1 is that, for all autocorrelators **R** that we consider, 4.1 leads to localized, translation invariant receptive fields. To see this note that 4.1 implies that **W** satisfies the more restricted equation $\mathbf{W} \cdot \mathbf{W} = \mathbf{R}$, which has (up to sign) a unique solution since the **U** symmetry has been eliminated. This means that if **R** is translation invariant so is **W**.[2] Furthermore, translation invariance of **W** allows us to go to frequency space and write $W^2(f) = R(f)$. Recall then that $W(f)$ is the inverse of the receptive field kernel $K(f)$, so $K(f) = \pm\sqrt{1/R(f)}$. This means that $K(f)$ will be localized so long as $R(f)$ has the property that it is a sufficiently smooth function of frequency f. One can show that for the receptive field to be localized to an approximate size D, the smoothness criterion for $K(f)$ [and thus implicitly for $R(f)$] is $[\partial K(f)/\partial f]/[D K(f)] \ll 1$. This smoothness condition, for the appropriate D, is satisfied by the autocorrelators $R(f)$ that we use here which are based on the properties of natural scenes.

Now that we know what condition 4.1 we wish the solution **W** to satisfy once it converges, the next step is to find a way to guarantee that the learning algorithm 3.4 will actually converge to the specific **W** satisfying 4.1, rather than to one of the many other **W** related to it through multiplication by some **U**. In the next section we introduce a procedure for doing so that is well known to physicists as "gauge-fixing" and that we call here "symmetry-fixing." [3] The discussion in that section is somewhat technical, so for the reader who is not interested in the details we state the conclusion here so that the next section can be skipped without loss of continuity: To guarantee that the system converges to a solution that satisfies 4.1 (i.e., localized solution) it turns out that it is *sufficient* to start the algorithm at time zero with the initial condition $\mathbf{W}(t=0) = \mathbf{1}$ (this is sufficient but may not be necessary). While this is a very simple boundary condition, it is not obvious that it alone ensures convergence to configurations satisfying both $\mathbf{W} \cdot \mathbf{W}^T = \mathbf{R}$ and $\mathbf{W} = \mathbf{W}^T$, which is what we prove in the next section.

5 Symmetry Fixing

Our approach here is to ask how the algorithm 3.4 can in general be forced to converge to a solution that satisfies some symmetry fixing constraint, say 4.1 that we argued in the last section ensures locality. To

---

[2] This follows since the solution to $\mathbf{W} \cdot \mathbf{W} = \mathbf{R}$ is unique. Therefore if a translation invariant solution is found it must be the only solution.

[3] An alternative way to fix the symmetry is to include in the developmental algorithm terms that attempt to produce statistical independence beyond pairwise decorrelation (there is no proof yet that any developmental algorithm with higher order terms converges). This is assuming, of course, that higher order correlations break the U symmetry, but this is often the case (see, e.g., Hopfield 1991).

accomplish this we study both the possibility of using special initial conditions [such as $\mathbf{W}(t = 0) = \mathbf{1}$] as well as the possibility of modifying the algorithm itself in a way that does not spoil its decorrelating or convergence properties. It will turn out that for the special case of the condition $\mathbf{W} = \mathbf{W}^T$, no modification of the algorithm is needed if one uses the initial condition $\mathbf{W}(t = 0) = \mathbf{1}$. However, to prove this requires that we look at the general symmetry fixing problem, where it *will* be necessary to modify the algorithm. One reason, also, that we explore the more general symmetry fixing problem is that the U symmetry is ubiquitous in the literature on decorrelating algorithms. Therefore, it is important to learn tools for handling this symmetry.

Generally speaking, symmetry fixing is a procedure that introduces extra control over the dynamics for $\mathbf{W}$ in a way that *automatically* forces the system to converge to the $\mathbf{W}$ satisfying the desired constraint. The extra control as we explain next is introduced by modifying 2.8 in a way that does not interfere with the convergence proof. The key to the modification of the dynamics comes from recognizing that not only the *solution* $\mathbf{W} \cdot \mathbf{W}^T = \mathbf{R}$ possesses the U symmetry, but also the dynamic equation 2.10, which is the fundamental equation ensuring convergence to the decorrelation solution, is invariant under the transformation $\mathbf{W} \rightarrow \mathbf{W} \cdot \mathbf{U}(t)$ for any time-dependent orthogonal matrix $\mathbf{U}(t)$. This means that multiplication of $\mathbf{W}(t)$ by a time-dependent orthogonal transformation does not interfere with the convergence proof. However, it does modify the dynamics in 2.8 since that equation is not invariant under this transformation. In fact under $\mathbf{W} \rightarrow \mathbf{W} \cdot \mathbf{U}(t)$ 2.8 transforms to

$$\tau \frac{d\mathbf{W}}{dt} = \mathbf{R} \cdot \left(\mathbf{W}^{-1}\right)^T - \mathbf{W} + \mathbf{W} \cdot \frac{d\mathbf{U}}{dt} \cdot \mathbf{U}^T \tag{5.1}$$

To see that the last term indeed drops out from the dynamic equation 2.10 for $\mathbf{W} \cdot \mathbf{W}^T$ we need only to note that $\mathbf{U} \cdot \left(d\mathbf{U}^T/dt\right) = -\left(d\mathbf{U}/dt\right) \cdot \mathbf{U}^T$, valid since $\mathbf{U} \cdot \mathbf{U}^T = \mathbf{1}$.

The next step is to show how the freedom to choose $\mathbf{U}(t)$ can be used to control the dynamics such that the system will converge to a $\mathbf{W}$ with a particular property, say $\mathbf{W}^T = \mathbf{W}$. One might attempt to satisfy this constraint 4.1 on the solution $\mathbf{W}$ by starting with initial conditions that satisfy it. However, the original dynamic equation 2.8 very quickly would evolve $\mathbf{W}(t)$ to configurations that violate 4.1. On the other hand, the modified equation 5.1 gives us the extra freedom to pick $\mathbf{U}(t)$ such that the property 4.1 is maintained at all time t.

For completeness we explicitly give the symmetry-fixing term in 5.1 that does maintain 4.1 for all time t, so long as $\mathbf{W}^T(0) = \mathbf{W}(0)$ at time $t = 0$. We give it in a basis where $\mathbf{W}$ is diagonal with eigenvalues λ_i:

$$\left(\frac{d\mathbf{U}}{dt} \cdot \mathbf{U}^T\right)_{ij} = \frac{1}{\lambda_i + \lambda_j}[\mathbf{R}, \mathbf{W}^{-1}]_{ij} \tag{5.2}$$

where the brackets denote the commutator defined for any two matrices A and B as $[A, B] = A \cdot B - B \cdot A$. One could try to simulate the dynamics in 5.1 with the explicit expression 5.2 included, however, this term appears too complex to be biologically plausible. However, if we choose the more restrictive initial condition for $W(0)$ to satisfy $[R, W^{-1}(0)] = 0$, in addition to $W(0) = W^T(0)$, then the necessary symmetry fixing term 5.2 vanishes on the first iteration, and can be shown to remain zero thereafter. So by going through the symmetry-fixing exercise we have identified a set of special initial conditions on W that do guarantee that 4.1 is maintained at all times, and moreover do so without modifying the original equation 2.8.

One choice of initial conditions that very simply satisfies both $[R, W^{-1}] = 0$ and $W = W^T$ is $W(0) = \mathbf{1}$, which is the condition we use in our simulations in the next section. Without the above analysis we would not have known a priori that this initial condition is sufficient to ensure that the solution the system converges to will satisfy $W = W^T$. This particular initial condition may be biologically plausible since it means that initially the neurons have no lateral links and that these links are developed as needed. Also, we have tested for the stability of this initial condition by starting the runs from configurations where the lateral links are nonvanishing but small, and we find small nonvanishing links do not disturb the convergence to the unique solution.

6 Simulations

To test the learning algorithm 3.4 we first applied it to a one-dimensional (1D) ensemble of inputs S_i, $i = 1, \ldots, n$ with $n = 64$. For simulation purposes, we imposed periodic boundary conditions on the 1D space and generated an ensemble of S_i with an autocorrelator R_{ij} whose Fourier transform (power spectrum) was $R(f) \sim 1/|f|^4$ but that had no higher order correlations. This particular $R(f)$ in one dimension was an arbitrary choice that happened to give clear results. By itself, however, this ensemble is not realistic since unlike real sensory signals it is noise free. So we added to the signal S_i noise with flat power spectrum $|N(f)|^2 = N^2$. This type of noise signal N_i is already spatially decorrelated having autocorrelator $\langle N_i N_j \rangle \sim \delta_{i,j}$.

Adding the random noise signal N_i also happens to serve a significant function by increasing the stability of the algorithm 3.4, although this might seem anti-intuitive. The source of the instability is that W^{-1} appearing in 2.8 (even though we implement 3.4) can eventually blow up if there are any very small eigenvalue modes in R, since ultimately $(W \cdot W^T)^{-1} \rightarrow R^{-1}$ according to 2.11. This small eigenvalue problem can be accentuated during the learning process while $W \cdot W^T$ is only approximately equal to R, so during learning W may have even smaller eigenvalues than it does once it converges. Adding noise with a flat spectrum eliminates this small eigenvalue problem by adding a constant to all the eigenvalues. In frequency space $R(f) \rightarrow R(f) + N^2$ so the eigenvalues can never get too small. In practice *any nonvanishing noise* N^2 assures stabilization. Thus the algorithm 3.4 applied to any realistic problem—which always has nonvanishing noise—will continue to be convergent. In our one-dimensional simulations we chose a signal to noise of four.

The parameter τ in 3.4 was chosen to be much larger than the characteristic time scale of the ensemble so that 3.4 could approximate the convergent algorithm 3.3. A general lower bound on τ is not possible since it is ensemble dependent and hence requires experimentation. We find that smooth convergence does require a relatively large τ compared to the size of the terms on the right-hand side of 3.4. In our one-dimensional simulations we chose $\tau = 5000$. Finally, we used the initial condition $W_{ij} = \delta_{ij}$, that as discussed in Section 3 is sufficient to eliminate the **U** symmetry. This then turns out to produce spatially local receptive fields $\mathbf{W}^{-1}$ as shown in Figure 2, which exhibits the converged solution for the 32nd neuron, W_{32j}^{-1}, after $20,000$ iterations.

Having demonstrated the viability of 3.4 through a one-dimensional example, the next step is to apply 3.4 to a two-dimensional ensemble with statistical properties close to those of a natural visual environment. Field (1987) argued, based on some experimentation with "natural" scenes, that natural environments have an approximately scale invariant spatial autocorrelator, which is equivalent to having a spatial power spectrum proportional to $|f|^{-2}$ for two-dimensional frequencies f. We have shown previously (Atick and Redlich 1992) that the retinal ganglion cell kernel $\mathbf{W}^{-1}$ acts to decorrelate the environmental signal—at least at low frequencies where the signal to noise is high—which in frequency space means $W^{-1}(f) \sim |f|$ so that $|W(f)|^2 = R(f)$. Here, the goal of the two-dimensional simulation is to demonstrate that this decorrelating kernel can be learned by a network implementing the developmental rule 3.4.

In two dimensions (2D) we generated an ensemble with power spectrum $|f|^{-2}$ and without higher order statistics. We again added random noise for a $S/N = 4$, chose the initial condition $\mathbf{W} = \mathbf{1}$, and found that $\tau = 20,000$ was sufficiently large to ensure smooth convergence. There was one major difference, however, between our one- and two-dimensional simulations that was necessitated by the need to reduce computation time in the two-dimensional case. In 2D it was computationally necessary to assume translation invariance of the solution W_{ij}, meaning assuming in advance that W_{ij} will take the form $W_{ij} = W(|i-j|)$ after convergence [note that the index i in 2D now denotes the two-dimensional vector $i = (i_x, i_y)$]. This is a valid assumption since, as discussed in Sections four and five, the initial condition $\mathbf{W} = \mathbf{1}$ implies $\mathbf{W} = \mathbf{W}^T$, which in turn implies translation invariance of $\mathbf{W}$, as long as the ensemble is chosen to be translation invariant. Restricting $\mathbf{W}$ to

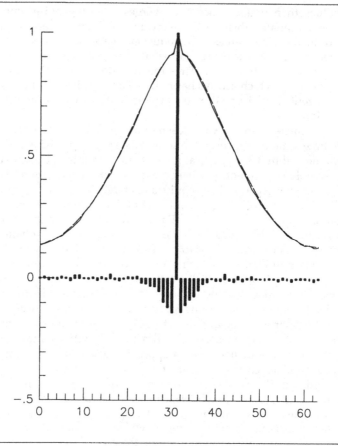

Figure 2: The one-dimensional receptive field, W_{32j}^{-1}, for the 32nd neuron after the algorithm converges (j running along the horizontal axis with 64 the total number of neurons). The receptive fields of other neurons are very similar. The dashed line is the autocorrelator $\langle S_i S_{32} \rangle$ averaged over the training data, while the solid curve is $(\mathbf{W} \cdot \mathbf{W}^T)_{i32}$, which is very close to the actual autocorrelator. The training was done with 20,000 iterations, $\tau = 5000$ and $S/N = 4$ starting with the initial condition $W_{ij}(t = 0) = \delta_{ij}$.

Figure 3: *Facing page.* Typical two-dimensional images used in training the network in 2D. Image B differs from image A only by the addition of a small amount of noise. These images have the property that their power spectrum is identical to that of natural scenes, namely $1/|\mathbf{f}|^2$. We have trained networks using these images instead of actual scenes for convenience only. The algorithm should converge to similar solutions if trained on actual natural scenes as long as the power spectrum is the same.

a

b

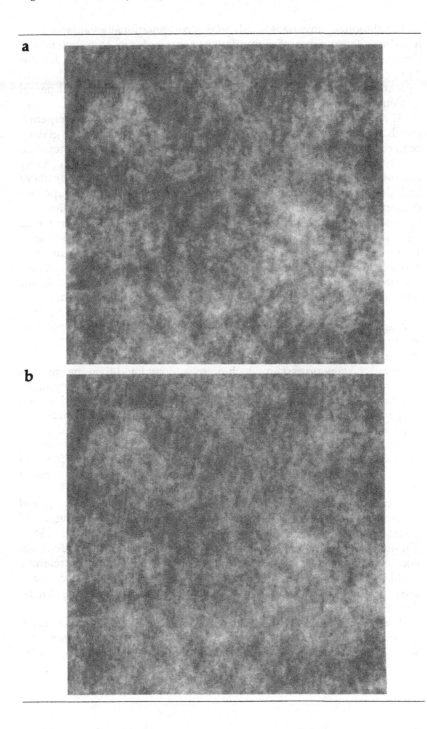

be translationally invariant in advance is computationally valuable since it reduces the number of computations from order n^2 to n, where n is the number of input signals (number of photoreceptors), which for our simulation was $n = 16 \times 16$. We should emphasize, though, that this restriction was purely for simulation purposes, and in an actual neural implementation of 3.4 there would be no need for it.

The result of the two-dimensional simulation following convergence, which took about 200,000 steps, is shown in Figure 4. It has the generic center-surround property of a ganglion cell, but does not correspond exactly to a ganglion cell receptive field. That is because it is a purely *decorrelating kernel*, whereas the true ganglion cell kernel both decorrelates and filters noise, as shown in Atick and Redlich (1992). In that paper we demonstrated that the total retinal kernel can be obtained by first low pass filtering the noisy input signal and then decorrelating the result. Here we have demonstrated that 3.4 can perform the decorrelation step. Therefore if one first low pass filters in exactly the same way as in Atick and Redlich (1992) (where we were careful to include the appropriate transmission noise following the lowpass stage) and then applies 3.4, one must arrive at the same realistic ganglion cell kernels found in that paper, since this effectively reproduces the steps outlined there. We also expect that applying 3.4 to natural scenes, since they have the same spectrum as our simulation scenes, would likewise produce results close to those shown here.

In a two-stage process in which noise is filtered and then the signal is decorrelated, it is also possible to derive the noise filter separately using a different learning algorithm. For example in Atick and Redlich (1991) we gave a convergent developmental rule for learning least mean square noise smoothing. (Such noise filtering algorithms differ from decorrelation algorithms such as 3.4 in that they require sufficient supervision to distinguish signal from noise.) Therefore, both noise filtering and decorrelation can be achieved developmentally in a two-step process in which first noise filtering and then decorrelation are learned. There are also information theoretic formalisms in which both noise filtering and decorrelation can be achieved through minimizing (or maximizing) a *single* information theoretic quantity (Atick and Redlich 1990; Linsker 1988). If a developmental algorithm could be found to perform this minimization (or maximization) then both goals, noise filtering and decorrelation, could be achieved through one learning stage. Linsker (1991) has made some progress in this direction, though his learning algorithm still requires a two-phase process.

We recently became aware of the Ph.D. thesis of Mark Plumbley (Engineering Dept., Cambridge University), where a proof of convergence for another decorrelating algorithm is presented, using a similar approach.

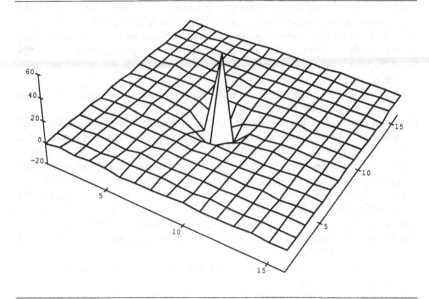

Figure 4: The receptive field found by the algorithm for the central neuron in two-dimensional 16×16 array of neurons. The receptive fields of other neurons are very similar. The training was done with $200,000$ iterations, $\tau = 20,000$, $S/N = 4$, and $\mathbf{W} = \mathbf{1}$ using images like those shown in Figure 3.

Acknowledgments

We would like to thank K. Miller for useful discussions and the Seaver Institute for its support.

References

Atick, J. J., and Redlich, A. N. 1990. Towards a theory of early visual processing. *Neural Comp.* **2**, 308–320.

Atick, J. J., and Redlich, A. N. 1991. Predicting ganglion and simple cell receptive field organizations. *Int. J. Neural Syst.* **1**, 305–315.

Atick, J. J., and Redlich, A. N. 1992. What does the retina know about natural scenes? *Neural Comp.* **4**, 196–210.

Barlow, H. B. 1989. Unsupervised learning. *Neural Comp.* **1**, 295–311.

Barlow, H. B., and Foldiak P. 1989. *The Computing Neuron*. Addison-Wesley, New York.

Barlow, H. B., Kaushal, T. P., and Mitchison, G. J. 1989. Finding minimum entropy codes. *Neural Comp.* **1**, 412–423.

Field, D. J. 1987. Relations between the statistics of natural images and the response properties of cortical cells. *J. Opt. Soc. Am. A* **4**, 2379–2394.

Foldiak, P. 1989. Adaptive network for optimal linear feature extraction. *Proc. IEEE/INNS Int. Joint Conf. Neural Networks*, Washington, DC, Vol. 1, 401–405.

Goodall, M. C. 1960. Performance of stochastic net. *Nature (London)* **185**, 557–558.

Hopfield, J. J. 1991. Olfactory computation and object perception. *Proc. Natl. Acad. Sci. U.S.A.* **88**, 6462–6466.

Kohonen, T., and Oja, E. 1976. Fast adaptive formation of orthogonalizing filters and associative memory in recurrent networks of neuron-like elements. *Biol. Cybern.* **21**, 85–95.

Linsker, R. 1986. From basic network principles to neural architecture: Emergence of spatial-opponent cells. *Proc. Natl. Acad. Sci. U.S.A.* **83**, 508–512.

Linsker, R. 1988. Self-organization in a perceptual network. *Computer* **21**, (March), 105–117.

Linsker, R. 1991. Talk at the 1991 meeting for the Society for Neuroscience.

Oja, E. 1982. A simplified neuron model as a principal component analyzer. *J. Math. Biol.* **15**, 267–273.

Rubner, J., and Schulten, K. 1990. Development of feature detectors by self-organization. *Biol. Cybern.* **62**, 193–199.

Sanger, T. D. 1989. Optimal unsupervised learning in a single-layer linear feedforward neural network. *Neural Networks* **2**, 459–473.

4

Emergence of Position-Independent Detectors of Sense of Rotation and Dilation with Hebbian Learning: An Analysis

Kechen Zhang
Martin I. Sereno
Margaret E. Sereno*
Department of Cognitive Science, University of California, San Diego, La Jolla, CA 92093-0515 USA

We previously demonstrated that it is possible to learn position-independent responses to rotation and dilation by filtering rotations and dilations with different centers through an input layer with MT-like speed and direction tuning curves and connecting them to an MST-like layer with simple Hebbian synapses (Sereno and Sereno 1991). By analyzing an idealized version of the network with broader, sinusoidal direction-tuning and linear speed-tuning, we show analytically that a Hebb rule trained with arbitrary rotation, dilation/contraction, and translation velocity fields yields units with weight fields that are a rotation plus a dilation or contraction field, and whose responses to a rotating or dilating/contracting disk are exactly position independent. Differences between the performance of this idealized model and our original model (and real MST neurons) are discussed.

1 Introduction ───

A major stream of motion information processing in the primate visual system goes from layer 4B in primary visual cortex (V1) to the middle temporal area (MT) and then to the medial superior temporal area (MST) (for reviews see Sereno and Allman 1991; Felleman and Van Essen 1991). Most neurons in area MT have moderate-sized receptive fields, and a subset is tuned to the local pattern velocity (Movshon *et al.* 1985). Neurons in the dorsal part of MST, by contrast, have much larger receptive fields and some are selective to higher order motion features—for example, rotation (either clockwise or counterclockwise, but not both), and dilation or contraction (but not both) on the frontoparallel plane (Saito *et al.* 1986; Sakata *et al.* 1986; Tanaka and Saito 1989; Tanaka *et al.* 1989; Duffy and Wurtz 1991a,b). Detecting rotation, dilation, and contraction provides useful information about an animal's motion relative to the environment or about the intrinsic motion of an object (Koenderink and

---

*Present address: Department of Psychology, University of Oregon, Eugene, OR 97403.

van Doorn 1975, 1976; Longuet-Higgins and Prazdny 1980; Koenderink 1986).

An interesting property is that some dorsal MST neurons give nearly identical responses to a rotation, or dilation or contraction, no matter where the center of the velocity flow is located. We sought to find a neural mechanism for this position invariance. To be selective to a rotation or dilation/contraction with a fixed center, the receptive field of an MST neuron need just be composed of the MT neurons whose preferred directions are arranged circularly or radially around that center (Saito et al. 1986). At first glance, this simple mechanism would not seem to be able to support an invariant response when the position of the center changes (Saito et al. 1986; Tanaka et al. 1989; Duffy and Wurtz 1991b).

Two previous proposals for a position-independent mechanism assume a homogeneous organization for an MST receptive field to ensure that all its subfields have identical structure and function. In one model, the local rotation and dilation of the velocity field is first derived and then summed up across space to get invariant responses (Duffy and Wurtz 1991b). This algorithm requires that MT neurons be selective to local rotation and dilation/contraction, which is generally not the case (Tanaka et al. 1986). Another model makes use of partially overlapping compartments in an MST receptive field (Saito et al. 1986). But this model needs a special surround effect in MT neurons to prevent many compartments from being activated simultaneously, the exact mechanism of which awaits further experimental proof.

A simpler yet counterintuitive solution was discovered in a computer simulation experiment using a feedforward network and unsupervised learning (Sereno and Sereno 1990, 1991). That work was based on a previous study in which Hebbian learning was used to find a solution to the aperture problem in a two-layer feedforward network corresponding to the connections from V1 → MT (Sereno 1989). When a similar network (with a larger interlayer divergence) representing MT → MST connections is trained with rotation, dilation, and contraction using a Hebb rule and input-layer units with MT-like tuning curves, MST-like units with position-independent responses emerge. Surprisingly, such rotation or dilation/contraction detectors turned out to have inhomogeneous receptive fields with a circular, spiral, or radial arrangement of local direction selectivity, just as in the simple mechanism mentioned before.

In this letter we analyze a modified version of the original model in Sereno and Sereno (1991). The input layer of the modified model has broader (cosine) tuning curves than in the original model (and broader than those of real MT neurons), but it allows us to derive explicit expressions for the course of learning empirically observed in the original model. The modified model gives rise to MST-like units that linearly decompose the flow field into flow field components—for example, a clockwise rotation-preferring unit will respond as well to the rotation in a clockwise spiral as to a pure clockwise rotation, ignoring any added dilation/contraction. By contrast, in our original model, the sharper tuning curves for the MT-like units result in MST-like units whose response falls off as other optic flow components are added. This smooth fall-off has also been observed with real MST neurons (Graziano *et al.* 1990; Orban *et al.* 1992). It is important to note, however, that the basic mechanism of position-invariant response to flow field stimuli (a position-*variant* direction-tuning template) is identical in both the idealized model with cosine tuning curves as well as the original model with narrower tuning curves. Linear decomposition might yet be found in areas beyond MST. It would be useful for filtering out certain movement components (e.g., translation) while exactly signaling the magnitude of others of interest (e.g., dilation). On the other hand, tighter input-layer tuning curves allow individual output layer units to code more information about a flow field (see Discussion).

2 A Mechanism for Position Independence

First, we show the basic principles for the position-independent responses, as initially revealed by computer simulation (and recently independently derived in similar form by Poggio *et al.* 1990, 1991). Let $\mathbf{v} = \mathbf{v}(\mathbf{r})$ be the velocity field on the image plane (frontoparallel plane), where the vector $\mathbf{r} = x\mathbf{i} + y\mathbf{j}$ denotes the position with $\mathbf{i}$ and $\mathbf{j}$ being the unit vectors of x and y axes. Consider MT-like units that are sensitive to the local stimulus velocities $\mathbf{v}$. Each MT-like unit has a *preferred direction*. Given $\mathbf{v}$ as the stimulus velocity at a fixed position, the response or activation a of the MT-like unit at that position is assumed to be proportional to the velocity component in the preferred direction, or

$$a = cv\cos(\theta - \phi) = c\mathbf{d}_\phi \cdot \mathbf{v} \tag{2.1}$$

where $v = |\mathbf{v}|$ is the stimulus speed, c is a constant coefficient representing the slope of the (linear) speed tuning, θ is the direction angle of $\mathbf{v}$, and $\mathbf{d}_\phi$ is the unit vector for the preferred direction angle ϕ. In other words, the unit has linear response to the speed v and a sinusoidal direction tuning curve with the maximum at the preferred direction ϕ (Fig. 1).

The artificial MT-like units resemble the real neurons in area MT of monkey in certain respects (Rodman and Albright 1987). For most MT neurons, speed does not alter the shape of direction tuning curves, which implies a multiplicative interaction of the speed tuning and the direction tuning as used in expression 2.1. The linear speed tuning is a reasonable approximation for small speeds, although the response is sometimes reduced when the speed exceeds an optimum value. The sinusoidal direction tuning is broader than a typical real MT neuron (Maunsell and Van Essen 1983). Also, the responses of real MT neurons to the antipreferred direction are usually smaller. We retain expression 2.1 for its simplicity and ease of analysis.

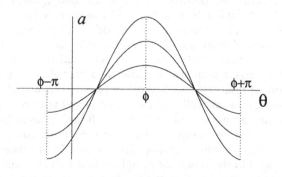

Figure 1: A family of direction tuning curves for different speeds.

Now consider an MST-like unit that receives inputs from many MT-like units. It is convenient to define the *weight vector field* of an MST-like unit. For any position on the image plane, we define the weight vector $\mathbf{w}$ at that point as

$$\mathbf{w} = cw\mathbf{d}_\phi \tag{2.2}$$

where $\mathbf{d}_\phi$ is the preferred direction of the MT-like unit at that position, w is the scalar weight for its connection to the MST-like unit, and c is the same constant coefficient as in 2.1. The total input I to the MST-like unit is assumed to be the weighted sum of the inputs from all the MT-like units within the receptive field of the MST-like unit:

$$I = \sum_r wa = \sum_r \mathbf{w} \cdot \mathbf{v} \tag{2.3}$$

where the simple relation (see equations 2.1 and 2.2) $wa = wc\mathbf{d}_\phi \cdot \mathbf{v} = \mathbf{w} \cdot \mathbf{v}$ has been used. The output of the MST-like unit is simply

$$O = \sigma(I)$$

where $\sigma(\ )$ is a sigmoid function.

If the weight vector field of an MST-like unit is itself a rotational field, namely,

$$\mathbf{w} = \boldsymbol{\Omega} \times \mathbf{r} = -\Omega y\mathbf{i} + \Omega x\mathbf{j} \tag{2.4}$$

where vector $\boldsymbol{\Omega} = \Omega\mathbf{k}$ can be regarded as the "angular velocity" for the weight vector field $\mathbf{w}$, with $\mathbf{k}$ being the unit vector of the z axis (perpendicular to the image plane), then we can prove that the MST-like unit's response O to a rotating disk of angular velocity $\boldsymbol{\omega} = \omega\mathbf{k}$ depends only on the angular speed ω of the stimulus but not on the location of the stimulus disk.

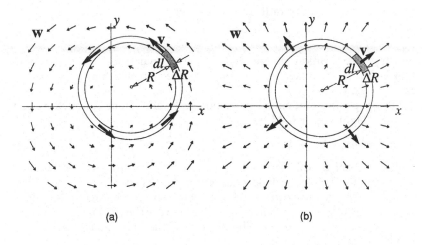

(a)   (b)

Figure 2: Response elicited by a rotating (a) or dilating (b) ring in a receptive field with circular or radial distribution of direction selectivity is independent of the position of the ring (see text).

To show this, decompose the stimulus disk into many concentric rings and calculate the response elicited by a single rotating ring of radius R and width ΔR (Fig. 2a). Let $\mathbf{v}$ be the velocity field of the stimulus ring, and $\Delta I = \sum \mathbf{w} \cdot \mathbf{v}$ be the increment to the total input to the MST-like unit contributed by all the MT-like units within the area covered by the ring. We treat the weight vector field $\mathbf{w} = \mathbf{w}(\mathbf{r})$ as depending continuously on the position $\mathbf{r}$. The number of units for a unit area on the image plane is assumed to be a constant, and is taken as unity for simplicity. Replacing the sum by the integration along the ring, we get

$$\Delta I = \Delta R \oint \mathbf{w} \cdot \mathbf{v}\, dl = v\Delta R \oint \mathbf{w} \cdot d\mathbf{l} = v\Delta R \int_S (\nabla \times \mathbf{w}) \cdot \mathbf{k}\, dS \qquad (2.5)$$

where $d\mathbf{l} = (\mathbf{v}/v)dl$ with $\mathbf{v}/v$ being the unit vector in the circular direction, and S is the area enclosed by the ring. The last equality is a direct application of Stokes' theorem, where dS is the area element. Since the weight vector field 2.4 has a constant curl $\nabla \times \mathbf{w} = (\partial w_y/\partial x - \partial w_x/\partial y)\mathbf{k} = 2\Omega\mathbf{k}$, the last integral in equation 2.5 is equal to $\int_S 2\Omega\, dS = 2\pi\Omega R^2$. Since the rotational speed v of the stimulus ring is proportional to its radius ($v = \omega R$), we finally obtain

$$\Delta I = 2\pi\omega\Omega R^3 \Delta R$$

which is independent of the position of the stimulus ring. The total response to the disk of radius ρ is therefore

$$O = \sigma(I) = \sigma\left(\pi\omega\Omega\rho^4/2\right)$$

which is also position independent. If the angular speed ω changes sign, that is, the disk rotates in the opposite direction, the total input I also changes sign.

To get position-independent responses to dilation or contraction, just let the weight vector field be

$$\mathbf{w} = \Lambda\mathbf{r} = \Lambda x\mathbf{i} + \Lambda y\mathbf{j} \tag{2.6}$$

which is itself a "dilation" when constant $\Lambda > 0$ and a "contraction" when $\Lambda < 0$. This vector field has constant divergence $\nabla \cdot \mathbf{w} = \partial w_x/\partial x + \partial w_y/\partial y = 2\Lambda$ (cf. the expression for constant curl above, except that div is a scalar). The response elicited by a dilating ring (Fig. 2b) is independent of the position of its center. The proof is similar, but Gauss' theorem is used to evaluate the integral:

$$\oint \mathbf{w} \cdot \mathbf{v}\,dl = v\oint \mathbf{w} \cdot \mathbf{n}\,dl = v\int_S \nabla \cdot \mathbf{w}\,dS = 2\pi\lambda\Lambda R^3$$

where $\mathbf{n} = \mathbf{v}/v$ is the unit vector in the radial direction of the ring, and $v = \lambda R$, where λ specifies the rate of dilation (as ω specifies the rotation speed). It follows that the response to a dilating disk is also position independent. In the case that the stimulus is a contraction, the input just changes sign.

This result can be intuitively appreciated by considering Figure 3. In (a), the stimulus is centered. Since the local stimulus direction $\mathbf{v}(\mathbf{r})$ always agrees with the weighted local preferred direction $\mathbf{w}_\phi(\mathbf{r})$ in the receptive field, the dot product between each pair is positive, though small. In (b), with the stimulus center situated to the right of the receptive field center, local direction selectivity and local stimulus direction clash near the center of the receptive field—the dot products there are actually negative; but the negative terms are compensated, exactly, as we have seen, by the larger positive dot products in the periphery of the receptive field.

3 Development of Weight Vector Field under a Hebb Rule _____

Now we consider the general manner in which weight vector field changes during Hebbian learning. At each position on the image plane we use a set of MT-like units with different preferred directions. Let $w_\phi(\mathbf{r})$ denote the weight of the MT-like unit at position $\mathbf{r}$ with preferred direction ϕ. As before, the response or activation of the MT-like unit to the velocity field $\mathbf{v}(\mathbf{r})$ is

$$a_\phi(\mathbf{r}) = c_\phi(\mathbf{r})\mathbf{d}_\phi \cdot \mathbf{v}(\mathbf{r}) \tag{3.1}$$

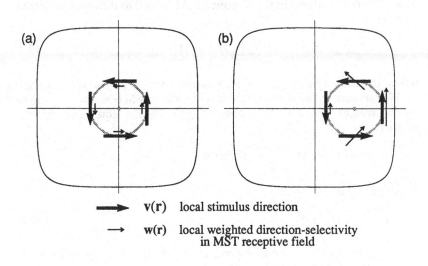

$\longrightarrow$ **v(r)**	local stimulus direction
$\rightarrow$ **w(r)**	local weighted direction-selectivity in MST receptive field

Figure 3: An intuitive interpretation of the mechanism for position independence. Negative dot products near the center of the receptive field in (b) are compensated by larger ones peripherally to give the same sum as in (a).

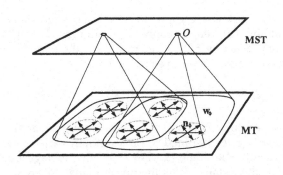

Figure 4: Each unit in the MST layer receives inputs from MT-like units at different positions and with different preferred directions (indicated by arrows).

and the weight vector is defined as $\mathbf{w}_\phi(\mathbf{r}) = c_\phi(\mathbf{r})w_\phi(\mathbf{r})\mathbf{d}_\phi$, with $\mathbf{d}_\phi$ again being the unit vector for the preferred direction of an MT-like unit. The total input I to the MST-like unit is the weighted sum of the responses from all MT-like units within the receptive field (Fig. 4), i.e., summing over different positions in the receptive field as well as different preferred directions:

$$I = \sum_{\mathbf{r}} \sum_{\phi} w_\phi(\mathbf{r}) a_\phi(\mathbf{r}) = \sum_{\mathbf{r}} \sum_{\phi} \mathbf{w}_\phi(\mathbf{r}) \cdot \mathbf{v}(\mathbf{r}) \qquad (3.2)$$

where the identity $w_\phi(\mathbf{r}) a_\phi(\mathbf{r}) = w_\phi(\mathbf{r}) c_\phi(\mathbf{r}) \mathbf{d}_\phi \cdot \mathbf{v}(\mathbf{r}) = \mathbf{w}_\phi(\mathbf{r}) \cdot \mathbf{v}(\mathbf{r})$ is used.

We can treat the system as if there were only one MT-like unit specified by the weight vector at each position (call this the equivalent weight vector)

$$\mathbf{w}(\mathbf{r}) := \sum_{\phi} \mathbf{w}_\phi(\mathbf{r}) = \sum_{\phi} c_\phi(\mathbf{r}) w_\phi(\mathbf{r}) \mathbf{d}_\phi$$

so we can write equation 3.2 as

$$I = \sum_{\mathbf{r}} \mathbf{w}(\mathbf{r}) \cdot \mathbf{v}(\mathbf{r}) \qquad (3.3)$$

which is exactly the same as expression 2.3 in the previous section. As before, the output of the MST-like unit is

$$O = \sigma(I)$$

Suppose the increment of the weight in each training step follows a simple Hebb rule

$$\Delta w_\phi(\mathbf{r}) = \epsilon a_\phi(\mathbf{r}) O \qquad (3.4)$$

In the present model no explicit distinction has been made between excitatory and inhibitory synaptic connections, and the weights are allowed to change sign. Since $\mathbf{w}(\mathbf{r}) = \sum_{\phi} c_\phi(\mathbf{r}) w_\phi(\mathbf{r}) \mathbf{d}_\phi$, the corresponding increment of the equivalent weight vector field is

$$\Delta \mathbf{w}(\mathbf{r}) = \sum_{\phi} c_\phi(\mathbf{r}) \Delta w_\phi(\mathbf{r}) \mathbf{d}_\phi = \sum_{\phi} \left[\epsilon c_\phi^2(\mathbf{r}) \mathbf{d}_\phi \cdot \mathbf{v}(\mathbf{r}) O \right] \mathbf{d}_\phi$$

where the last equality is obtained by substituting equation 3.1 into 3.4. The coefficient $c_\phi(\mathbf{r})$ is assumed to be a random variable with uniform distribution across the angle ϕ. Let $\bar{c}^2$ be the average of $c_\phi^2(\mathbf{r})$. It is assumed to be a constant across the image plane. As an approximation for large number of units, we have

$$\Delta \mathbf{w}(\mathbf{r}) = \bar{c}^2 \sum_{\phi} [\mathbf{d}_\phi \cdot \epsilon O \mathbf{v}(\mathbf{r})] \mathbf{d}_\phi \qquad (3.5)$$

To simplify this expression, first note that if there are $n (\geq 3)$ unit vectors $\{\mathbf{d}_\phi\}$ distributed evenly around the unit circle, then

$$\sum_{\phi} (\mathbf{d}_\phi \cdot \mathbf{V}) \mathbf{d}_\phi = \frac{n}{2} \mathbf{V} \qquad (3.6)$$

holds for all vector $\mathbf{V}$. For a proof, write each vector as a complex number, namely, $\mathbf{V} = \rho e^{i\theta}$ and $\mathbf{d}_\phi = e^{i\phi}$, where θ is the direction angle of $\mathbf{V}$ and $\rho = |\mathbf{V}|$ is the radius. Because $\mathbf{d}_\phi \cdot \mathbf{V} = \rho \cos(\theta - \phi) = \frac{1}{2}\rho \left(e^{i(\theta - \phi)} + e^{-i(\theta - \phi)} \right)$ is a real number, we have

$$\sum_\phi (\mathbf{d}_\phi \cdot \mathbf{V})\mathbf{d}_\phi = \sum_\phi \frac{1}{2}\rho(e^{i\theta}e^{-i\phi} + e^{-i\theta}e^{i\phi})e^{i\phi} = \frac{n}{2}\rho e^{i\theta} + \frac{1}{2}\rho e^{-i\theta} \sum_\phi e^{2i\phi}$$

Since ϕ is evenly distributed around the circle, $\sum_\phi e^{2i\phi} = 0$. This proves equation 3.6.

Assuming that the preferred directions of the MT-like units at each spatial position are evenly distributed, we can employ formula 3.6 by identifying $\mathbf{V}$ with $\bar{c}^2\epsilon O\mathbf{v}(\mathbf{r})$ so that equation 3.5 can be rewritten as

$$\Delta \mathbf{w}(\mathbf{r}) = \frac{1}{2}n\epsilon\bar{c}^2 O\mathbf{v}(\mathbf{r}) \tag{3.7}$$

where n is the number of the MT-like units at each position. This increment is caused by a single training step with the velocity field $\mathbf{v}(\mathbf{r})$. After training with a sequence of velocity fields, the equivalent weight vector field adds up to

$$\mathbf{w}(\mathbf{r}) = \mathbf{w}_0(\mathbf{r}) + \frac{1}{2}n\epsilon\bar{c}^2 \sum_t O\mathbf{v}(\mathbf{r}) \tag{3.8}$$

where $t(= 0, 1, 2, \ldots)$ stands for all time steps in the training and $\mathbf{w}_0(\mathbf{r})$ is the initial weight vector. In conclusion, the final equivalent weight vector field is just proportional to the sum of the training velocity fields weighted by the corresponding responses of the MST-like unit.

4 Training with Translation, Rotation, Dilation, and Contraction _____

We are now ready to consider the training with translation, rotation, dilation, and contraction velocity fields. To begin with, suppose for a single training step the velocity field is a rotation centered at $\mathbf{r}_c$

$$\mathbf{v}(\mathbf{r}) = \omega \times (\mathbf{r} - \mathbf{r}_c) \tag{4.1}$$

and in different steps both the angular velocity ω and the center $\mathbf{r}_c$ vary randomly. Substituting equation 4.1 into 3.8 and ignoring the initial weight vector for its smallness, we obtain the final weight vector field

$$\mathbf{w}(\mathbf{r}) = \eta \sum_t O\mathbf{v}(\mathbf{r}) = \eta \left(\sum_t O\omega \right) \times \mathbf{r} - \eta \sum_t (O\omega \times \mathbf{r}_c)$$

where $\eta = n\epsilon\bar{c}^2/2$ is a constant. This can be identified with the rotational field

$$\mathbf{w}(\mathbf{r}) = \Omega \times (\mathbf{r} - \mathbf{r}_0) \tag{4.2}$$

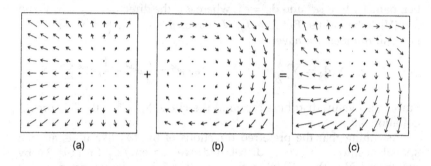

(a)   (b)   (c)

Figure 5: The final weight vector field is generally composed of a rotation field (a) and a dilation or contraction field (b). The result (c) is a spiral field.

where the weight field "angular velocity" Ω and the weight field center r_0 are defined by $\Omega := \eta \sum_t O\omega$ and $\Omega \times r_0 := \eta \sum_t (O\omega \times r_c)$. The latter equation has a unique solution of r_0 as long as $\Omega \neq 0$. In the special case $\Omega = 0$, $w(r)$ is a constant vector field (translation).

Similarly, training with dilation or contraction

$$v(r) = \lambda(r - r_c)$$

with rate λ and center r_c varying in time will lead to the final weight vector field

$$w(r) = \Lambda(r - r_0) \tag{4.3}$$

where $\Lambda := \eta \sum_t O\lambda$ and $\Lambda r_0 := \eta \sum_t O\lambda r_c$. This is either a dilation ($\Lambda > 0$) or a contraction ($\Lambda < 0$). In the special case $\Lambda = 0$, $w(r)$ is a constant (translation).

Note that expressions 4.2 and 4.3 are just what are required for position-independent responses (cf. equations 2.4 and 2.6). It should be realized that the center r_0 does not affect the curl and divergence of a vector field, and thus does not affect our previous conclusions.

For training with a mixture of translations, rotations, dilations, and contractions, it is readily shown by similar argument that the final weight vector field takes the form

$$w(r) = \Omega \times (r - a) + \Lambda(r - b) + c$$

It can always be written equivalently as

$$w(r) = \Omega \times (r - r_0) + \Lambda(r - r_0)$$

which is a spiral centered at r_0 (Fig. 5). An MST-like unit with a spiral weight vector field has position-independent responses to a particular sense of rotation as well as to either a dilation or contraction.

Even if the training velocity fields have a zero average, for example, clockwise and counterclockwise rotations have an equal chance of appearing, the weight vector field is still expected to grow with time. We consider the simple case where all rotations and dilations/contractions are centered at the same point so that the development of the two corresponding components is strictly independent. Consider the initial stage of development for training with, say, rotation fields alone. Now we need consider only the linear range of the sigmoid function σ, and for simplicity we assume $O = I$. According to equations 3.7 and 3.3, at time step $t + 1$

$$\mathbf{w}_{t+1} = \mathbf{w}_t + \eta O_t \mathbf{v}_t = \mathbf{w}_t + \eta \left(\sum_{\mathbf{r}} \mathbf{w}_t \cdot \mathbf{v}_t \right) \mathbf{v}_t$$

where the subscripts refer to time. Thus

$$O_{t+1} = \sum_{\mathbf{r}} \mathbf{w}_{t+1} \cdot \mathbf{v}_{t+1} = \sum_{\mathbf{r}} \mathbf{w}_t \cdot \mathbf{v}_{t+1} + \eta \left(\sum_{\mathbf{r}} \mathbf{w}_t \cdot \mathbf{v}_t \right) \left(\sum_{\mathbf{r}} \mathbf{v}_t \cdot \mathbf{v}_{t+1} \right)$$

It can be expressed as

$$O_{t+1} \doteq A \Omega_t \omega_{t+1} + \eta (A \Omega_t \omega_t)(A \omega_t \omega_{t+1}) \tag{4.4}$$

where Ω_t and ω_t are the angular speeds for the vector fields $\mathbf{w}_t$ and $\mathbf{v}_t$ at time t, respectively, and A is a constant depending on the size and shape of the receptive field as well as the position of the rotation center.

Imagine an ensemble of parallel training sessions starting from different initial weights and using different rotation sequences of random angular speeds, which are independent of each other while having identical statistics. We take the ensemble average on both sides of equation 4.4 to get $\langle O_{t+1} \rangle = A \langle \Omega_t \rangle \langle \omega \rangle + \eta A^2 \langle \Omega_t \rangle \langle \omega^2 \rangle \langle \omega \rangle$, where the subscript for the angular speed ω is dropped because the statistics of ω does not change over time. If $\langle \omega \rangle = 0$, then $\langle O_{t+1} \rangle = 0$ for all t. However, taking the ensemble average after squaring equation 4.4 and using $\langle O_t^2 \rangle = A^2 \langle \Omega_t^2 \rangle \langle \omega^2 \rangle$, we can obtain

$$\langle O_{t+1}^2 \rangle = (1 + 2\eta \mathcal{E} + \alpha \eta^2 \mathcal{E}^2) \langle O_t^2 \rangle \tag{4.5}$$

where

$$\mathcal{E} := A \langle \omega^2 \rangle = \left\langle \sum_{\mathbf{r}} \mathbf{v} \cdot \mathbf{v} \right\rangle$$

$$\alpha := \langle \omega^4 \rangle / \langle \omega^2 \rangle^2$$

are constants. When ω is drawn from a gaussian distribution of zero mean, for instance, $\alpha = 3$. Applying equation 4.5 iteratively yields $\langle O_{t+1}^2 \rangle = e^{t/\tau} \langle O_1^2 \rangle$, where constant

$$\tau := 1/\ln(1 + 2\eta\mathcal{E} + \alpha\eta^2\mathcal{E}^2)$$

Because $O_1 = \sum_r \mathbf{w}_1 \cdot \mathbf{v}_1$ and $\mathbf{w}_1 = \mathbf{w}_0 + \eta O_0 \mathbf{v}_0 \approx \eta O_0 \mathbf{v}_0 = \eta(\sum_r \mathbf{w}_0 \cdot \mathbf{v}_0)\mathbf{v}_0$, by similar arguments as above we can get $\langle O_1^2 \rangle = \alpha\eta^2\mathcal{E}^2 \langle O_0^2 \rangle$. Hence

$$\langle O_t^2 \rangle = \alpha\eta^2\mathcal{E}^2 e^{(t-1)/\tau} \langle O_0^2 \rangle \tag{4.6}$$

Consequently, when many MST-like units develop in parallel starting from random initial weights, the responses (either positive or negative) to rotation and to dilation/contraction are expected to grow exponentially in the initial stage of development. The variety of the initial responses leads to a continuous spectrum of selectivity to rotation and dilation/contraction, which is what has actually been found in the neurophysiological experiments (Duffy and Wurtz 1991a; Andersen et al. 1991).

5 Discussion

The model provides a unified, albeit simplified, account for several essential properties of MST neurons and how they might develop. These properties include selectivity to rotation, dilation, and contraction, the position independence of the responses (Saito et al. 1986; Tanaka and Saito 1989; Tanaka et al. 1989; Duffy and Wurtz 1991a,b), the selectivity to spiral velocity fields (Graziano et al. 1990; Andersen et al. 1991), and the continuous spectrum of selectivity (Duffy and Wurtz 1991a; Andersen et al. 1991). The model's response saturates at higher speeds (as a result of the sigmoid function) as does the response of real neurons (Orban et al. 1992).

In addition to rotation and dilation/contraction, shear also naturally arises in the optic flow (Koenderink 1986). Since the linear combination of shear fields is still a shear, according to equation 3.8 the weight vector field itself will also have a shear component. Consistent with the model, neurons selective to shear components were also found in the cortical areas including MST (Lagae et al. 1991).

This model differs somewhat from the original model in Sereno and Sereno (1991) and from real MST neurons in that it "linearly decomposes" the velocity field—that is, an MST-like unit will respond exclusively to the, say, rotational component of a flow field, regardless of the magnitude of the radial component. Since a cosine tuning curve means that the input unit sees exactly the vector component of the local stimulus movement in the preferred (here rotational) direction, it leads to linear decomposition. With narrower tuning curves, the response of individual MST-like units provides more information about the exact composition of the flow field—for example, the extent to which it approximates a pure rotation; nevertheless, approximate position independence with narrower tuning curves is still explained by a direction-template mechanism like that described above.

Roughly speaking, learning with a simple Hebb rule tends to maximize the total response by gradient ascent and thus tune the net to the input patterns that frequently occur. Consider the output

$$O = \sigma(I) = \sigma \left(\sum_i w_i I_i \right)$$

The Hebb rule

$$\Delta w_i \propto I_i O$$

is always of the same sign as the gradient of the function $E = \frac{1}{2}O^2$:

$$\frac{\partial E}{\partial w_i} = O \frac{\partial O}{\partial w_i} = I_i O \sigma'(I)$$

because the derivative σ' is always positive. As a consequence, there should be a general tendency for local direction selectivity to be aligned with the direction of the stimulus velocity.

Recently, it was demonstrated that although dilation-sensitive MSTd neurons are basically position invariant in their responses, they often respond best to dilations centered at a particular location in the receptive field (often not the receptive field center) (Duffy and Wurtz 1991c). Similar results were obtained in the simulations in Sereno and Sereno (1991) using MT-like (narrower) input-layer tuning curves. It may be advantageous to retain information about *combinations* of flow field components— here, dilation and translation—in single units since these combinations can have particular behavioral relevance—for example, in signaling direction of heading (Perrone 1992). More realistic peaked (instead of linear) speed tuning curves (Maunsell and Van Essen 1983) in the MT-like input layer could potentially sharpen the response to particular flow components since local speeds may be changed from the optimum as flow field components are added. Cross-direction inhibition (known to occur in MT: Snowden *et al.* 1991) could also be incorporated, effectively deleting portions of the flow field containing conflicting local motion signals. This could improve performance with more complex, real-world motion arrays.

The rotation, dilation, and contraction velocity fields required for training are readily produced when an animal is moving around in a rigid environment. Exposure to such velocity fields may be crucial in order for a young animal to develop rotation and dilation cells in its visual system. Human babies, for instance, can distinguish a rotation field from a random velocity field only after several months of visual experience (Spitz *et al.* 1988). This could be tested by recording from MST in infant monkeys.

Feedforward networks using Hebb rules have been shown to be capable of producing detectors selective to a hierarchy of features like those found in the successive stages of visual processing: center-surround units like those in the LGN (Linsker 1986a), orientation-selective units like simple cells in V1 (Linsker 1986b), pattern motion units like some cells in MT (Sereno 1989), and finally position-independent rotation and dilation units like cells in dorsal MST (Sereno and Sereno 1991). The visual system may use simple local learning rules and a richly textured environment to build up complex filters in stages. This strategy could drastically reduce the amount of supervision that is required later on (cf. Geman *et al.* 1992) as the visual system learns to recognize objects and direct navigation and manipulation.

Note Added in Proof

Recently, Gallant *et al.* (1993) found that neurons in V4 respond selectively, and in a position-invariant way to static patterns containing concentric, radiating, shearing, or spiral contours. The main outlines of our analysis could be extended to explain the selectivity and development of these neurons by substituting an orientation-selective input layer for the direction-selective input layer considered here.

Acknowledgments

M. E. S. was supported by a postdoctoral fellowship, K. Z. by a graduate fellowship, and M. I. S. by a research award from the McDonnell-Pew Center for Cognitive Neuroscience at San Diego. We thank an anonymous reviewer for helpful comments.

References

Andersen, R., Graziano, M., and Snowden, R. 1991. Selectivity of area MST neurons for expansion/contraction and rotation motions. *Invest. Ophthal. Vis. Sci., Abstr.* **32**, 823.
Duffy, C. J., and Wurtz, R. H. 1991a. Sensitivity of MST neurons to optic flow stimuli. I. A continuum of response selectivity to large-field stimuli. *J. Neurophysiol.* **65**, 1329–1345.
Duffy, C. J., and Wurtz, R. H. 1991b. Sensitivity of MST neurons to optic flow stimuli. II. Mechanisms of response selectivity revealed by small-field stimuli. *J. Neurophysiol.* **65**, 1346–1359.
Duffy, C. J., and Wurtz, R. H. 1991c. MSTd neuronal sensitivity to heading of motion in optic flow fields. *Soc. Neurosci. Abstr.* **17**, 441.
Felleman, D., and Van Essen, D. C. 1991. Distributed hierarchical processing in primate cerebral cortex. *Cerebral Cortex* **1**, 1–47.

Gallant, J. L., Braun, J., and Van Essen, D. C. 1993. Selectivity for polar, hyperbolic, and Cartesian gratings in macaque visual cortex. *Science* **259**, 100–103.

Geman, S., Bienenstock, E., and Doursat, R. 1992. Neural networks and the bias/variance dilemma. *Neural Comp.* **4**, 1–58.

Graziano, M. S. A., Andersen, R. A., and Snowden, R. 1990. Stimulus selectivity of neurons in macaque MST. *Soc. Neurosci. Abstr.* **16**, 7.

Koenderink, J. J. 1986. Optic flow. *Vision Res.* **26**, 161–180.

Koenderink, J. J., and van Doorn, A. J. 1975. Invariant properties of the motion parallax field due to the movement of rigid bodies relative to an observer. *Opt. Acta* **22**, 773–791.

Koenderink, J. J., and van Doorn, A. J. 1976. Local structure of movement parallax of the plane. *J. Opt. Soc. Am.* **66**, 717–723.

Lagae, L., Xiao, D., Ralguel, S., Maes, H., and Orban, G. A. 1991. Position invariance of optic flow component selectivity differentiates monkey MST and FST cells from MT cells. *Invest. Ophthal. Vis. Sci., Abstr.* **32**, 823.

Linsker, R. 1986a. From basic network principles to neural architecture: emergence of spatial-opponent cells. *Proc. Natl. Acad. Sci. U.S.A.* **83**, 7508–7512.

Linsker, R. 1986b. From basic network principles to neural architecture: emergence of orientation-selective cells. *Proc. Natl. Acad. Sci. U.S.A.* **83**, 8390–8394.

Longuet-Higgins, H. C., and Prazdny, K. 1980. The interpretation of a moving retinal image. *Proc. R. Soc. London B* **208**, 385–397.

Maunsell, J. H. R., and Van Essen, D. C. 1983. Functional properties of neurons in middle temporal visual area (MT) of the macaque monkey: I. Selectivity for stimulus direction, speed and orientation. *J. Neurophysiol.* **49**, 1127–1147.

Movshon, J. A., Adelson, E. H., Gizzi, M. S., and Newsome, W. T. 1985. Analysis of moving visual patterns. In *Pattern Recognition Mechanisms*, C. Chagas, R. Gattass, and C. Gross, eds., pp. 117–151. Springer-Verlag, New York.

Orban, G. A., Lagae, L., Verri, A., Raiguel, S., Xiao, D., Maes, H., and Torre, V. 1992. First-order analysis of optical flow in monkey brain. *Proc. Natl. Acad. Sci. U.S.A.* **89**, 2595–2599.

Perrone, J. A. 1992. Model for the computation of self-motion in biological systems. *J. Opt. Soc. Am. A* **9**, 177–194.

Poggio, T., Verri, A., and Torre, V. 1990. *Does cortical area MST know Green theorems?* Instituto per la Ricerca Scientifica e Technologica Tech. Rep. No. 9008-07, 1–8.

Poggio, T., Verri, A., and Torre, V. 1991. Green theorems and qualitative properties of the optical flow. *MIT A.I. Memo*, No. 1289, 1–6.

Rodman, H. R., and Albright, T. D. 1987. Coding of visual stimulus velocity in area MT of the macaque. *Vision Res.* **27**, 2035–2048.

Saito, H., Yukie, M., Tanaka, K., Hikosaka, K., Fukada, Y., and Iwai, E. 1986. Integration of direction signals of image motion in the superior temporal sulcus of the macaque monkey. *J. Neurosci.* **6**, 145–157.

Sakata, H., Shibutani, H., Ito, Y., and Tsurugai, K. 1986. Parietal cortical neurons responding to rotary movement of visual stimulus in space. *Exp. Brain Res.* **61**, 658–663.

Sereno, M. I. 1989. Learning the solution to the aperture problem for pattern

62 Kechen Zhang, Martin I. Sereno, and Margaret E. Sereno

motion with a Hebb rule. In *Advances in Neural Information Processing System I*, D. S. Touretzky, ed., pp. 468–476. Morgan Kaufmann, San Mateo, CA.

Sereno, M. I., and Allman, J. M. 1991. Cortical visual areas in mammals. In *The Neural Basis of Visual Function*, A. G. Leventhal, ed., pp. 160–172. Macmillan, London.

Sereno, M. I., and Sereno, M. E. 1990. Learning to discriminate senses of rotation and dilation with a Hebb rule. *Invest. Ophthal. Vis. Sci., Abstr.* **31**, 528.

Sereno, M. I., and Sereno, M. E. 1991. Learning to see rotation and dilation with a Hebb rule. In *Advances in Neural Information Processing Systems 3*, R. P. Lippmann, J. Moody, and D. S. Touretzky, eds., pp. 320–326. Morgan Kaufmann, San Mateo, CA.

Snowden, R. J., Treue, S., Erickson, R. G., and Andersen, R. A. 1991. The response of area MT and V1 neurons to transparent motion. *J. Neurosci.* **11**, 2768–2785.

Spitz, R. V., Stiles-Davis, J., and Siegel, R. M. 1988. Infant perception of rotation from rigid structure-from-motion displays. *Soc. Neurosci. Abstr.* **14**, 1244.

Tanaka, K., and Saito, H.-A. 1989. Analysis of motion of the visual field by direction, expansion/contraction, and rotation cells clustered in the dorsal part of the medial superior temporal area of the macaque monkey. *J. Neurophysiol.* **62**, 626–641.

Tanaka, K., Hikosaka, K., Saito, H.-A., Yukie, M., Fukada, Y., and Iwai, E. 1986. Analysis of local and wide-field movements in the superior temporal visual areas of the macaque monkey. *J. Neurosci.* **6**, 134–144.

Tanaka, K., Fukada, Y., and Saito, H.-A. 1989. Underlying mechanisms of the response specificity of expansion/contraction and rotation cells in the dorsal part of the medial superior temporal area of the macaque monkey. *J. Neurophysiol.* **62**, 642–656.

5

Learning Invariance from Transformation Sequences

Peter Földiák
Physiological Laboratory, University of Cambridge,
Downing Street, Cambridge CB2 3EG, U.K.

The visual system can reliably identify objects even when the retinal image is transformed considerably by commonly occurring changes in the environment. A local learning rule is proposed, which allows a network to learn to generalize across such transformations. During the learning phase, the network is exposed to temporal sequences of patterns undergoing the transformation. An application of the algorithm is presented in which the network learns invariance to shift in retinal position. Such a principle may be involved in the development of the characteristic shift invariance property of complex cells in the primary visual cortex, and also in the development of more complicated invariance properties of neurons in higher visual areas.

1 Introduction

How can we consistently recognize objects when changes in the viewing angle, eye position, distance, size, orientation, relative position, or deformations of the object itself (e.g., of a newspaper or a gymnast) can change their retinal projections so significantly? The visual system must contain knowledge about such transformations in order to be able to generalize correctly. Part of this knowledge is probably determined genetically, but it is also likely that the visual system learns from its sensory experience, which contains plenty of examples of such transformations. Electrophysiological experiments suggest that the invariance properties of perception may be due to the receptive field characteristics of individual cells in the visual system. Complex cells in the primary visual cortex exhibit approximate invariance to position within a limited range (Hubel and Wiesel 1962), while cells in higher visual areas in the temporal cortex show more complex forms of invariance to rotation, color, size, and distance, and they also have much larger receptive fields (Gross and Mishkin 1977, Perrett *et al.* 1982). The simplest model of a neuron, which takes a weighted sum of its inputs, shows a form of generalization in which patterns that differ on only a small number of input lines generate similar outputs. For such a unit, patterns are similar when they are close in Hamming distance. Any simple transformation, like a shift in position or a rotation, can cause a great difference in Hamming distance, so this simple unit tends to respond to the transformed image very differently and generalizes poorly across the transformation. The solution to this problem is therefore likely to require either a more complex model of a neuron, or a network of simple units.

2 Shift Invariance

Fukushima (1980) proposed a solution to the positional invariance problem by a network consisting of alternating feature detector ("S" or simple) and invariance ("C" or complex) layers. Feature detectors in the "S" layer are replicated in many different positions, while the outputs of detectors of the same feature are pooled from different positions in the "C" layers. The presence of the feature in any position within a limited region can therefore activate the appropriate "C" unit. This idea is consistent with models of complex cells in the primary visual cortex (Hubel and Wiesel 1962; Spitzer and Hochstein 1985) in that they assume that complex cells receive their major inputs from simple cells or simple-cell-like subunits selective for the same orientation in different positions. In Fukushima's model, the pair of feature detecting and invariance layers is repeated in a hierarchical way, gradually giving rise to more selectivity and a larger range of positional invariance. In the top layer, units are completely indifferent to the position of the pattern, while they are still sensitive to the approximate relative position of its components. In this way, not only shift invariance, but some degree of distortion tolerance is achieved as well. This architecture has successfully been applied both by Fukushima (1980) and LeCun et al. (1989) in pattern recognition problems. LeCun et al. achieve reliable recognition of handwritten digits (zip codes) by using such architectural constraints to reduce the number of free parameters that need to be adjusted. Some of the principles presented in these networks may also be extremely helpful in modeling the visual system. The implementation of some of their essential assumptions in biological neural networks, however, seems very difficult. Apart from the question of the biological plausibility of the backpropagation algorithm used in LeCun et al.'s model, both models assume that the feature detectors are connected to "complex" units in a fixed way, and that all the simple units that are connected to a complex unit have the same input weight vector (except for a shift in position). Therefore whenever the weights of one of the "simple" units are modified (e.g., by a Hebbian mechanism), the corresponding weights of all the other simple units connected to the same complex unit need to be modified in exactly the same way ("weight sharing"). This operation is nonlocal for the synapses of all the units except for the one that was originally modified. A "learn now" signal broadcast by the complex unit to all its simple units would not solve this problem either, as the shifted version of the input, which would be necessary for local learning, is not available for the simple units.

3 A Learning Rule

An arrangement is needed in which detectors of the same feature all
connect to the same complex unit. However, instead of requiring simple
units permanently connected to a complex unit (a "family") to develop
in an identical way, the same goal can be achieved by letting simple
units develop independently and then allowing similar ones to connect
adaptively to a complex unit (form "clubs"). A learning rule is therefore needed to specify these modifiable simple-to-complex connections.
A simple Hebbian rule, which depends only on instantaneous activations, does not work here as it only detects overlapping patterns in the
input and picks up correlations between input units. If the input to the
simple layer contains an example of the feature at only one spatial position at any moment then there will never be significant overlap between
detectors of that feature in different positions. The absence of positive
correlations would prevent those units being connected to the same output. The solution proposed here is a modified Hebbian rule in which the
modification of the synaptic strength at time step t is proportional not to
the pre- and post-synaptic activity, but instead to the presynaptic activity
(x) and to an average value, a trace of the postsynaptic activity ($\bar{y}$). A
second, decay term is added in order to keep the weight vector bounded:

$$\Delta w_{ij}^{(t)} = \alpha \bar{y}_i^{(t)}(x_j^{(t)} - w_{ij}^{(t)})$$

where

$$\bar{y}_i^{(t)} = (1 - \delta)\bar{y}_i^{(t-1)} + \delta y_i^{(t)}$$

A similar trace mechanism has been proposed by Klopf (1982) and
used in models of classical conditioning by Sutton and Barto (1981). A
trace is a running average of the activation of the unit, which has the effect that activity at one moment will influence learning at a later moment.
This temporal low-pass filtering of the activity embodies the assumption
that the desired features are stable in the environment. As the trace depends on the activity of only one unit, the modified rule is still local.
One possibility is that such a trace is implemented in a biological neuron
by a chemical concentration that follows cell activity.

4 Simulation

The development of the connections between the simple and complex
units is simulated in an example in which the goal is to learn shift invariance. In the simple layer there are position-dependent line detectors,
one unit for each of 4 orientations in the 64 positions on an 8×8 grid.
There are only 4 units in the complex layer, fully connected to the simple
units. During training, moving lines selected at random from four orientations and two directions are swept across a model retina, which gives

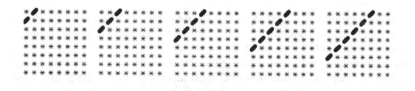

Figure 1: Five consecutive frames from one of the sequences used as input. Each line segment represents a simple unit of the corresponding orientation and position. Thick segments are active ($x_j = 1$), thin ones are inactive units ($x_j = 0$). The trace is maintained between sweeps.

rise to activation of the simple units of the appropriate orientation in different positions at different moments in time (Fig. 1). Such activation can either be the result of eye movements, object motion in the environment, or it may even be present during early development as there is evidence for waves of activity in the developing mammalian retina (Meister *et al.* 1990). The activation of these simple units is the input to the network. If an active simple unit succeeds in exciting one of the four complex units, then the trace of that complex unit gets enhanced for a period of time comparable to the duration of the sweep across the receptive fields of the simple units. Therefore all the connections from the simple units that get activated during the rest of that sweep get strengthened according to the modified Hebb rule. Simple units of only one orientation get activated during a sweep, causing simple units of only one orientation to connect to any given complex unit. To prevent more than one complex unit from responding to the same orientation, some kind of competitive, inhibitory interaction is necessary between the complex units. In some previous simulations an adaptive competitive scheme, decorrelation, was used (Barlow and Földiák 1989; Földiák 1990), which is thought to be advantageous for other reasons. For the sake of clarity, however, the simplest possible competitive scheme (Rumelhart and Zipser 1985) was used in the simulation described here. Each unit took a sum of its inputs weighted by the connection strengths. The output y_k of the unit with the maximal weighted sum was set to 1, while the outputs of the rest of the units were set to 0:

$$y_k = \begin{cases} 1 & \text{if argmax}_i(\sum_j w_{ij}x_j) = k \\ 0 & \text{otherwise} \end{cases}$$

Figure 2a shows the initially random connections between the simple and the complex units, while Figure 2b shows the connections after training with 500 sweeps across the retina.

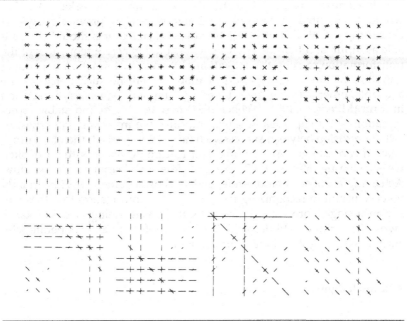

Figure 2: Connection patterns of the four complex units (a) before training and (b) after training on 500 line sweeps across the retina. The length of each segment indicates the strength of the connection from the simple unit of the corresponding position and orientation to the complex unit. Initial weights were chosen from a uniform distribution on $[0, 0.1]$. $\alpha = 0.02$, $\delta = 0.2$. (c) The result of training without trace ($\delta = 1$).

5 Discussion

The simple example given above is not intended to be a realistic model of complex cell development, since unoriented input to complex cells was ignored and simple units were considered merely as line detectors. By using a more realistic model of simple cells, the above principle would be able to predict that simple cells of the same spatial frequency and orientation but of different phase tuning (dark/bright line centre, even/odd symmetry) connect to the same complex cell, which would therefore lose sensitivity to phase. A further consequence would be that simple cells tuned to different spatial frequencies would segregate on different complex cells. The application of this algorithm to more complicated or abstract invariances (e.g., 3D rotations or deformations) would perhaps be even more interesting as it is even harder to see how they could be specified without some kind of learning; the way in which such invariance properties could be wired in is much less obvious than in the case of positional invariance in Fukushima's or LeCun's networks. All that would be required by the proposed algorithm from previous stages of processing is that the transformation-dependent features should be available as input, and that the environment should generate sequences of the transformation causing the activation of these transformation-dependent detectors within a short period of time. Where no such detectors are available, other learning rules, based on temporal sequences or variation in form (Mitchison 1991, Webber 1991) may be able to find stable representations. If a supervision signal indicates the invariant properties, or self-supervision between successive time steps is applied, then backpropagation can also give rise to invariant feature detectors without explicit weight sharing (Hinton 1987). Nevertheless such learning is rather slow. Achieving a transformation-independent representation would certainly be very useful in recognizing patterns, yet the information that these invariance stages throw away may be vital in performing visual tasks. A "where" system would probably have to supplement and cooperate with such a "what" system in an intricate way.

Acknowledgments

I would like to thank Prof. H. B. Barlow, Prof. F. H. C. Crick, Dr. A. R. Gardner-Medwin, Prof. G. E. Hinton, and Dr. G. J. Mitchison for their useful comments. This work was supported by an Overseas Research Studentship, a research studentship from Churchill College, Cambridge, and SERC Grants GR/E43003 and GR/F34152.

References

Barlow, H. B., and Földiák, P. 1989. Adaptation and decorrelation in the cortex. In *The Computing Neuron*, R. M. Durbin, C. Miall, and G. J. Mitchison, eds., Chap. 4, pp. 54–72. Addison-Wesley, Wokingham.

Földiák, P. 1990. Forming sparse representations by local anti-Hebbian learning. *Biol. Cybernet.* **64**, 165–170.

Fukushima, K. 1980. Neocognitron: A self-organizing neural network model for a mechanism of pattern recognition unaffected by shift in position. *Biol. Cybernet.* **36**, 193–202.

Gross, C. G., and Mishkin, M. 1977. The neural basis of stimulus equivalence across retinal translation. In *Lateralization in the Nervous System*, S. Harnad, R. Doty, J. Jaynes, L. Goldstein, and G. Krauthamer, eds., pp. 109–122. Academic Press, New York.

Hinton, G. E. 1987. Learning translation invariant recognition in a massively parallel network. In *PARLE: Parallel Architectures and Languages Europe*, G. Goos and J. Hartmanis, eds., pp. 1–13. Lecture Notes in Computer Science, Springer-Verlag, Berlin.

Hubel, D. H., and Wiesel, T. N. 1962. Receptive fields, binocular interaction and functional architecture in the cat's visual cortex. *J. Physiol.* **160**, 106–154.

Klopf, A. H. 1982. *The Hedonistic Neuron: A Theory of Memory, Learning, and Intelligence.* Hemisphere, Washington, DC.

LeCun, Y., Boser, B., Denker, J. S., Henderson, D., Howard, R. E., Hubbard, W., and Jackel, L. D. 1989. Backpropagation applied to handwritten zip code recognition. *Neural Comp.* **1**, 541–551.

Meister, M., Wong, R. O. L., Baylor, D. A., and Shatz, C. J. 1990. Synchronous bursting activity in ganglion cells of the developing mammalian retina. *Investi. Ophthalmol. Visual Sci.* (suppl.) **31**, 115.

Mitchison, G. J. 1991. Removing time variation with the anti-Hebbian synapse. *Neural Comp.*, in press.

Perrett, D. I., Rolls, E. T., and Caan, W. 1982. Visual neurons responsive to faces in the monkey temporal cortex. *Exp. Brain Res.* **47**, 329–342.

Rumelhart, D. E., and Zipser, D. 1985. Feature discovery by competitive learning. *Cog. Sci.* **9**, 75–112.

Spitzer, H., and Hochstein, S. 1985. A complex-cell receptive-field model. *J. Neurophysiol.* **53**, 1266–1286.

Sutton, R. S., and Barto, A. G. 1981. Toward a modern theory of adaptive networks: Expectation and prediction. *Psychol. Rev.* **88**, 135–170.

Webber, C. J. St. C. 1991. Self-organization of position- and deformation-tolerant neural representations. *Network* **2**, 43–61.

Learning Perceptually Salient Visual Parameters Using Spatiotemporal Smoothness Constraints

James V. Stone[1]
School of Cognitive and Computing Sciences,
University of Sussex, Sussex BN1 9QH, UK

A model is presented for unsupervised learning of low level vision tasks, such as the extraction of surface depth. A key assumption is that perceptually salient visual parameters (e.g., surface depth) vary smoothly over time. This assumption is used to derive a learning rule that maximizes the long-term variance of each unit's outputs, whilst simultaneously minimizing its short-term variance. The length of the half-life associated with each of these variances is not critical to the success of the algorithm. The learning rule involves a linear combination of anti-Hebbian and Hebbian weight changes, over short and long time scales, respectively. This maximizes the information throughput with respect to low–frequency parameters implicit in the input sequence. The model is used to learn stereo disparity from temporal sequences of random-dot and gray-level stereograms containing synthetically generated subpixel disparities. The presence of temporal discontinuities in disparity does not prevent learning or generalization to previously unseen image sequences. The implications of this class of unsupervised methods for learning in perceptual systems are discussed.

1 Introduction

The ability to learn perceptually salient visual parameters — surface orientation, curvature, depth, texture, and motion — is a prerequisite for the more familiar tasks (e.g. object recognition, catching prey) associated with biological vision. This paper addresses the question: What strategies enable neurons to learn these parameters from a spatiotemporal sequence of images, without the aid of an external teacher?

According to Gibson (1979), the problem of vision consists of obtaining invariant structure from continually changing sensations. Whereas Gibson's intuitively appealing approach has been well received by perceptual psychologists, the lack of a detailed theory has ensured that this approach has received little empirical vindication from computer vision.

---

[1]Present address: Psychology Building, Western Bank, University of Sheffield, Sheffield S10 2TP, UK.

However, the potential of Gibson's ideas has recently begun to be realized as a series of connectionist models (Phillips, *et al.* 1995; Becker and Hinton 1992; Becker 1992; Zemel and Hinton 1991; Foldiak 1991; Schraudolph and Sejnowski 1991; Mitchison 1991). In particular, the IMAX models (Becker and Hinton 1992; Zemel and Hinton 1991; Becker 1992, 1996) have been instrumental in drawing attention to the possibility of learning perceptually salient parameters using unsupervised learning methods.

The model described in this paper is different from these models, although it shares with them a common assumption: models of perceptual processes can be derived from an analysis of the types of spatial and temporal changes immanent in the structure of the physical world. For example, a learning mechanism might discover perceptually salient visual parameters by taking advantage of quite general properties (such as spatial and temporal smoothness) of the physical world. These properties are not peculiar to any single physical environment so that such a mechanism should be able to extract a variety of perceptually salient parameters (e.g., three-dimensional orientation and shape) via different sensory modalities (vision, speech, touch), and in a range of physical environments.

2 Unsupervised Learning of Visual Parameters

Learning in artificial neural networks consists of two broad classes, supervised and unsupervised. Supervised learning requires access to a vector-valued error signal (as in backpropagation) and therefore may not considered as biologically plausible [although reinforcement learning (Sutton 1988) via scalar-valued error signals is clearly more realistic]. Unsupervised learning methods perform a type of cluster analysis on a given set of inputs. However, almost all unsupervised methods form clusters on the basis of only the low order statistics of their inputs. Accordingly, in the absence of hand-crafted architectures (Linsker 1988), networks that perform unsupervised learning tend to "discover" parameters that are linear functions of their inputs (e.g., Oja 1982).

The data compression of inputs performed by linear systems reduces the redundancy of the transformed input data. While such a process might be considered to be desirable during the early stages of perceptual processing (Barlow 1972), it is not obvious how such a mechanism could give rise to the complex response characteristics typical of neurons in visual area V2 and in the inferotemporal cortex. These "high order" neurons have outputs that respond selectively to disparity(V2) (Poggio *et al.* 1985), facial expression (Heywood and Cowey 1992), and even "moving light displays"[2] (Perret *et al.* 1990) of human walkers, which are defined

---

[2]Typically, a light is attached to each major joint of a moving person in a darkened room, so that only the motion of the joints is visible (Johansson 1973).

principally in terms of their spatiotemporal characteristics (Perret *et al.* 1990). The response properties of such neurons cannot be modeled using linear systems, unless the input representation is hand-crafted to ensure that inputs are linearly separable. While such an approach may be fruitful for restricted domains, it is unlikely to yield solutions of general utility.

Both Mitchison (1991) and Schraudolph and Sejnowski (1991) make use of an anti-Hebbian learning rule in an explicit attempt to minimize the variance of the outputs of units. The authors aim to discover invariant properties of the input data. Mitchison's model is linear, which restricts it to computing linear functions of its inputs. The network described in Schraudolph and Sejnowski (1991) is nonlinear, and appears to benefit from hierarchical learning through successive layers of units. However, the methods described in Mitchison (1991) and Schraudolph and Sejnowski (1991) both require weight normalisation.

In Foldiak (1991) and Barrow and Bray (1992), a temporal trace mechanism is used with a Hebbian rule to discover temporally related inputs. Each unit becomes sensitive to lines at a particular orientation, but the precise position of these lines is ignored. However, as pointed out by Becker (1992 p. 363), the input representation used in Foldiak (1991) ensures that lines at different orientations are linearly separable sets of vectors. This is also true of the work described in Barrow and Bray (1992).

In Becker and Hinton (1992) the IMAX method was introduced. IMAX models work by attempting to maximize the mutual information between different output units (Becker and Hinton 1992; Zemel and Hinton 1991), or between outputs of each of a number of units over successive time steps (Becker 1992). However, these models suffer from several drawbacks. The IMAX merit function has a high proportion of poor local optima. In Becker and Hinton (1992) this problem was ameliorated by using a hand-crafted weight-sharing architecture. In Becker (1992) the "tendency to become trapped in poor local optima" (p. 367) was addressed by introducing a user-defined regularization parameter to prevent weights from becoming too large. The IMAX models require that the training data are presented to the network twice per weight update, whereas a biologically plausible model should only use quantities that can be computed on-line. The computationally expensive weight update process used by IMAX requires large amounts of processing time, which, in Zemel and Hinton (1991), increases with the cube of the number of independent visual parameters (e.g., size, position, orientation) implicit in the input data.

More recently, Phillips *et al.* (1992) emphasized how different sensory modalities, or streams within modalities, often signal aspects of the input that are correlated (e.g., the sound and sight of a word being spoken). Using an unsupervised algorithm, they demonstrate that the correlations between different streams of synthetic data can be used to discover the

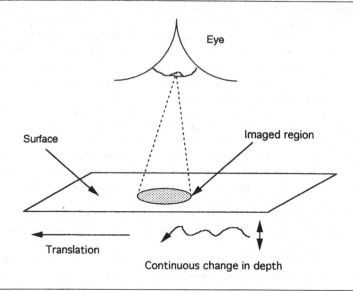

Figure 1: Schematic diagram of how surface moves over time. Surface depth varies continuously as the surface translates at a constant velocity parallel to the image plane.

features that are related across streams as well as discovering the relations between them.

3 Learning Using Spatiotemporal Constraints

The input to a perceptual system can be characterized as a vector in a high-dimensional space. In humans, there are approximately 10^6 fibers in the optic nerve, so that the retinal image can be considered as a vector with 10^6 components. As the retinal image changes over time, this *image vector* describes a trajectory through the high-dimensional space. However, this vector is generated by events in the physical world, and can therefore be described in terms of a small number of parameters (e.g., surface depth). It is these parameters that are useful to an organism. A large part of the problem of perception consists of extracting these physical parameters implicit in the changing image vector.

Consider a sequence of images of an oriented, planar, textured surface that is moving relative to a fixed camera (see Fig. 1). Between two consecutive image frames the distance to the surface changes by a small amount. Simultaneous with this small change in surface depth, a relatively large change in the intensity of individual pixels can occur. For example, a one-pixel shift in camera position can dramatically alter the intensity of individual image pixels, yet the corresponding change in the depth of the imaged surface is usually small. Thus, for a moving camera or surface, there is a difference between the rate of change of the intensity of individual pixels and the corresponding rate of change of parameters associated with the imaged surface. A perceptually salient parameter is therefore characterized by variability over time, but the rate of change of the parameter is usually small, relative to that of the intensity of individual image pixels. More importantly, a sequence of images defines an ordered set in which neighboring images are derived from similar physical scenarios, and that the temporal proximity of images provides a *temporal binding* of parameter values. It is this temporal binding that permits us to legitimately cluster temporally proximal images together, and thereby discover which invariances they share.

It is possible to constrain the learning process such that a sequence of outputs is forced to possess the general characteristics of perceptually salient parameters (e.g., temporal smoothness). This can be achieved without specifying the required output value for any given input. Using an unsupervised method, the value of each output is essentially arbitrary, but each output is uniquely and systematically associated with a particular input parameter value. An "economical" way for a model to generate such a set of outputs is to adapt its connection weights so that the outputs specify some perceptually salient parameter implicit in the model's inputs. That is, it is possible to place quite general constraints (e.g., temporal smoothness) on the outputs, such that the "easiest" way for a model to satisfy these constraints is to compute the value of a perceptually salient parameter. Such constraints do not determine which particular parameter should be learned, nor the output value for any given input. Instead, these constraints specify only that particular types of relations must hold between successive outputs. Finally, although a learning method may be based on an assumption of temporal smoothness, violations of the smoothness assumption can be tolerated without compromising learning of perceptual parameters (see Experiment 2.3).

4 The Learning Method

A model that uses a type of *temporal smoothness* constraint can be made to learn visual parameters. The degree of smoothness of the output or *state* of a model unit can be measured in terms of the "temporally local," or *short-term*, variance associated with a sequence of output values. A sequence of states defines a curve that is maximally smooth if the variance of this curve is minimal (the straighter the curve, the smoother the output). However, minimizing only the short-term variance has a trivial solution. This consists of setting all model weights to zero, generating a horizontal output curve. This is consistent with one characteristic (smoothness) of perceptually salient parameters, but it is not very useful. Moreover, it does not conform to the other characteristic, variability over time. The output can be made to reflect both smoothness *and* variability by forcing it to have a small short-term variance, and a large *long-term* variance. Accordingly, the variance of the output over small periods should be small, relative to its variance over longer periods.

The general strategy just described can be implemented using a multilayer model. Units in the input, hidden, and output layers are labeled i, j, and k, respectively. Input and output layers have linear units, and the hidden layer has *tanh* units. The state of an output unit u_k at each time t is $z_{kt} = \sum_j w_{jk} z_{jt}$, where w_{jk} is the value of a weighted connection from the jth hidden unit to u, and z_{jt} is the state of the jth hidden unit.

The desired behaviour in z_k can be obtained by altering interunit connection weights such that z_k has a large long-term variance V, and a small short-term variance U. These requirements can be embodied in a merit function (the k subscripts have been omitted here):

$$F = \log \frac{V}{U} = \log \frac{1/2 \sum_{t=1}^{T} (\bar{z}_t - z_t)^2}{1/2 \sum_{t=1}^{T} (\tilde{z}_t - z_t)^2} \tag{4.1}$$

The $\frac{1}{2}$s are formally redundant, but have been introduced to simplify the derivatives of U and V. The cumulative states $\tilde{z}_t$ and $\bar{z}_t$ are both exponentially weighted sums of states z:

$$\tilde{z}_t = \lambda_S \tilde{z}_t + (1 - \lambda_S) z_{(t-1)} : \quad 0 \le \lambda_S \le 1 \tag{4.2}$$

$$\bar{z}_t = \lambda_L \bar{z}_t + (1 - \lambda_L) z_{(t-1)} : \quad 0 \le \lambda_L \le 1 \tag{4.3}$$

Where λ_L and λ_S are time decay constants. The half-life h_L of λ_L is much longer (typically 100 times longer) than the corresponding half-life h_S of λ_S.

Note that 4.1 is invariant with respect to the magnitude of z, and therefore with respect to the magnitude of the weights. Therefore, no weight normalization is required. In the experiments described below, the pattern of weights altered during learning, but variation in the magnitude of weights was relatively small.

The derivative of F with respect to output weights results in a learning rule that is a linear combination of Hebbian and anti-Hebbian weight update, over long and short time scales, respectively.[3] Given a hidden unit with output state z_{jt}, short-term mean $\tilde{z}_{jt}$, and long-term mean $\bar{z}_{jt}$, which projects to an output unit with state z_{kt}, short-term mean $\tilde{z}_{kt}$, and long-term mean $\bar{z}_{kt}$:[4]

$$\frac{\partial F}{\partial w_{jk}} = \frac{1}{V} \sum_t (\bar{z}_{kt} - z_{kt})(\bar{z}_{jt} - z_{jt}) - \frac{1}{U} \sum_t (\tilde{z}_{kt} - z_{kt})(\tilde{z}_{jt} - z_{jt}) \tag{4.4}$$

---

[3]Thanks to Harry Barrow and Alistair Bray for pointing this out.

[4]For hidden unit weights, additional terms resulting from the *tanh* hidden unit activation function are required (see Appendix A).

The Hebbian and anti-Hebbian components are given by the first and second terms (respectively) on the right-hand side of 4.4. The pre- and postsynaptic means used in conventional Hebbian learning rules (e.g., Sejnowski 1977) have been replaced by the exponentially weighted means, $\bar{z}_{jt}$ and $\bar{z}_{kt}$ (respectively) in the Hebbian part of 4.4, and by $\hat{z}_{jt}$ and $\hat{z}_{kt}$ in the anti-Hebbian part of 4.4. In contrast, the rule described in Bienstock *et al.* (1982) uses the exponentially weighted mean of only the postsynaptic output to modulate learning, and this learning is *either* Hebbian or anti-Hebbian, depending on the state of the post-synaptic unit. In summary, the rule defined in 4.4 uses the exponentially weighted mean of both the pre- *and* postsynaptic states to modulate both the Hebbian *and* anti-Hebbian learning applied to every weight.

The learning algorithm consists of computing the derivative of F with respect to every weight in the model to locate a maximum in F. The derivatives of F with respect to weights between the input and hidden unit layers are required. These derivatives are computed using the chain rule (but not the learning method) described in Rumelhart *et al.* (1986). The cumulative result of these computations is used to alter weights only after the entire sequence of inputs has been presented. However, storage requirements are minimal because all quantities can be computed incrementally (see Appendix A). This can also permit weights to be updated after the presentation of each input, as demonstrated in Stone and Bray (1995).

A conjugate gradient method (Williams 1991) was used to maximize F.[5] Each iteration, or line search, involves quadratic interpolation in a given conjugate search direction, so that each line search requires the derivative of F at two points along the current search direction.

Note that, whereas weight changes depend on the history of inputs to a unit, a unit's state z is a function only of the current input. An information-theoretic interpretation of F is given in Appendix B.

5 Experiments

5.1 Model Architecture. The model consists of three layers of units, as shown in Figure 2. Units in each layer are connected to every unit in the next layer. The first layer consists of 20 linear input units, arranged in two rows. The hidden layer consists of a fixed number of between 3 and 10 units. The state of a unit in the hidden layer is $z = tanh(x)$, where x is the total input to a hidden layer unit from units in the input layer. The input to the jth hidden unit is $x_j = \sum_i (w_{ij} z_i + \theta_j)$, where w_{ij} is the value of a weighted connection from the ith input unit to the jth hidden unit, and z_i is the state of the ith input unit. All and only units in the hidden layer

---

[5]In results not reported here, an iterative weight update rule that took steps of size $\eta \, \partial F / \partial w$ (where η was adjusted automatically) was about 10 times slower than the conjugate gradient method.

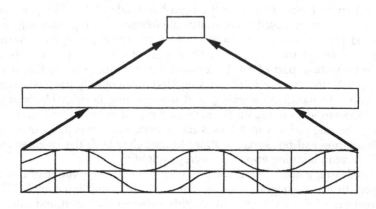

Figure 2: Network architecture. The network has 20 input units, arranged in two rows of 10, between 3 and 10 *tanh* hidden units, and one linear output unit. At each time step, a pair of one-dimensional stereo images is presented at the input layer.

have a bias weight θ from a unit with constant output of 1. These bias weights are adapted in the same way as all other weights. The output layer consists of a single linear unit, as described in the previous section.

5.2 Experiment Series 1: Random Dot Stereograms.

5.2.1 Input Data. The input data consisted of a temporal sequence of one-dimensional random dot stereograms. The sequence of stereograms was derived by simulating the motion of a planar surface which was both translating at a fixed velocity while oscillating in depth (see Fig. 1). The image dot-density was 0.167 dots/pixel throughout the sequence of stereograms, and each stereogram was presented for one time step.

The amount of linear shift or *disparity* between the left and right images of each stereo pair varied between ±1 image pixel. The disparity values were generated by convolving a one-dimensional circular array of 1000 random numbers with a gaussian of standard deviation of 100, and then normalizing these values to lie between ±1.

The one-dimensional random dot "surface" from which images were derived was constructed by placing 1s randomly in an array. The gray-levels of two adjacent image pixels were derived from the means of two nonoverlapping surface regions, in which each region contained 10 surface elements. Image subsampling of the surface gray-levels allowed subpixel disparities to be generated. For example, if members of a stereo pair were derived from surface regions that overlapped by one surface element (=0.1 of a pixel width) then the images had a disparity of 0.1 pixels. The gray-level profiles of a sample of typical stereo pairs are shown in Figure 3.

The smoothing effects of the optics of the eye were simulated by smoothing the image gray-levels. To save computer time, this image smoothing was achieved by smoothing the surface gray-levels (using a gaussian with a standard deviation of 10 surface elements). The set of surface gray-levels was then normalized to have zero mean and unit variance.

To simulate the translation of the surface, the first image I_1 of a pair was moved along the surface by 20 surface elements (=2 image pixels) at each time step, and the gray-levels of the surface were read into the image array (with 10 surface elements to each image pixel). The second image I_2 of a pair was aligned with I_1, and then shifted along the surface according to the current disparity value, which varied between ±1 pixel (equivalent to ±10 surface elements, see above).

5.2.2 Network Parameter Values. The half-life h_S of λ_S in 4.2 was set to 32 time steps. In this set of experiments, the long-term variance was set to the variance of z, so that $\bar{z}$ was equal to the mean state of a unit. This produced results which are not noticeably different from the method described above, and which was implemented for the second series of experiments (see below). As stated previously, each of the 1000 stereo pairs had a disparity that was determined by a circular array of 1000 smoothly varying disparity values. This circular array permitted $\bar{z}_t$ to be computed for $t < 1$. The initial weights were set to random values between ±0.3.

5.3 Experiment 1.1: Discovering Stereo Disparity. The following results were obtained by maximizing F using a conjugate gradient method (Williams 1991). The model was tested on stereo pairs of images (see Fig. 1, 2, and 3).

5.3.1 Results. The number of hidden units was reduced between different runs to discover the minimum number required to solve the task. If between 4 and 10 hidden units were used then the model always succeeded within 100 conjugate gradient line searches, with $|r| > 0.9$, where r is the correlation between the output unit state z and stereo disparity. Using less than four hidden units did not always result in convergence within 100 line searches (see Experiments 1.5 and 2.2 for convergence results).

5.4 Experiment 1.2: Hidden Unit Weight Vectors. A network with three hidden units was used for further analysis. After 100 conjugate

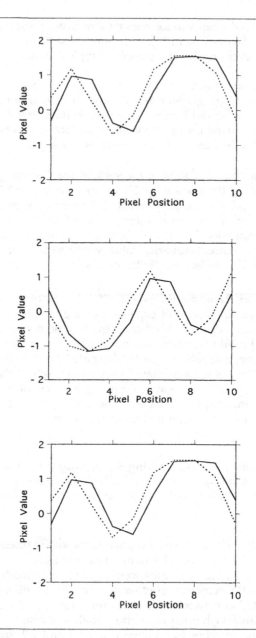

Figure 3: Examples of random-dot input image pairs. Each graph shows the overlaid gray-levels of one image pair. The gray-levels of the left (– – –) and right (———) images are plotted for each of the 10 pixel positions of a stereo pair. Each image was obtained by subsampling a gray-level random-dot surface (see text).

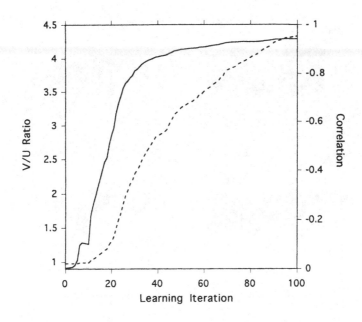

Figure 4: Graph of learning iteration number versus V/U ratio (- - -) and correlation r (——) between output unit state z and disparity during conjugate gradient learning.

gradient iterations $r = -0.943$ (see Fig. 4). Output curves plotted during the learning process are given in Figure 5. The output unit state after 100 iterations was plotted against the time-varying disparity in Figure 6. Results using a surface on which every element has a random gray-level (instead of the random dots used here) are similar to those reported here (see Stone 1995).

Note that the correlation r between unit outputs and disparity is negative for some of the results presented here. It is not necessary, nor even desirable, that r should be positive. If we consider the output unit as part of an integrated system that computes the values of different visual parameters then it is necessary only that a unit is able to signal to other units information regarding some aspect of the input. This can be achieved equally well with either a high magnitude negative or positive value of r.

The weight vector of each of the three hidden units after 100 conjugate gradient line searches is shown in Figure 7. In each graph, the weighting given to corresponding pixels of a stereo pair is shown on a common (pixel position) x-axis. Thus, the 20-dimensional weight vector

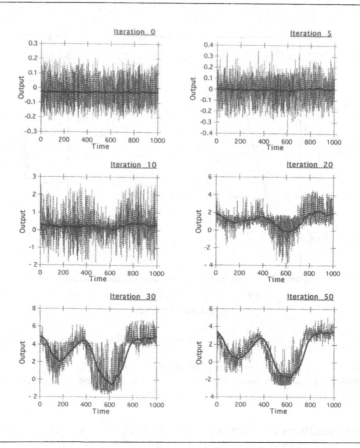

Figure 5: Graphs of output unit state z (– – –) and $\tilde{z}$ (▬▬) versus time at different learning iterations. At each of 1000 time steps the network was presented with a stereo pair of images. The disparity of these input images varied over time as depicted in Figure 6.

of each unit is shown as two overlaid 10-dimensional weight vectors. The weight values between each hidden unit and the output unit are $\{-2.563, 2.607, -2.796\}$ for units labeled 1, 2, and 3, respectively, in Figures 7 and 8.

For each hidden unit, the disparity of every image pair from the training set was plotted against the corresponding hidden unit state (see Fig. 8). Units 1 and 3 appear to have antisymmetric response profiles. This is consistent with their weight vector profiles.

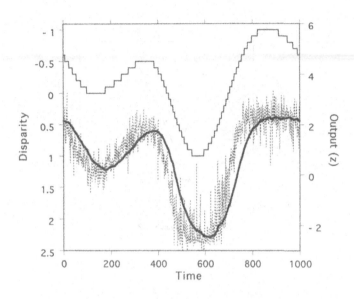

Figure 6: Graph of output unit state z (– – –), $\tilde{z}$ (━━), and stereo disparity (———
) versus time after 100 conjugate gradient line searches. The jagged appearance
of the latter is due to the fact that the smallest change in the disparity of input
image pairs is 0.1 of a pixel (see section on Input Data).

5.5 Experiment 1.3: No Hidden Units. As expected for a system
that attempts to discover a nonlinear input/output mapping, learning
without a hidden layer of units failed to compute disparity. With the
output unit connected directly to the input layer, correlations of $|r| > 0.01$
were not exceeded over 10 different simulations with different initial
random weights.

5.6 Experiment 1.4: Generalization. If the model has learned disparity (and not some spurious correlate of disparity) then it should generalize to new stereo data sets, without any learning of these new sets.
Accordingly, the network described in Experiment 1.2 with a correlation
$r = -0.943$ was tested with test data consisting of 1000 stereo pairs. These
were obtained from a new surface constructed in the same manner as was
used for the original data set. During testing, the disparity varied exactly
as before, but now each image pair was derived from a random point on
the surface. (This tested the ability of the system to estimate disparity
independently of the particular gray-level profiles in each image pair).
Using these data the correlation was $r = -0.937$.

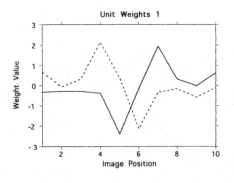

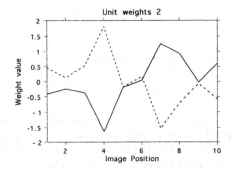

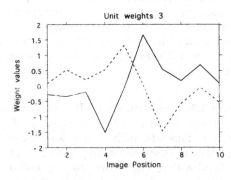

Figure 7: Weight vectors of the three hidden units. Weight values projecting from left (——) and right (– – –) images of a stereo pair to one hidden unit are shown in each graph.

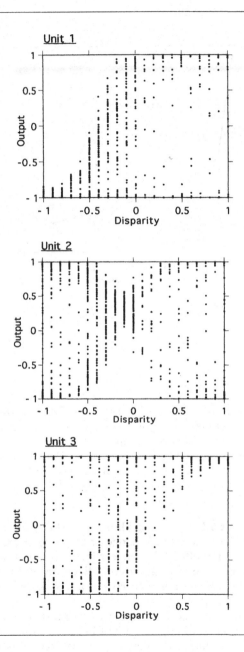

Figure 8: Scattergrams of hidden unit state versus stereo disparity for 1000 image pairs. Each graph shows the scattergram of a single hidden unit. (The vertical striations are an artifact of the disparity values which varied in intervals of 0.1 of a pixel.)

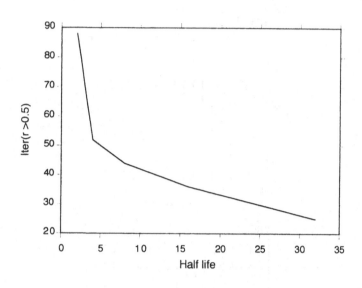

Figure 9: Graph of number of iterations required to exceed $r = 0.5$ versus half-life h_S of λ_S.

Note that the rate at which disparity varies has no effect on this test correlation. This is because, while *learning* depends upon current and previous states, the *state z* of a unit at any time depends only upon the current input. Thus, after learning, the model can detect disparities irrespective of the rate at which disparity varies in the input.

5.7 Experiment 1.5: Effect of Half-Life. The relation between the half-life h_S of λ_S and the rate of change of disparity clearly has implications for learning. The effect of h_S on learning was tested, with 10 hidden units, using the random-dot data used in Experiment 1.1. Within limits, the value of h_S was found not to be critical to the success of the learning method.

The magnitude of the correlation between unit state and disparity was $|r| < 0.9$ only for simulations with a half-life $h_S < 2$ time steps. A graph of h_S versus the number of conjugate gradient iterations required such that $|r| > 0.5$ (denoted by $[iter(|r| > 0.5)]$) is shown in Figure 9. A graph of h_S versus $[iter(|r| > 0.5)]^{-2}$ gives a straight line with a correlation of 0.986 for $h_S = \{2, 4, 8, 16, 32\}$. In all cases, additional learning resulted in a final value of $|r| > 0.9$. A network with three hidden units gave qualitatively similar, but less systematic, results.

Setting h_S too high can increase the rate at which the function F is maximized without resulting in a high correlation r. For values of $h_S >$ 32, the function F was maximized, but a graph of z versus time yielded a bell-shaped curve. In this case, each value of z corresponded to two values of disparity.

As can be seen from Figure 9, h_S acts somewhat like an *annealing parameter*, smoothing out local maxima in F at high values of h_S. This is true in general, but is more apparent if (as above) $h_L = \infty$ so that V is the variance of z. Now, as $h_S \to \infty$, so $U \to V$, and therefore $V/U \to 1$, for any weight values. As in Hopfield (1984), Durbin and Willshaw (1987), and Stone (1992), at high "temperatures" (high values of h_S) the energy surface defined by F is convex, and there exists a single maximum. As the temperature is reduced, the energy function becomes increasingly nonconvex. A series of decreasing temperatures is associated with a corresponding series of increasingly nonconvex energy functions. At each temperature, the maximum of the current energy function can be used as the starting point to search for the maximum of the next function (associated with a new, lower temperature). This brief sketch is consistent with results given in Figure 9, which shows an inverse square relation between h and the rate of convergence.

Annealing methods are well suited to error surfaces containing many local extrema. For the tasks tested in this paper, only a slight advantage was observed when h_S was annealed in a variety of tests. This suggests that the error surface defined by F has relatively few local extrema. However, it may be that annealing h_S provides significant improvements in the rate of convergence and in the ability to find deep extrema for more complex tasks.

5.8 Experiment 1.6: Hierarchical Learning. If we associate a function $F_j = \log(V_j/U_j)$ with each hidden unit u_j in the hidden layer then each unit can independently and simultaneously adjust its weights to maximize its F_j. Note that F_j is defined only in terms of the states of unit u_j. We can then freeze the input-hidden unit weights, and maximize F (as above) with respect to the hidden-output weights.

This hierarchical learning method does not require the backpropagation of an error signal between successive unit layers. Instead, each weight of each unit u_j is updated according to the derivative of F_j with respect to that weight. Neither this nor the method described above requires a conjugate gradient method, though learning is about 10 times faster if conjugate gradients are used.

The correlations between the outputs of individual hidden units and disparity were $\{0.60, 0.44, 0.45, 0.59, -0.09, 0.47, 0.46, -0.60, 0.55, -0.40\}$.

Typically, each unit state varied monotonically over a small range of disparities, and was almost constant outside of that range.

Using the hierarchical learning method, the correlation between the single output unit state z and disparity for the test data was $r = -0.74$, with 10 units in the hidden layer. This was achieved after 10 conjugate-gradient updates of weights between the hidden and output unit layer only.

The highest value of r from the hidden units was 0.6. From a statistical perspective, this hidden unit accounts for 0.36 ($= 0.6^2$) of the variance in disparity. This contrasts with a value $r = -0.74$ of the output unit which accounts for 0.55 ($= -0.74^2$) of the variance. Therefore, a linear combination of outputs of hidden units (as implemented via the addition of an output unit) accounts for about 1.5 times the amount of variance in disparity than is accounted for by any single hidden unit.

The network used in these experiments did not use any form of competition between hidden units. It is possible that such a mechanism might force each unit to become sensitive to a small range of parameter values in a more efficient manner than was obtained here.

5.9 Experiment Series 2: Gray-Level Images.

5.9.1 Input Data. The input data were derived from a gray-level image (see Fig. 10), using 1000 synthetically generated disparity values (see below). The image in Figure 10 was convolved with a difference of gaussian (DOG) filter to reduce the range of spatial frequencies present in the image. This procedure also simulates the action of retinal ganglion cells with center–surround receptive fields. The ratio of gaussian standard deviations was 1.6, with the smaller gaussian having a standard deviation of 2 pixels.

One image I_1 of a stereo pair was copied from a 10-pixel image strip of Figure 10. The position of this strip was advanced by two pixels per time step. The position of the second image I_2 of a pair was the same as I_1, except for a linear shift given by the current value of disparity (subpixel shifts were obtained by linear interpolation of gray-levels in Fig. 10). Each input image was normalized to have zero mean and unit variance. The disparity varied sinusoidally over time with a period of 1000 time steps between ± 1 pixels. This ensured that the value of disparity at $t = 0$ is equal to the disparity at $t = 1000$.

The fact that disparity was defined by a circular array of continuously varying values was used to initialize the value of $\tilde{z}_{k0}$ as follows. The 1000 stereo pairs data were presented to the network once, then the value of $\tilde{z}_{k0}$ was set to $\tilde{z}_{k1000}$. In contrast, it would require several complete presentations of the data set to achieve a stable value for $\bar{z}_{k0}$ because it has a long half-life (3200 time steps). To a first approximation, this stable value is equal to the mean of z. Accordingly, the initial value of $\bar{z}_{k0}$ was

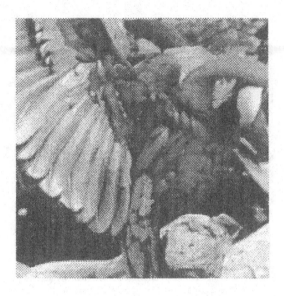

Figure 10: Parrot image used for learning.

set to the mean value of z after one complete presentation of the set of 1000 stereo pairs.[6]

5.9.2 Parameter Values. The values of the half-lives h_S and h_L were set to 32 and 3200 time steps, respectively. The network had 10 hidden units. Unless stated otherwise, parameter values were the same as in previous experiments.

5.10 Experiment 2.1: Gray-Level Images. After 10 conjugate gradient iterations the correlation was $r = -0.546$, and by 60 iterations it was $r = -0.971$. The set of weights learned by this network at 60 iterations was used to test its performance (without further learning) on data derived from the test image shown in Figure 11. This data was generated using the same temporal sequence of disparities as was used during learning. For data derived from this test image, $r = -0.959$.

5.11 Experiment 2.2: Convergence and Local Optima. This experiment was designed to test the reliability and speed of convergence of the

---

[6]For optimization techniques (as in Williams 1991) that take large steps on the error surface defined by F, $\dot{z}_{k0}$ and $\ddot{z}_{k0}$ should be reinitialized at the start of each iteration.

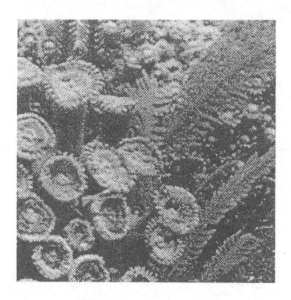

Figure 11: Coral image used for testing.

learning method. Experiment 2.1 was repeated 100 times, with each run being terminated when $|r| > 0.9$. All 100 runs converged with $|r| > 0.9$. The median number of iterations required such that $|r| > 0.9$ was 69, with a minimum of 31 and a maximum of 132 iterations.

Overall, these results indicate that at least for the task demonstrated here, the function F has a low proportion of poor local maxima. This, in turn, suggests that the "energy landscape" defined by F is relatively smooth, allowing it to be traversed by simple search techniques. More importantly, it suggests that maxima are reliably associated with model weight values that enable the detection of perceptually salient parameters.

5.12 Experiment 2.3: Discontinuous Stereo Disparity. A critical assumption of the method is that the perceptual parameter implicit in the input data varies smoothly over time. Obviously, smoothness is defined relative to a particular temporal scale, parameterized by the half-life h_S in the model. However, given a particular temporal scale, how do discontinuities affect learning? The effect of discontinuities in stereo disparity on learning is shown in Figure 12. The sequence of 1000 disparities was obtained by taking the 1000 sinusoidally varying disparity values used

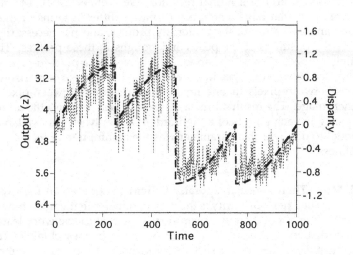

Figure 12: Graph of state z (- - -) and disparity (▬ ▬ ▬) versus time after learning with temporal discontinuities in disparity.

so far in this series of experiments, and swapping the positions of four subsequences of 250 disparity values with each other. After 100 conjugate gradient learning iterations with 10 hidden units, $r = -0.916$ for the training set derived from Figure 10, and $r = -0.901$ on a test set derived from Figure 11. Clearly, a small proportion of discontinuities in an otherwise smoothly changing parameter does not seriously compromise the learning method.

6 Discussion

The sequences of synthetic stereograms used in this paper differ from stereograms obtained from a natural scene in the following ways: (1) the disparity is constant across the input array, (2) no discontinuities in disparity occur within any stereo pair, and, (3) stereo disparity is the only quantity that varies smoothly over time. Given these limitations, the main contribution of this paper is to demonstrate that a learning rule, based on a generic assumption about temporal smoothness, can be used to reliably learn a nontrivial function (stereo disparity).

The stereo disparity task learned is a hyperacuity task. That is, the amount of disparity is less than the width of a receptor (pixel). This is consistent with psychophysical studies that demonstrate that subjects can discriminate disparities as small as 2 sec of arc, less than one-tenth of the width (30 sec of arc) of a retinal receptor (Westheimer 1994). Members of a stereo pair that have a subpixel disparity differ in terms of the local slope and curvature of their intensity profiles, and not necessarily in terms of the positions of the peaks and troughs in these profiles. Thus, detecting subpixel disparities cannot be achieved by a pixel-to-pixel correspondence between images in a stereo pair. It requires comparisons of relations-between-pixels in one image with relations-between-pixels in the other image. The resultant meta-relation, which specifies the amount of disparity in each pair, is of a high order. The only means available to the model to discover this parameter was the assumption of its temporal smoothness.

6.1 More Than One Perceptually Salient Parameter. In the experiments described here, disparity is the only parameter that varies smoothly over time. It may not therefore seem surprising that the network learned to detect disparity. Given a sequence of stereo images obtained from a moving pair of cameras, a system based on this type of smoothness assumption is likely to discover simple parameters in preference to disparity. For example, like disparity, luminance tends to vary smoothly across time and space. However, with regard to the human visual system, simple parameters such as luminance are not a major determinant of neuronal activity in area V1, because only a relatively small amount of luminance information is preserved (Nicolls, *et al.* 1992, p. 630). So, although such simple parameters could present problems for an artificial neural network, these problems may not be encountered in the central nervous system.

If more than one "nonsimple" perceptually salient parameter (e.g., depth, color, motion) is implicit in the input sequence then these may be kept separate in a network architecture, which is analogous to the separate processing streams in the human visual system. For example, information regarding parameters such as color and motion are thought to be transmitted by distinct retinal ganglion cells, and this information remains segregated within the LGN and V1 (Livingstone and Hubel 1988). Thus, discovering a perceptual parameter derived from one (or more) of these processing streams is not necessarily precluded by the presence of many perceptual parameters in the retinal image.

6.2 Effect of Half-Life. The assumption of temporal smoothness was implemented via a time decay constant λ_S with half-life h_S. Consider a model in which each output unit has a different value of h_S. Choosing a value for h_S implicitly specifies a temporal "grain size," and therefore restricts learning to parameters that change at a particular rate. Perceptually salient events (such as motion) occur within a relatively small range of temporal windows. At rates of change that are either too high or too low, events cannot be detected by a given unit. Between these two extremes, different units have temporal tuning characteristics (defined by their respective half-lives h_S) that ensure that a range of rates of perceptual change can be detected by some subpopulation of units. Just as an array of differently tuned spatial receptive fields can be used to recognize spatial patterns characteristic of certain parameter values [e.g., surface orientation (Stone and Isard 1995)], so an array of differently tuned temporal receptive fields may be used recognize temporal patterns characteristic of human walkers [e.g., Johansson figures (Johansson 1973)]. The value chosen for h_S was important (though not critical) for learning to succeed. However, for any "reasonable" rate of change of disparity, some units in a population tuned to different temporal frequencies would learn disparity.

6.3 Violating the Temporal Smoothness Assumption. Even if we accept that temporal smoothness is defined relative to a particular value of h_S, it might be argued that perceptually salient parameters do not always vary smoothly over time. In the perceptual world, violations of the smoothness assumption are not hard to find. However, such violations do not necessarily undermine the model's performance. This is because, in practice, the learning method requires only that discontinuities in parameter values are *rare*, relative to gradual changes over time. In the example presented earlier, four discontinuities every 1000 time steps did not disrupt the learning process, because most of the input data remained consistent with the smoothness assumption. Thus, the model does not require that perceptually salient parameters change smoothly at all times, but (more realistically) that such parameters change smoothly *most* of the time.

6.4 Detecting Perceptual Parameters with Different Half-Lives. In Hinton (1989a, p. 208) it was suggested that if the hidden units of an autoencoder network were constrained to vary their states slowly over time then they might encode invariant input parameters such as object identity, and, in Hinton (1989b), that conventional hidden units could be used to encode transient quantities such as object position. However, it may be unrealistic to expect the physical world to partition neatly into invariant (e.g., object identity) and transient (e.g., object position) parameter types. One alternative would be to encode parameters with varying degrees of temporal transience using units with different half-lives. It might then be expected that units with long half-lives would reflect invariant input parameters such as object identity, units with shorter half-lives might encode color (for instance, if a single type of object were presented in many colors), and those with even shorter half-lives might encode transient parameters such as the position of that object.

6.5 Interpreting z. The output z can be interpreted as a noisy version of the temporal average $\bar{z}$ (see Appendix B). As can be seen, $\bar{z}$ provides a more accurate measure of disparity than z. Although z is labeled as the output of a unit, the precise correspondence between units and neurons has not been specified. If such a correspondence were to be established then it is likely that $\bar{z}$ would be equated with the neuron membrane potential because it is commonly assumed that a neuron behaves like a leaky integrator. This results in a membrane potential that, like $\bar{z}$, tends to decay exponentially with time.

6.6 A Spatial Analogue. It is noteworthy that there exists a spatial analogue to the temporal method presented here. Rather than defining V and U over time, these can be defined over a spatial array of units, so that $\bar{z}$ and $\bar{z}$ are short-range and long-range spatial means, respectively (Eglen *et al.* 1996). In this case, maximizing F forces neighboring units to have similar outputs (low U), but units separated by large distances are forced to have dissimilar outputs (high V). It may be possible to use this method to model the topology-preserving mappings of V1 and V2 in which the value of a perceptual parameter varies smoothly across an array of units.

This paper is not intended to suggest that all human perceptual development can be modeled using a generic neocortical learning strategy. However, it is proposed that, in evolutionary terms, a small class of generic learning strategies could have acted as an economical foundation for building neocortical systems to analyse perceptual inputs.

7 Conclusion

Marr's observation that "the world is continuous almost everywhere" (Marr 1982) has been applied to the temporal domain, in which it is assumed that (to paraphrase Marr) the world is continuous almost every*when*. This assumption was used to derive a learning method that, when presented with a sequence of stereo images of a moving surface, discovered precisely that parameter (stereo disparity) that described the behavior of the imaged surface through time.

The model may lend itself to the self-organized construction of hierarchical systems, in which successive layers compute increasingly higher order parameters, with the highest layers performing object recognition.

Whatever the limitations of the particular model presented in this paper, any learning system that does not take advantage of the temporal continuity of perceptual parameters implicit in its input discards a powerful and general heuristic for discovering perceptually salient properties of the physical world.

Appendix A: The Learning Algorithm _____

The learning algorithm relies upon batch update of a weight vector $\mathbf{w}$, which contains all weights in the network. At each time step t, a stereo pair is presented at the input layer, and the derivative of F with respect to every weight in the network is computed and added to a cumulative weight derivative vector $\nabla F_{\mathbf{w}}$. This derivative vector is used to update $\mathbf{w}$ only after all $T = 1000$ stereo pairs have been presented at the input units. The same set of stereo pairs is repeatedly presented in the same order during learning. Storage requirements are minimal because all quantities required for learning can be computed incrementally.

Notation. Units in the input, hidden and output layers are indexed by subscripts i, j, and k, respectively. For example, a weight that connects hidden unit u_j to output unit u_k is denoted w_{jk}. The state z_{kt} of u_k at time t is $z_{kt} = \sum_j w_{jk} z_{jt}$, where z_{jt} is the state of u_j. Input and output layer units have linear activation functions, whereas hidden units have a nonlinear (*tanh*) activation functions. Weights connecting input to hidden units, and hidden to output units, are referred to as *lower* and *upper* weights, respectively.

The function to be maximized is $F = \log V/U$, where

$$U = 1/2 \sum_{t=1}^{T} (\tilde{z}_{kt} - z_{kt})^2$$

$$V = 1/2 \sum_{t=1}^{T} (\bar{z}_{kt} - z_{kt})^2$$

V is the long-term variance of z_k, U is the short-term variance of z_k, and T is the period over which they are defined (numerically equal to the number of inputs here). Both V and U are defined in terms of exponentially weighted means of z_k. The weighted means $\tilde{z}_k$ and $\bar{z}_k$ differ only in terms of their respective exponential rates of decay:

$$\tilde{z}_{kt} = \lambda_S \tilde{z}_{k(t-1)} + (1 - \lambda_S) z_{k(t-1)} : \qquad 0 \le \lambda_S \le 1 \tag{A.1}$$

$$\bar{z}_{kt} = \lambda_L \bar{z}_{k(t-1)} + (1 - \lambda_L) z_{k(t-1)} : \qquad 0 \le \lambda_L \le 1 \tag{A.2}$$

where λ_S and λ_L are decay constants with half-lives of h_S and h_L, respectively, with $h_L \gg h_S$. The formula for obtaining a value of λ for a given half-life h is $\lambda = 2^{1/h}$. (Note that $z_{k(t-1)}$ contributes to $\tilde{z}_{kt}$ and $\bar{z}_{kt}$, but not to $\tilde{z}_{k(t-1)}$ and $\bar{z}_{k(t-1)}$.)

Evaluating $\partial F/\partial w$. The derivative of F with respect to any weight w is

$$\frac{\partial F}{\partial w} = \frac{1}{V} \frac{\partial V}{\partial w} - \frac{1}{U} \frac{\partial U}{\partial w} \tag{A.3}$$

The identical form of U and V permits us to derive $\partial U/\partial w$ for lower and upper weights, from which corresponding equations for V can be obtained by substitution.

The incremental computation of U up to time t is

$$U(t) = U(t-1) + 1/2 \, (\tilde{z}_{kt} - z_{kt})^2 \qquad \text{(A.4)}$$

Therefore the derivative of $U(t)$ with respect to any weight w is

$$\frac{\partial U(t)}{\partial w} = \frac{\partial U(t-1)}{\partial w} + (\tilde{z}_{kt} - z_{kt}) \left(\frac{\partial \tilde{z}_{kt}}{\partial w} - \frac{\partial z_{kt}}{\partial w} \right) \qquad \text{(A.5)}$$

Where, from A.1:

$$\frac{\partial \tilde{z}_{kt}}{\partial w} = \lambda_S \frac{\partial \tilde{z}_{k(t-1)}}{\partial w} + (1 - \lambda_S) \frac{\partial z_{k(t-1)}}{\partial w} \qquad \text{(A.6)}$$

Thus, the incremental computation of A.5 depends upon evaluation of $\partial z_{kt}/\partial w$ in A.5 and $\partial z_{k(t-1)}/\partial w$ in A.6, for both upper and lower weights. Equations for $\partial z_{kt}/\partial w$ (for upper and lower weights) will be derived next, from which equations for $\partial z_{k(t-1)}/\partial w$ can be obtained by substitution.

Evaluating $\partial z_{kt}/\partial w_{jk}$. In the case of an upper weight w_{jk} projecting to an output unit u_k:

$$z_{kt} = \sum_j w_{jk} \, z_{jt} \qquad \text{(A.7)}$$

where z_{jt} is the state of the jth hidden unit at time t, so that

$$\frac{\partial z_{kt}}{\partial w_{jk}} = z_{jt} \qquad \text{(A.8)}$$

Evaluating $\partial z_{kt}/\partial w_{ij}$. Equation A.7 can be rewritten in terms of a lower weight w_{ij}, which projects to a hidden unit u_j:

$$z_{kt} = \sum_j w_{jk} \, tanh \left(\sum_i w_{ij} z_{it} \right) \qquad \text{(A.9)}$$

where z_{it} is the state of the ith input unit at time t. The derivative of z_{kt} with respect to w_{ij} is

$$\frac{\partial z_{kt}}{\partial w_{ij}} = w_{jk}(1 - z_{jt}^2) \, z_{it}$$

For an upper weight, this yields

$$\frac{\partial U(t)}{\partial w_{jk}} = \frac{\partial U(t-1)}{\partial w_{jk}} + (\tilde{z}_{kt} - z_{kt}) \left[\lambda_S \frac{\partial \tilde{z}_{k(t-1)}}{\partial w_{jk}} + (1 - \lambda_S) z_{j(t-1)} - z_{jt} \right]$$

where $\partial \tilde{z}_{k(t-1)}/\partial w$ is recursively defined as in A.6. The corresponding derivative for a lower weight is

$$\frac{\partial U(t)}{\partial w_{ij}} = \frac{\partial U(t-1)}{\partial w_{ij}} + (\tilde{z}_{kt} - z_{kt})$$

$$\times \left[\lambda_S \frac{\partial \tilde{z}_{k(t-1)}}{\partial w_{ij}} + w_{jk} \left[(1-\lambda_S)\,(1-z_{j(t-1)}^2)z_{i(t-1)} - (1-z_{jt}^2)z_{it} \right] \right]$$

Thus A.5 can be incrementally evaluated up to any time t. Corresponding equations for $\partial V/\partial w$ can be obtained by substitution in the derivation of $\partial U/\partial w$. The quantities U and V are by definition simple to compute incrementally. Therefore, A.3 can be computed on-line. For results presented in this paper, weights were adapted only after weight derivatives obtained with 1000 inputs had been accumulated. On-line weight update is possible, if, at each time step t, the cumulative values of $U(t)$ and $V(t)$ are good estimates of $U(T)$ and $V(T)$, respectively. This was achieved (for a different learning task) in Stone and Bray (1995) by defining $U(t)$ and $V(t)$ as exponentially weighted moving averages:

$$U(t) = \gamma U(t-1) + 1/2\,(1-\gamma)(\tilde{z}_t - z_t)^2 \qquad (A.10)$$
$$V(t) = \gamma V(t-1) + 1/2\,(1-\gamma)(\tilde{z}_t - z_t)^2 \qquad (A.11)$$

where $\gamma \gg \lambda_L$.

Appendix B: An Information-Theoretic Interpretation

Mutual Information. Consider a gaussian signal $X = S$, and a noisy version $Y = (S + N)$ of S that has been corrupted by additive gaussian noise N. It can be shown (Reza 1961) that the mutual information $I(X;Y)$ between $X = S$ and $Y = (S + N)$ is the log of the ratio of two variances; that of $Y = (S + N)$ and of $(Y - X) = N$:

$$I(X;Y) = 1/2 \log \frac{Var(Y)}{Var(Y - X)}$$

$$= 1/2 \log \frac{Var(S + N)}{Var(N)} \qquad (B.1)$$

Where Var denotes variance.

Relation to the Learning Algorithm.[7] The network can be considered in terms of maximizing information with respect to a low frequency (nonlinear) function of the input sequence.

The exponentially weighted quantity $\tilde{z}$ is a low-pass version of z, and we can therefore view $\tilde{z}$ as the result of passing z through a filter G with an exponentially decaying impulse response. The effective cutoff frequency f_c of this filter is defined by the time constant λ_S of its exponential decay.

---

[7]This analysis was suggested by Mark Plumbley of Kings College, London.

If G is an ideal low-pass filter[8] then the information capacity I_G of G is given by the rate of information transmitted about components of z below f_c. The quantity I_G is given by the difference between the rate of information transmission I_z about z and the rate of information transmission I_{zhi} about components of z which are above f_c:

$$I_G = I_z - I_{zhi} \tag{B.2}$$

If z has bandwidth B_z and G has noise variance n then the variance of the noise added to z as it passes through G is nB_z. If the variance of z is V then, from B.1

$$I_z = 1/2 \log \frac{V_z}{nB_z} \tag{B.3}$$

If z_{hi} has bandwidth B_{hi} then the variance of the noise added to z_{hi} as it passes through G is nB_{hi}. If the variance of z_{hi} is V_{hi} then the high pass signal z_{hi} can be transmitted through G using capacity

$$I_{zhi} = 1/2 \log \frac{V_{hi}}{nB_{hi}} \tag{B.4}$$

Substituting B.3 and B.4 in B.2, and rearranging:

$$I_G = 1/2 \log \frac{V_z}{V_{hi}} - K \tag{B.5}$$

where $K = 1/2 \log(B_z/z_{hi})$, which is a constant defined by the filter decay constant λ_S. The quantity $V_{hi} = Var(z_{hi}) = Var(\tilde{z} - z_t)$, where Var denotes variance. If we assume that z_{hi} has zero mean then $V_{hi} = 2U$, as defined in A.1, and B.5 can be rewritten as

$$I_G = 1/2 \log \left(\frac{V}{U} \right) - K \tag{B.6}$$

$$I_G = 1/2 F - K \tag{B.7}$$

Thus, in maximizing F, the learning algorithm adjusts network weights so as to maximize information transmission regarding a low frequency, nonlinear function of the sequence of input vectors.

Acknowledgments

Thanks to R. Lister, S. Isard, T. Collett, J. Budd, N. Hunkin, C. North, and G. Hinton for comments on drafts of this paper, and to D. Willshaw, A. Bray, and H. Barrow for useful discussions. Thanks also to S. Becker, M. Plumbley, and P. Williams for useful discussions on the information-theoretic interpretation given in Appendix B. Thanks to the anonymous referees, one of whom suggested the idea of an information-theoretic interpretation. This research was supported by a Joint Council Initiative grant awarded to J. Stone, T. Collett, and D. Willshaw.

---

[8]An ideal low-pass filter passes only those frequency components below its cut-off frequency f_c.

References

Barlow, H. 1972. Single units and sensation: A neuron doctrine for perceptual psychology? *Perception* 1, 371–394.

Barrow, H. G., and Bray, A. J. 1992. A model of adaptive development of complex cortical cells. In *Artificial Neural Networks II: Proceedings of the International Conference on Artificial Neural Networks*, I. Aleksander and J. Taylor, eds. Elsevier, Amsterdam.

Becker, S. 1992. Learning to categorize objects using temporal coherence. In *Neural Information Processing Systems 4*, J. E. Moody and R. Lippmann, eds., pp. 361–368. Morgan Kaufmann, San Mateo, CA.

Becker, S. 1996. Mutual information maximization: Models of cortical self-organisation. *Network: Computation in Neural Systems*, 7(1), 7–31.

Becker, S., and Hinton, G. 1992. Self-organizing neural network that discovers surfaces in random-dot stereograms. *Nature (London)* 335, 161–163.

Bienstock, E., Cooper, L., and Munro, P. 1982. Theory for the development of neuron selectivity: Orientation specificity and binocular interaction in visual cortex. *J. Neurosci.* 2, 32–48.

Durbin, R., and Willshaw, D. 1987. An analogue approach to the travelling salesman problem using an elastic net method. *Nature (London)* 326(6114), 689–691.

Eglen, S., Stone, J., and Barrow, H. 1996. *Learning Perceptual Invariances: A Spatial Model*. Tech. Rep. 404, Cognitive and Computing Sciences, University of Sussex.

Foldiak, P. 1991. Learning invariance from transformation sequences. *Neural Comp.* 3(2), 194–200.

Gibson, J. 1979. *The Ecological Approach to Visual Perception*. Houghton Mifflin, Boston.

Heywood, C., and Cowey, A. 1992. The role the 'face-cell' area in the discrimination and recognition of faces by monkey. *Phil. Transact. Royal Soc. London(B)* 335, 31–38.

Hinton, G. 1989a. Connectionist learning procedures. *Artif. Intell.* 40(1-3), 185–234.

Hinton, G. 1989b. Unsupervised learning procedures. *First Sun Annual Lecture*. Manchester University, Audio tape recording.

Hopfield, J. 1984. Neurons with graded response have collective computational properties like those of two-state neurons. *Proc. Natl. Acad. Sci. U.S.A.* 81, 3088–3092.

Johansson, G. 1973. Visual perception of biological motion and a model for its analysis. *Percept. Psychophys.* 14, 201–21.

Linsker, R. 1988. Self-organization in perceptual network. *Computer* 105–117.

Livingstone, M., and Hubel, D. 1988. Segregation of form, color, movement, and depth: Anatomy, physiology and perception. *Science* 240, 740–749.

Marr, D. 1982. *Vision*. Freeman, New York.

Mitchison, G. 1991. Removing time variation with the anti-hebbian differential synapse. *Neural Comp.* 3, 312–320.

Nicolls, J., Martin, A., and Wallace, B. 1992. *From Neuron to Brain*. Sinauer Associates, Sunderland, MA.

Oja, E. 1982. A simplified neuron model as a principal component analyzer. *J. Math. Biol.* **15**(3), 267–273.

Perrett, D., Harries, M., Mistlin, A., and Chitty, A. 1990. Three stages in the classification of body movements by visual neurons. In *Images and Understanding: Thoughts about Images, Ideas about Understanding*, H. Barlow, C. Blakemore and M. Weston-Smith, eds. Cambridge University Press, Cambridge.

Phillips, W., Kay, J., and Smyth, D. 1995. The discovery of structure by multistream networks of local processors with contextual guidance. *Network* **6**, 225–246.

Poggio, G., Motter, B., Squatrito, S., and Trotter, Y. 1985. Responses of neurons in visual cortex (v1 and v2) of the alert macaque to dynamic random-dot stereograms. *Vis. Res.* **25**(3), 397–406.

Reza, F. 1961. *Information Theory*. McGraw-Hill, New York.

Rumelhart, D., Hinton, G., and Williams, R. 1986. Learning representations by back-propagating errors. *Nature (London)*, **323**, 533–536.

Schraudolph, N., and Sejnowski, T. 1991. Competitive anti-hebbian learning of invariants. *NIPS4*, 1017–1024.

Sejnowski, T. 1977. Storing covariance with nonlinearly interacting neurons. *J. Math. Biol.* **4**(4), 303–321.

Stone, J. V. 1992. The optimal elastic net: Finding solutions to the travelling salesman problem. *Proc. Int. Conf. Artif. Neural Networks*, 170–174.

Stone, J. V. 1995. Learning spatio-temporal invariances. In *Neural Computation and Psychology Proceedings*, L. S. Smith and P. J. B. Hancock, eds., pp. 75–85. Springer-Verlag, Berlin.

Stone, J. V., and Bray, A. 1995. A learning rule for extracting spatio-temporal invariances. *Network*, **6**(3), 1–8.

Stone, J. V., and Isard, S. 1995. Adaptive scale filtering: A general method for obtaining shape from texture. *IEEE PAMI*, **17**(7), 713–718.

Sutton, R. 1988. Learning to predict by the methods of temporal differences. *Machine Learn.* **3**, 9–44.

Westheimer, G. 1994. The ferrier lecture, 1992. Seeing depth with two eyes: Stereopsis. *Proc. Royal Soc. London B*, **257**, 205–214.

Williams, P. 1991. A Marquardt algorithm for choosing the step-size in backpropagation learning with conjugate gradients. Cognitive science research paper CSRP 229, University of Sussex.

Zemel, R., and Hinton, G. 1991. *Discovering Viewpoint Invariant Relationships That Characterize Objects*. Tech. Rep., Department of Computer Science, University of Toronto, Toronto.

7

What Is the Goal of Sensory Coding?

David J. Field
Department of Psychology, Cornell University, Ithaca, NY 14850 USA

A number of recent attempts have been made to describe early sensory coding in terms of a general information processing strategy. In this paper, two strategies are contrasted. Both strategies take advantage of the redundancy in the environment to produce more effective representations. The first is described as a "compact" coding scheme. A compact code performs a transform that allows the input to be represented with a reduced number of vectors (cells) with minimal RMS error. This approach has recently become popular in the neural network literature and is related to a process called Principal Components Analysis (PCA). A number of recent papers have suggested that the optimal "compact" code for representing natural scenes will have units with receptive field profiles much like those found in the retina and primary visual cortex. However, in this paper, it is proposed that compact coding schemes are insufficient to account for the receptive field properties of cells in the mammalian visual pathway. In contrast, it is proposed that the visual system is near to optimal in representing natural scenes only if optimality is defined in terms of "sparse distributed" coding. In a sparse distributed code, all cells in the code have an equal response probability across the class of images but have a low response probability for any single image. In such a code, the dimensionality is not reduced. Rather, the redundancy of the input is transformed into the redundancy of the firing pattern of cells. It is proposed that the signature for a sparse code is found in the fourth moment of the response distribution (i.e., the kurtosis). In measurements with 55 calibrated natural scenes, the kurtosis was found to peak when the bandwidths of the visual code matched those of cells in the mammalian visual cortex. Codes resembling "wavelet transforms" are proposed to be effective because the response histograms of such codes are sparse (i.e., show high kurtosis) when presented with natural scenes. It is proposed that the structure of the image that allows sparse coding is found in the phase spectrum of the image. It is suggested that natural scenes, to a first approximation, can be considered as a sum of self-similar local functions (the inverse of a wavelet). Possible reasons for why sensory systems would evolve toward sparse coding are presented.

1 Introduction

Although we know a great deal about how sensory systems code information, there remains considerable debate regarding the goal of this coding. In many studies, there is an implicit assumption that there is no single goal. It is assumed that sensory systems solve a wide range of tasks important to the animal and since the range of tasks varies widely, one would not expect to see any common "theme" across the different coding strategies. A second approach, which serves as the basis for the ideas presented in this paper, proposes that it is possible to describe sensory coding in terms of a general information processing strategy. By this tradition, it is presumed that redundancy in different sensory environments can be represented within a single framework and that the goal of sensory coding is to transform the redundancy to provide some advantage to later stages of processing. In this paper, two information processing strategies are contrasted. Both of these approaches take advantage of the redundancy in the input to produce more effective representations of the environment. However, the two approaches achieve different goals and depend on different forms of redundancy.

The first of these, which will be described as "compact coding," has gained considerable attention in the neural network literature and serves as the basis of much of the work in image compression. This approach suggests that the principal goal of visual coding is to reduce the redundancy of the visual representation. Many of these ideas can be traced backed to Barlow's theories of redundancy reduction (e.g., Barlow 1961). Recently, a number of studies have proposed that spatial coding by the mammalian visual system is well described by codes that make use of the correlations to reduce the redundancy of the sensory representation (e.g., Atick and Redlich 1990, 1992; Atick 1992; Barlow and Foldiak 1989; Daugman 1988, 1991; Linsker 1988; Foldiak 1990; Sanger 1989).

This approach to coding is illustrated in Figure 1A. In a compact code, the goal is to represent all the likely inputs with a relatively small number of vectors (e.g., cells) with minimal loss in the description of the input. In such a code, the dimensionality of the representation is reduced, resulting in a code where only a subset of the possible inputs can be accurately represented. The code is effective when this subset is capable of representing the probable inputs to the code. In the next section, we will see how this approach reduces redundancy.

The second approach suggests that the principal goal of sensory coding is to produce a sparse-distributed representation of the sensory input. This approach has been specifically proposed with respect to visual code and the representations of natural scenes (Field 1987, 1989, 1993; Zetzsche 1990). However, several authors have noted that codes that produce sparse outputs may provide several advantages for representing sensory information (e.g., Barlow 1972, 1985; Palm 1980; Baum et al. 1988). Unfortunately, in much of this work, the distinction between sparse and

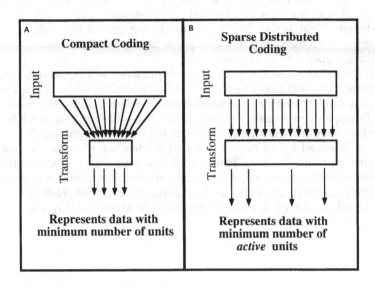

Figure 1: Two methods of taking advantage of redundancy in a sensory environment. In the compact coding approach (A), the code transforms the vector space to allow the data to be represented by a smaller number of vectors with only minimal loss in the representation (i.e., dimensionality is reduced). In a sparse coding scheme (B), the code transforms the vector space to allow the input to be represented with a minimum number of active cells. In a sparse coding scheme, the dimensionality is not reduced. Rather, the redundancy in the input is transformed into the redundancy in the firing rate of the cells (i.e., the response histogram) to produce a code where the response probability for any particular cell is relatively low.

compact codes has not been clear. Therefore, in this paper, much of the discussion will be devoted to the differences and requirements for each type of coding.

In a sparse-distributed code, the dimensionality of the representation is maintained (the number of cells remains roughly constant and may even increase). However, the number of cells responding to any particular instance of the input is minimized. Over the population of likely inputs, every cell has the same probability of producing a response (i.e., distributed) but that probability is low for any given cell (i.e., sparse). In sparse-distributed coding, the goal is to obtain a code where only a few cells respond to any given input. However, across the population of images the information is distributed across all of the cells. As we will see in the next section, this coding scheme does not reduce redundancy.

Rather, high-order redundancy is transformed into redundancy of the firing patterns of the cells (i.e., the response histograms) as was proposed previously (Field 1987). By this approach, the goal of the coding is to maximize the redundancy of the response histograms by minimizing the statistical dependencies between units.

In the following sections, these two approaches will be analyzed and contrasted. We will begin by looking at the type of redundancy required for producing a compact code and discuss the relations between this code and Principal Components Analysis (PCA). We will then look at the type of redundancy and the type of transform required for a sparse code. This will be followed by an experiment that models the response of visual neurons to natural scenes. Throughout this paper, we will concentrate on the response properties of cells in the mammalian visual system and the statistical relations found in the natural environment. However, the general ideas can be applied to any sensory system and any sensory environment.

2 State Space

One effective method for describing redundancy in a data set is to consider the "state space" of possible inputs. The state space (sometimes called vector space or phase space) describes the space of all possible states. This approach provides a useful means of showing how different coding schemes take advantage of the various forms of redundancy present in a population of inputs. Although the notion of state space has proved popular in descriptions of chaotic interactions and learning in neural networks (e.g., Churchland and Sejnowski 1992 for an introduction), it is not widely discussed in theories of visual coding.

To describe the state space of an image set, one can use the pixel amplitudes to represent the coordinate axes of the space. For any n-pixel image, one requires an n-dimensional space to represent the set of all possible images. Every possible image (e.g., a particular face, tree, etc.) is represented in terms of its unique location in the space. For example, white noise patterns (i.e., patterns with random pixel intensities) represent random locations in that n-dimensional space. Therefore, if we let the space become filled with examples of such white noise patterns, then all regions of the space would be filled equally—that is, the probability density will be uniform throughout the state space.

However, most naturally occurring phenomena are not random. Any redundancy that occurs in a data population implies that the population does not fill the state space uniformly. Natural scenes, for example, are statistically very different from white noise patterns and we would therefore not expect the state space of natural scenes to have the same probability density. Consider the case of a 256×256 pixel image. The state space of all possible images at this resolution requires a 65,536-

dimensional space where the amplitudes of each of the pixels represent the axes of the space. As one can imagine, the probability of seeing something resembling a natural scene when presented with white noise patterns is extremely low. This implies that in the state space of all possible 256×256 images, natural scenes occupy an extremely small area of the space.

To develop an understanding of the functional properties of the mammalian visual system, a number of recent studies have proposed that one must understand the statistical regularity of the mammalian visual environment and its relation to the visual code (e.g., Field 1987, 1989, 1993; Atick and Redlich 1990, 1992; Bialek *et al.* 1991; Eckert and Buchsbaum 1993; Hancock *et al.* 1992; van Hateren 1992; Kersten 1987). In terms of the state space, every statistical regularity that one finds in the visual environment provides a clue about the location and shape describing the probability density of natural scenes within the state space. Our visual environment is highly structured. The physics of how objects and surfaces reflect light forces the probability density into highly constrained forms. We will see that much of the debate about the goal of visual coding depends on the particular shape that is produced with data from the sensory system's typical environment. It will be argued that the state space describing the probability density of natural scenes is highly predictable but does not have the shape that is widely presumed.

Similarly, the spatial response properties of a cell (e.g., the receptive field) can also be described in terms of locations in the state space that will produce a response. For example, a cell with a linear response can be represented by a vector extending from the origin of the state space in a direction that depends uniquely on the particular receptive field profile. Every distinguishable receptive field profile is represented in terms of a unique direction in the state space. Thus, an array of cells can be considered as an array of vectors each pointing to unique locations in the state space.

If the local amplitudes of a waveform (e.g., the pixels) represent the coordinate axes of the state space, then an ortho-normal transform (e.g., a Fourier transform) can be represented by a rotation and/or translation of the coordinate axes.[1] This concept of treating a transform as a rotation of the coordinate axes will prove important in the discussions below. Ortho-normal transforms represent the special class of transforms where the vectors remain of normal length

$$|V_i| = 1$$

and the vectors remain orthogonal.

$$V_i \cdot V_j = 0$$

---

[1] Technically, an ortho-normal transform performs an "isometric" transform on the state space (i.e., it is form preserving).

It is unlikely that the visual system's transform is either completely orthogonal or normal, but this will not affect the main points of the discussion presented in this paper. To a first approximation, a sensory code can be thought of as rotation of the coordinate axes of the state space. The response properties of any particular cell (e.g., the receptive field) describe the direction of the vector in the state space. The collection of cells mapping out the visual field forms an array of vectors mapping out the state space.

To understand the goal of sensory coding, it is proposed that one must determine the relation between the directions of the vectors (i.e., the response properties of the cells) and the "state space" of typical inputs for that sensory system. Throughout this paper, terms such as "the form of the state space" or "the state space of input" will be used. This represents a shorthand for "the regions within the state space where images have a relatively high probability." The state space always represents the space of all possible images. However, "state space of natural scenes" will refer to the region within this space that describes where natural scenes are likely to fall.

This study will investigate the relation between the spatial response properties of some of the cells in the visual pathway (e.g., the vectors described by the receptive field profiles) and the state space populated by natural scenes. The redundancy in the environment can take several forms. In the next sections, two forms of redundancy will be considered and we will explore two types of transform that can take advantage of this redundancy.

2.1 Correlations in State-Space. Let us consider a very simple example where a data set consists of only two independent variables (e.g., the intensities of two neighboring pixels). Figure 2 shows an example of the state space of a collection of two pixel images where the horizontal

---

Figure 2: *Facing page.* (a) An example of a two-dimensional state space. In this example, we have assumed that the axes represent the intensities of two pixels. The ellipse represents a population of probable inputs showing that Pixel A and Pixel B are highly correlated. However, in this example, there is little redundancy in the response histograms of the two pixels. Each shows a gaussian distribution with a relatively large variance. The histogram of activity for the two pixels is found by projecting the state space onto the two axes. (b) The transform where the new basis functions are represented by a rotation of the coordinate axes. In this new coordinate system, most of the variance in the data can be represented with only a single coefficient (A'). Removing B' from the code produces only minimal loss. This rotation of the coordinate system to allow the vectors to be aligned with the principal axes of the data is what is achieved with the process called Principal Component Analysis (PCA).

axis represents the intensity of Pixel A and the vertical axis represents the intensity of Pixel B. Any two-pixel image is represented as a unique point in the two-dimensional state space.

Figure 2a provides an example of one form of redundancy. In this case, the population of images produces a correlation in the outputs of the two pixels. Although the pixels are correlated, each pixel is contributing equal information about the image. In this case, it has been assumed that

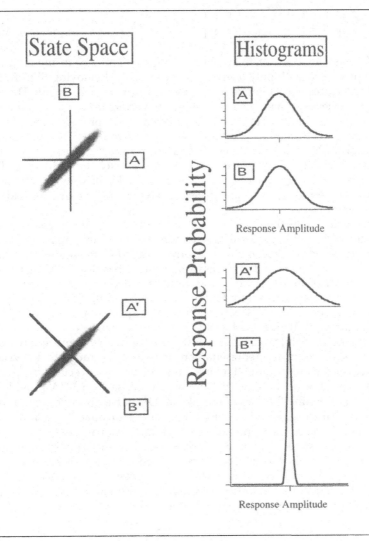

the response behavior is normally distributed about the two axes. The histogram of activity (i.e., the probability distribution function) for the two pixels is found by projecting the state space onto the two axes. In this case, the activity of each pixel is normally distributed and the two have equal variance.

It is possible to transform the coordinate system to take advantage of the redundancy. Figure 2b shows the transform where the new basis functions are represented by a simple rotation of the coordinate axes where $A' = A + B$ and $B' = A - B$. To keep the basis vectors of normal length, the transform is

$$\begin{bmatrix} A' \\ B' \end{bmatrix} = \begin{bmatrix} \frac{1}{\sqrt{2}} & -\frac{1}{\sqrt{2}} \\ \frac{1}{\sqrt{2}} & \frac{1}{\sqrt{2}} \end{bmatrix} \begin{bmatrix} A \\ B \end{bmatrix} \tag{2.1}$$

In this new coordinate system, most of the variance in the data can be represented with only a single coefficient (A'). Removing B' from the code produces only minimal loss in the description of the input. This rotation of the coordinate system to allow the vectors to be aligned with the principal axes of the data is what is achieved with a process called Principal Component Analysis (PCA)—sometimes called the Karhounen–Loeve transform. Principal component analysis computes the eigenvalues of the covariance matrix (e.g., the covariance of the pixels in an image). The corresponding eigenvectors represent a hierarchy of orthogonal coefficients where the highest valued vectors account for the greatest part of the covariance.

By using only these highest valued vectors, the state space can be represented with a subset of the vectors and only minimal loss in the representation as measured in RMS error. As shown in Figure 2, the variance in A' has increased and the variance in B' has decreased markedly. Now, most of the variance of the input is coded in A'. In general, by removing those vectors with low variance, we end up with a state space that is "more packed." Thus, the new state space has less redundancy. Redundancy reduction is achieved by removing regions of the state space where the probability density is low. One can either remove low variance vectors from the representation or reduce the range that a vector can cover (i.e., reduce the dynamic range of the basis vector).

If we think of the data as forming an ellipse then PCA provides a method of finding the axes of the ellipse. Of course, this two-point transform is a rather restricted example. If one hopes to model the redundancy of natural scenes then one needs a high-dimensional space to describe the possible states. An n-pixel image requires an n-dimensional state space. Although the different forms of redundancy can become quite complex, it is not necessarily difficult to describe. It is possible to generalize the ellipse shown in Figure 3 to high dimensions where the region of high-probability images (i.e., high density) is described by

$$ax_0^2 + bx_1^2 + cx_2^2 + dx_3^2 + ex_4^2 + \cdots <= k \tag{2.2}$$

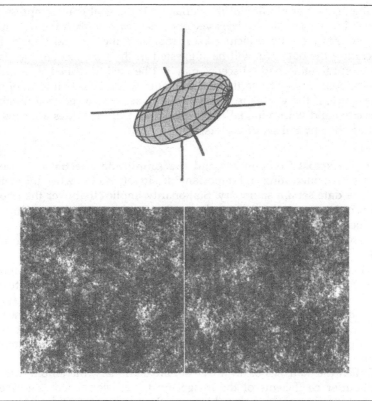

Figure 3: Ellipse and two filtered images. Examples of two images created by multiplying the spectrum of white noise (flat spectrum) by $1/f$. With images like this, all the redundancy is captured in the Fourier amplitude spectrum. The state space of images created in this fashion form a high-dimensional ellipse as described in equation 2.2. The axes of the ellipse are aligned with the vectors in the Fourier transform. Thus, the "principal components" and the vectors of Fourier transform are equivalent.

where

$$a \geq b \geq c \geq d \geq e \cdots$$

and $x_1, x_2, x_3 \ldots$ represent the axes of the ellipsoid. Whatever direction the axes are pointing, PCA can use the correlations in the data to find the directions of these axes and produce the vectors that correspond to the axes of the ellipsoid. The advantage of these particular vectors is that they provide a means of compressing image data with minimal RMS error. Just as the axes of the ellipse are ordered in equation 2.2, the eigenvectors are ordered in a sequence where the first few vectors account for the highest proportion of the variance. If the goal is to compress an n-pixel image set using only m vectors where $m < n$, then the principal components (i.e., the principal axes) represent the optimal vectors for describing the data. As will be suggested in the next section, the state space representing natural scenes may not be well described by a high-dimensional ellipse. Nevertheless, no matter what the actual form of the state space, if the goal is to transmit a data set with a reduced number of vectors and with minimal RMS error, then PCA provides a means of finding the optimal set of vectors.[2]

2.2 Principal Components and the Amplitude Spectra of Natural Scenes. An interesting and important idea involves PCA when the statistics of a data set are stationary. Stationarity implies that over the population of images in the data set (e.g., all natural scenes), the statistics at one location are no different than at any other location.

Across all images $P(x_i \mid x_{i+1}, x_{i+2}, \ldots) = P(x_j \mid x_{j+1}, x_{j+2}, \ldots)$ for all i and j.

This is a fairly reasonable assumption with natural scenes since it implies that there are no "special" locations in an image where the statistics tend to be different (e.g., the camera does not have a preferred direction). It should be noted that stationarity is not a description of the presence or lack of local features in an image. Rather, stationarity implies that over the population, all features have the same probability of occurring in one location versus another.

When the statistics of an image set are stationary, the amplitudes of the Fourier coefficients of the image must be uncorrelated (e.g., Field 1989). Indeed, any two filters that are orthogonal over translation:

$$g(x) \cdot h(x - x_0) = 0 \qquad \text{for all } x_0$$

will have uncorrelated outputs in the presence of data with stationary statistics (Field 1993). Since this holds for the Fourier coefficients, the amplitudes of the Fourier coefficients will be uncorrelated.

This means that when the statistics of a data set are stationary then all the redundancy reflected in the correlations between pixels is captured by the amplitude spectra of the data. This should not be surprising since the Fourier transform of the autocorrelation function is equal to the power spectrum. Therefore, with stationary statistics, the amplitude spectrum describes the principal axes (i.e., the principal components) of the data in the state space (Pratt 1978). With stationary data, the phase spectra of the data are irrelevant to the directions of the principal axes.

As noted previously (Field 1987), an image that is scale invariant will have a well-ordered amplitude spectrum. For a two-dimensional image,

---

[2]It should be noted that PCA finds only the optimal linear solution. It is always possible that for a given data set there exists a nonlinear transform that will provide better compression than the vectors provided by PCA.

the amplitudes will fall inversely with frequency (i.e., a $1/f$ spectrum). Natural scenes have been shown to have spectra that fall as roughly $1/f$ (Burton and Moorhead 1987; Field 1987, 1993; Tolhurst *et al.* 1992). If we accept that the statistics of natural images are stationary, then the $1/f$ amplitude spectrum provides a complete description of the correlations in natural scenes. The amplitude spectrum certainly does not provide a complete description of the redundancy in natural scenes, but it does describe the relative amplitudes of the principal axes.

We can ask what an image would look like if all the redundancy in the image set was described by a $1/f$ amplitude spectrum. Or in terms of the state space, we can ask what images would look like if the probability density was described by a high-dimensional ellipsoid where the principal axes of the ellipsoid are the Fourier transform. Figure 3 shows examples of two such images. They are created by multiplying the spectrum of white noise (flat spectrum) by $1/f$. Although these images have amplitude spectra similar to natural scenes (and therefore the same principal components), they clearly do not look like real scenes. They do not contain any of the local structure like edges and lines found in the natural environment. As proposed in the next section, images that have such local structure are not described well by a high-dimensional ellipsoid.

A number of recent studies have discussed the similarities between the principal components of natural scenes and the receptive fields of cells in the visual pathway (Bossomaier and Snyder 1986; Atick and Redlich ,1990, 1992; Atick 1992; Hancock *et al.* 1992; Baddeley and Hancock 1991; MacKay and Miller 1990; Derrico and Buchsbaum 1991). And there have been a number of studies that have shown that under the right constraints, units in competitive networks can develop large oriented receptive fields (e.g., Lehky and Sejnowski 1990; Linsker 1988; Sanger 1989). Indeed, it has been noted that networks like Linsker's work off the induced correlations caused by the overlapping receptive fields in the network and the network produces results similar to the principal components (MacKay and Miller 1990). And it has been noted that Hebbian learning can, under the right conditions, find the principal components (Oja 1982; Foldiak 1989; Sanger 1989).

This appears to pose a dilemma. If the principal components of images with stationary statistics are equivalent to the Fourier transform, shouldn't the derived receptive field profiles of the appropriate Hebbian network look like the Fourier transform if presented with natural scenes? Not necessarily. The two-dimensional Fourier transform of natural scenes shows considerable symmetry. The amplitude spectra of natural scenes fall as approximately $1/f$ at all orientations. Therefore, at any frequency there exists a range of orientations that are likely to have similar amplitude. When a number of Fourier coefficients have the same amplitude, there will exist a wide range of linear combinations that will account for equal amounts of the covariance (i.e., the solution is degenerate). Therefore, linear combinations of these equivariant vectors will also account for equal amounts of the covariance.

Recently, Baddeley and Hancock (1991) and Hancock *et al.* (1992) calculated the principal components of a number of natural scenes directly. When gaussian windowed, the first few coefficients do show some resemblance to cortical receptive fields—but this is expected since a gaussian-windowed low-frequency sinusoid (the first Fourier coefficients with the greatest amplitude) will produce the popular "Gabor function" shown to provide good models of cortical receptive fields (e.g., Field and Tolhurst 1986). Past the first 3 or 4 Fourier coefficients, the receptive field profiles no longer look like cortical receptive field profiles. Instead, the profiles are substantially different from those found in the mammalian visual system.

Figure 4B shows an example of the two-dimensional amplitude spectrum of a natural scene. On average, a ring of frequencies around the origin will have the same amplitude. This produces degeneracy in the set of possible solutions. The principal components can consist of any linear combination of these frequencies. That is, an equivalent solution for the principal components may consist of an ortho-normal transformation of these vectors. Figure 4C shows four spatial frequencies that would be expected to account for equal amounts of the covariance in natural scenes. The four lower "receptive fields" represent a rotation of the other receptive fields. For a natural scene with a $1/f$ spectrum and stationary statistics, the vectors in either 4C or 4D will serve equally well as principal components. Thus, even if the statistics of the input are stationary, the Fourier transform is not necessarily the only solution.

It is important to recognize that if the statistics of the input are stationary then there is no reason for Principal Components Analysis to produce localized receptive fields. In Fourier terms, a function is localized because the phases of the different frequencies are aligned at the point where the function is localized. Cortical simple cells, for example, have been shown to have a high degree of phase alignment at the center of the receptive field (Field and Tolhurst 1986). The large low-frequency receptive fields may contain only a few spectral components. However, the small high-frequency receptive fields have relatively broad bandwidths and hence have a large number of spectral components, all aligned near the center of the receptive field. Randomizing the phases of a localized function will distribute the energy across the image. Since the covariance matrix does not capture the phases (if the statistics are stationary), Principal Components Analysis cannot produce localized receptive fields.

If the primary constraints of the code are to represent the input with reduced dimensionality, then the codes should not be capable of producing the small high-frequency orientation selective receptive fields. Atick

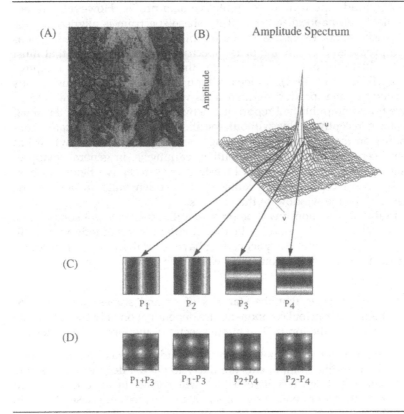

Figure 4: An example of a scene (A) and its two-dimensional amplitude spectrum (B). For a population of images scenes with stationary statistics, the amplitude spectrum describes the principal components. However, in the two-dimensional amplitude spectrum of natural scenes there is considerable symmetry with similar frequencies at different orientations likely to have the same amplitude (C). This means that appropriate combinations of the Fourier coefficients with equal amplitude will account for equal amounts of the covariance. (D) An example of a rotation of the Fourier vectors that should account for equal amounts of the covariance. With stationary statistics, the phase of the phase spectrum of the input is irrelevant to the principal components. Thus, Principal Components Analysis (PCA) cannot result in localized receptive fields without forcing constraints on the phase.

and Redlich (1990, 1992) have suggested that the spatial frequency tuning of retinal ganglion cells is well matched to the combination of amplitude spectra of natural scenes and high-frequency quantal limitations found in the natural environment. This is an important finding with regards to the amplitude spectrum of the receptive field profile. However, a receptive field will be localized only if its phase spectrum is aligned, so this approach cannot explain why the receptive fields are localized. It has been proposed that it is the phase spectrum of natural scenes that must be considered if one is to account for the localized nature of receptive fields (Field 1989, 1993). Indeed, although there are numerous reports of networks that produce hidden units with oriented receptive fields, I have found no published report of a network that can produce the small localized receptive fields without specifically forcing these locality constraints on the network (e.g., forcing a small gaussian window). It has even been suggested that competitive learning is, in general, inappropriate for producing the small high-frequency receptive fields (Webber 1991). The receptive field profiles of the hidden units are always the same size as the window of the network.

In the next section it will be proposed that the principal components of natural images do not describe the important forms of redundancy. To summarize, PCA and compact coding have several problems in accounting for receptive field profiles of cells in the retina and primary visual cortex.

1. If one accepts that the statistics of natural scenes are stationary, then the principal components are dependent on only the amplitude spectra of the input. The phase spectra of the inputs are irrelevant.

2. Because of the symmetry in the amplitude spectra of natural scenes, the principal components are likely to have a degenerate solution. The resulting "receptive fields" will consist of an unconstrained collection of orientation components with random phase. This will be most apparent at higher frequencies where there exists a wide range of orientation components at each frequency.

3. A function is localized only when the phases of the Fourier coefficients are aligned. Thus, when the statistics are stationary, the Principal Components Analysis will not produce localized receptive fields because the phase spectrum is not constrained.

4. Since the principal components are not dependent on the phase spectra of the input, the principal components will not reflect the presence of local structure in the data.

In the next section, it will be proposed that the shape of the state space describing natural scenes is not elliptical and this nonelliptical state space provides a clue as to why the mammalian visual system represents spatial data as it does. To account for receptive field profiles in primary visual cortex, we consider a different theory regarding the goal of visual coding and we consider a different form of redundancy found in natural scenes.

However, before discussing sparse coding techniques, it should be noted that the PCA represents an important technique for reducing the number of vectors describing the input—when it is possible. For example, in the color domain, it has been found that the first three principal components can account for much of the variance in the spectra of naturally occurring reflectances. This has led investigators to suggest that the three cone types found in primate vision provide an efficient description of our chromatic environment (e.g., Buchsbaum and Gottschalk 1983; Maloney 1986).

In general, the principal components can be used to determine which dimensions of the state space are needed to represent the data. If a reduced dimensionality is possible, the principal components will be able to tell you that. However, once the dimensions have been decided, it is proposed that other factors must be considered to determine the best choice of vectors to describe that space.

2.3 State Spaces That Allow Sparse Coding. Consider a two-pixel data set with redundancy like that shown in Figure 5. The data are redundant since the state space is not filled uniformly. However, this data set has some interesting properties. We can think of this data set as a collection of two types of images: one set with pixels that have high positive correlation and one set with high negative correlation.

For this data set, there will be no correlation between Pixel A and Pixel B. Furthermore, there is no "high-order" redundancy since there are only two vectors. This is an example of a type of second-order redundancy that is not captured by correlations. However, the same transformation performed as before (i.e., a rotation) produces a marked change in the histograms of the basis functions A' and B'. This particular data set allows a "sparse" response output. Although the variance of each basis function remains constant, the histogram describing the output of each basis function has changed considerably. After the transformation, vector A' is high or vector B' is high but they are never high at the same time. The histograms of each vector show a dramatic change. Relative to a normal distribution, there is a higher probability of no response and a higher probability of a high response, but a reduction in the probability of a mid-level response.

This change in shape can be represented in terms of the kurtosis of the distribution where the kurtosis is defined as the fourth moment according to

$$K = 1/n \sum [(x - x)^4/\sigma^4] - 3 \tag{2.3}$$

Figure 6 provides an example of distributions with various degrees of kurtosis. In a sparse code, any given input can be described by only a subset of cells, but that subset changes from input to input. Since only a small number of vectors describe any given image, any particular vector should have a high probability of no activity (when other vectors describe the image) and a higher probability of a large response (when the vector is part of the family of vectors describing the image). Thus, a sparse code

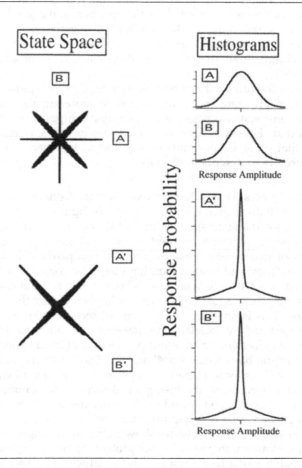

Figure 5: As in Figure 2, this shows an example of the state space of a population of two-pixel images. The data set are redundant since the state space is not filled uniformly. However, with these data, there are no correlations in the data and, therefore, there are no principal axes that can account for a major component of the variance. In such a data set, there is no way to take advantage of the redundancy by reducing the dimensionality. The right of the figure shows how the response distribution changes if the vector space is transformed to allow the vectors to be aligned with the axes of the data. In this case, each of the vectors maintains the same variance. However, the shape of the distribution is no longer gaussian (high entropy). Instead, the response distribution shows a high degree of kurtosis (lower entropy–higher redundancy).

Kurtosis

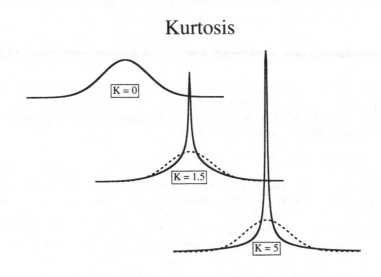

Figure 6: Examples of three levels of kurtosis. Each of the distributions has the same variance. A gaussian distribution has minimal redundancy (highest entropy) for a fixed variance. The higher the kurtosis, the higher the redundancy. With high kurtosis, there is a higher probability of a low response or a high response with a reduced probability of a mid-level response.

should have response distributions with high kurtosis. Although kurtosis appears to capture this property of a distribution with both high and low variances, one should not presume that kurtosis necessarily represents the optimal measure for defining a sparse code. At this time, we consider it a "useful measure." We will return to this point later.

As we move to higher dimensions (e.g., images with a larger number of pixels), we might consider the case where only one basis vector is active at a time (e.g., vector 1 or vector 2 or vector 3 ...):

$$ax_1 \cup ax_2 \cup ax_3 \cup ax_4 \ldots \tag{2.4}$$

In this case, each image can be described by a single vector and the number of images equals the number of vectors. However, this is a rather extreme case and is certainly an unreasonable description of most data sets, especially natural scenes.

When we go to higher dimensions, there exist a wide range of possible shapes that allow sparse coding. Overall, the shape must require a large set of vectors to describe entire population of possible inputs, but require a subset of vectors to describe any particular input.

$$\text{Image} = \sum_i^n aV_i \qquad \text{where } n < m \tag{2.5}$$

where m is the number of dimensions required to represent all images in the population (e.g., all natural scenes).

For example, with a three-pixel image where only two pixels are nonzero at a time, it is possible to have:

$$ax_1 + bx_2 \cup ax_2 + bx_3 \cup ax_1 + bx_3 \tag{2.6}$$

This state space consists of three orthogonal planes. If the data fall in these three planes with equal probability, then there will be no correlations in the data and therefore the principal components will not provide the axes of the planes (indeed, there are no *principal* axes of the state space). However, by choosing vectors aligned with the planes (e.g., x_1, x_2, x_3), it is possible to have a code in which only two vectors are nonzero for any input. In some situations, the principal components may even point in the wrong direction for achieving a sparse code. Figure 7A shows an example where the data fall along slightly nonorthogonal lines. In this case, there is a positive correlation in pixels. As with the ellipse shown in 7B, the principal components lie along the diagonals rather than the axes of the data. However, selecting vectors aligned with the data can produce histograms with positive kurtosis even though these are nonorthogonal. Indeed, it is important to recognize that the optimal sparse representation of a data set is not necessarily an ortho-normal representation.

Figure 7C shows a three-dimensional variation that has some interesting properties. If the state space forms a hollow three-dimensional cone like that shown, the first principal component will fall along the major axis of the cone. Indeed, Figure 7D shows an ellipsoid with the same principal axes as 7C. However, in the case of the ellipsoid, all the redundancy is captured by the principal components (i.e., the principal axes define the ellipse). In the case of the cone, the principal components fail to exploit some of the most interesting aspects of the data.

The reason for using the cone as an analogy is that the vectors along the tangents of the cone extending from the origin can allow a sparse representation but the probability distribution is locally continuous. Also, we have found that the cone provides a reasonable description of how a localized function (e.g., a gaussian blob) will be distributed within the state space when the feature is varied in position and amplitude. However, a three-dimensional state space cannot begin to describe the full complexity of the redundancy in natural scenes, so the cone should be considered as only a crude example. The precise form within the state space is not critical to the argument. For a sparse code to be possible, a

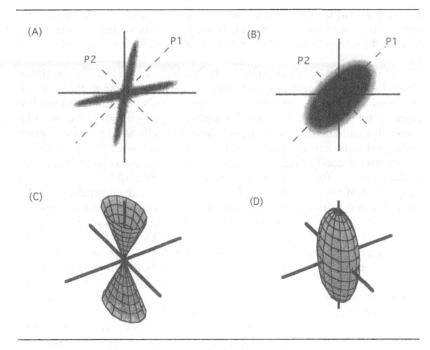

Figure 7: (A) An example of a data distribution where the principal components lie along the diagonal but where such components are ineffective at producing a sparse code. (B) A data set with the same principal components (an ellipse). (C, D) Two three-dimensional examples of state spaces that have the same principal components. State spaces like that shown in A and C allow sparse coding. State spaces like B and D do not. It is suggested that the local structure available in natural scenes produces a high-dimensional state space analogous to this cone rather than the ellipse.

large set of vectors must be required to describe all points on the form (all possible images) but the form must require only a subset of vectors to describe any particular point in the space (any particular image)—equation 2.5.

There will always exist a wide range of shapes of the probability density function that can result in the same principal components. The possibility of finding a sparse code depends on this shape. For an ellipsoid, it is not possible to produce a sparse output. In this paper, it is proposed that the signature of a sparse code is found in the kurtosis of the response distribution. A high kurtosis signifies that a large proportion of the cells is inactive (low variance) with a small proportion of the cells describing the contents of the image (high variance). However, an effective sparse code is not determined solely by the data or solely by the vectors but by the relation between the data and the vectors. In the next section we take a closer look at the vectors described by the receptive field profiles of two types of visual cells and look at their relation to natural scenes.

Before we begin this description, it should be noted that the results of several studies suggest that cells with properties similar to those in the mammalian visual cortex will show high kurtosis in response to natural scenes. In Field (1987), visual codes with a range of different bandwidths were studied to determine how populations of cells would respond when presented with natural scenes. It was found that when the parameters of the visual code matched the properties of simple cells in the mammalian visual cortex, a small proportion of cells could describe a high proportion of the variance in a given image. When the parameters of the code differed from those of the mammalian visual system, the response histograms for any given image were more equally distributed. The published response histograms by both Zetzsche (1990) and Daugman (1988) also suggest that codes based on the properties of the mammalian visual system will show positive kurtosis in response to natural scenes. Burt and Adelson (1983) noted that the histograms of their "Laplacian pyramids" showed a concentration near zero when presented with their images and suggested that this property could be used for an efficient coding strategy. In this paper, it is emphasized that these histograms have these shapes because of the particular relation between the code and the properties of the images. In particular, when the input has stationary statistics, it is the phase spectrum that describes the redundancy required for sparse coding.

In previous work by the author (Field 1993) complex correlations in natural scenes were studied to determine the extent to which the phases were aligned across the different frequency bands. The extent of the phase alignment across neighboring frequency bands was found to be proportional to frequency (i.e., at high frequencies, the phases were aligned across a broader range of frequencies). In other words, at low frequencies, local structure tends to be spatially extended while at high frequencies the local structure tends to be more spatially limited. It was noted that this particular alignment in phases would be expected if these scenes were scale invariant with regards to both their amplitude spectra and their phase spectra. It was proposed that, to a first approximation, natural scenes should be considered as a sum of bandlimited, self-similar "phase structures" (points of phase alignment). The spectral extent of this phase alignment was found to be well matched to the bandwidths of cortical simple/complex cells (Field 1989, 1993) and it was suggested this property is what allowed the visual system to produce a sparse output. We will return to this discussion when we consider synthetic images that produce high kurtosis in wavelet transforms. First, however, this study considers a more direct test of sparse coding by looking at the kurtosis of the response distributions of two types of visual cells when presented with natural scenes.

3 Receptive Fields in the Mammalian Visual Pathway as Vectors ____

Just as it is possible to rotate the coordinate axes in a wide variety of ways, there exist a wide range of transforms that are capable of representing the information in an n-dimensional data space. The Fourier transform represents one example of a rotation. Gabor (1946) described a family of transforms that were capable of representing one-dimensional waveforms. These ideas were extended by Kulikowski *et al.* (1982) to include transforms in which the bandwidths increase proportionally to frequency. Such transforms, which have recently become known as "wavelet transforms" (e.g., Mallatt 1989), consist of arrays of self-similar basis functions that differ only by translations, dilations, and rotations of a single function. Although much of the work on wavelet transforms has been devoted to the development of ortho-normal bases (e.g., Adelson *et al.* 1987; Daubechies 1988) the coding with these transforms has found a wide variety of applications (e.g., Farge *et al.* 1993) from image processing to the representation of turbulence. For our purposes, however, it is important to recognize that such transforms can be considered as rotations of the coordinate system.

Figure 8 shows one part of a two-dimensional implementation of a wavelet transform. Wavelets based on the gaussian modulated sinusoid (i.e., Gabor functions) have proved to be popular models of the visual cortex (Watson 1983; Daugman 1985; Field 1987). Although the Gabor function has found some support in the physiology (Webster and DeValois 1985; Field and Tolhurst 1986; Jones and Palmer 1987), other functions have been proposed such as the Cauchy (Klein and Levi 1985) and the log-Gabor used in this study (Field 1987). Transforms based on these functions capture some of the basic properties of cells in the mammalian visual cortex. (1) The receptive fields are localized in space and are band-pass in frequency but overlap in both space and frequency. (2) The spatial frequency bandwidths are constant when measured on logarithmic axes (in octaves) resulting in a set of self-similar receptive fields. (3) They are orientation selective. These basic properties provide the basis for a number of models of visual coding and the model used in this study does not have any major components that differ from previous models (e.g., Watson 1983; Daugman 1985; Field 1987).

It is important to recognize that these transforms are not ortho-normal. First, the basis functions are not quite orthogonal. Second, in this study (as in Field 1987) the vector length of the transform increases with frequency (i.e., the peak of the spatial frequency response is constant and the bandwidth increases). As previously noted, this results in a code with distributed activity in the presence of images with $1/f$ spectra like that found in natural scenes (Field 1987; see Brady and Field 1993 for a discussion of vector length). This means that the variance of the filtered images will be roughly the same magnitude at the different frequencies.

It must also be emphasized that the functions used in this study to model visual neurons are highly idealized versions of actual cells. Both the models of retinal neurons and cortical simple cells involve codes in which all the cells have the same logarithmic bandwidth. Visual neurons are known to show a range of bandwidths which average around 1.5 octaves but become somewhat narrower at higher frequencies (e.g., Tolhurst and Thompson 1982; DeValois *et al.* 1982). However, the most important difference is that the "cells" in this study do not have many of the known nonlinearities found in cortical simple cells (e.g., end-stopping, cross-orientation inhibition, etc.). Indeed, the response histograms are allowed to go negative in our modeled cells while actual cortical cells can produce only the positive component of the histogram. We will return to this discussion of nonlinearities later. However, it should be remembered that the simple cells that are modeled are only rough approximations to the cells that are actually found in the visual cortex.

The codes in this study represent images with arrays of basis functions that are localized in the two-dimensional frequency plane as well as the two-dimensional image plane. Figure 8 shows one example of the division of the two-dimensional frequency plane and the corresponding

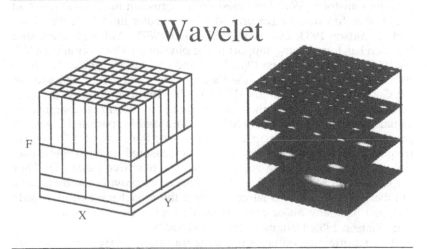

Wavelet

Figure 8: Two-dimensional wavelet. Three-dimensional information diagrams for a two-dimensional wavelet. The information diagrams are actually four-dimensional (u, v, x, y) but we have limited the diagram to the representation of a single orientation, to allow a graphic description.

representation in space for one orientation and one phase. Each basis function is thus localized in the four dimensions of x, y, u, v. In this particular description, the spatial sampling grid is rectangular, but this is not a requirement. One requires a four-dimensional plot to cover the full 2-D space by 2-D frequency trade-off, but this is difficult to depict graphically. If we consider only a single orientation for the purposes of the display, it is possible to show the space-frequency trade-off using the representations shown in the figure.

A comment should also be made with regards to the phase spectra of these filters. In line with previous studies (Field 1987, 1989, 1993), the oriented wavelet transform uses a pair of even- and odd-symmetric filters (i.e., filters in quadrature) at each location. Since these receptive fields are localized, they can be defined in Fourier terms by an alignment in the phase at the center of the receptive field (e.g., Field and Tolhurst 1986; Field 1993). Even complex cells have localized receptive fields, so to some extent, they must also be phase selective. One recent model of complex cells describes the response of a complex cell as a vector sum of two quadrature-phase cortical cells (Field 1987; Morrone and Burr 1988). By this model, complex cells detect an alignment of phases at particular locations of the visual field but the response does not depend on the absolute phase of that alignment (e.g., sine versus cosine). However, in this study the intention is not to model all of the various forms of nonlinearity found in the mammalian visual system. Rather, the goal is to show that the basic properties of visual neurons (i.e., orientation tuning, spatial frequency tuning, and position selectivity) produce a sparse representation of natural scenes.

4 Kurtosis in the Response to Natural Scenes

In the previous sections, it was proposed that if the visual system is producing a sparse representation of the environment then the histograms describing the response of the visual system should have a high kurtosis. In this section, these two approaches will be contrasted by investigating the histograms of the cells in several visual codes.

4.1 Method.

Images. The images used in the following sections consist of digitized photographs of the natural environment. They consist of 55 scenes, six of which are shown in Figure 9. The only photographic restriction was that the images have no man-made features (buildings, signs, etc.) since these tend to have different statistical structures (e.g., a higher probability of long straight edges). Images were photographed with Ilford XP1 film using a 35-mm camera. Photographic negatives were scanned using a Barneyscan digitizer that provided a resolution of 512×512 pixels per

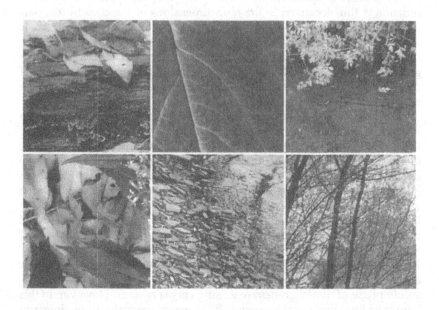

Figure 9: Examples of six images used in this study. Each of the images was calibrated for the intensity response of the film.

picture with 256 gray levels. The images were calibrated for luminance using Munsell swatches allowing the pixel values to have a linear relation to the image intensities in the original scene. The optics of the camera were taken into account by determining the response to thin lines and correcting for the changes produced in the amplitude spectrum (i.e., the modulation transfer function). Before analysis, the log of the image was determined and the calculations were based on this simple nonlinear transform of the image. This allows the units to respond in terms of contrast (i.e., ratios of intensities) rather than to intensity differences (i.e., amplitude) since:

$$\log(a) - \log(b) = \log(a/b) \qquad (4.1)$$

This is believed to produce a more accurate representation of cells in the visual pathway since cells are know to produce a more linear response to contrast (e.g., see Shapley and Lennie 1985) rather than amplitude. It was also found that the pixel histograms of some of the images had spuriously high kurtosis values (several images had $K > 20$ before the log transform) because of a few bright points in the image such as bright sky filtering through a tree. One should note film normally uses a compressive gamma, so studies that do not calibrate their film end up with similar high-intensity compression without intending to do so. Also, this collection of images did not contain large blank regions (e.g., an image of half sky). Such images result in a large number of inactive cells that will also increase the kurtosis for any code using local operators. These efforts were made to minimize any biases that might have been present in our image collection and allow a more accurate comparison of the different codes.

4.2 Population Activity. Population measures were based on the outputs of arrays of cells determined by convolving the images with the appropriate filters. The methodology is similar to that of Field (1987). However, in this study results are provided for a fixed number of spatial frequencies and orientations. Two types of filters are compared. The first is a center surround operator made from a difference of gaussians (DOG) where the surround has three times the width of the center.

$$g(x,y) = 9e^{-(x^2+y^2)/2(\sigma)^2} - e^{-(x^2+y^2)/2(3\sigma)^2} \qquad (4.2)$$

For the DOG calculations, each image was convolved with two filter sizes (the spectrum peaked at 20 and 40 cycles/picture). The second type is the oriented "log-Gabor" described previously (Field 1987). Radially the function has a log-normal spectrum:

$$G(k) = e^{-\ln(k/k_0)^2/2[\ln(\sigma/k_0)]^2} \qquad (4.3)$$

and is gaussian along the orthogonal axis.

As in Field (1987) the local phase was represented by a pair of filters in quadrature (i.e., even-symmetric and odd-symmetric). Thus, each image was convolved with filters at two spatial frequencies ($k_0 = 20$ and 40 cycles/picture), four orientations (10, 55, 100, and 145°), and two phases. For each bandwidth selected, this requires $2 \times 2 \times 4 = 16$ convolutions per image to obtain the total response histograms at the 8 spectral locations. Although these codes do not provide a complete representation of the image, the results provide a relatively direct method of comparing the population responses of different codes and eliminate problems of filters near the edges of the spectrum.

With the wavelet codes, different spatial frequency bandwidths are compared. With the orientation bandwidth set to 40° orientation tuning (full width at half height), the spatial frequency bandwidth was set to one of 8 spatial frequency bandwidths ranging from 0.5 to 8.0 octaves in logarithmic steps where the bandwidth is defined as

$$B_{oct} = \ln_2(k_2/k_1) \qquad (4.4)$$

where k_1 and k_2 define the lower and upper frequencies defining the width at half-height.

For each image and each bandwidth, the kurtosis of the distribution was determined by calculating the histogram of the pixels from the 16 filtered images. Near the edges of each of the filtered images, the response of any basis function can produce spurious results. To remove these effects, only the data from the central 180×180 region was used in the analysis. Thus for each image, the histograms were based on a total of $16 \times 180 \times 180 = 518,400$ samples for the wavelet and $2 \times 180 \times 180 = 97,200$ samples for the DOG. One should note that these samples are not completely independent samples since the images are not sampled in proportion to the size of the basis function as in Field (1987). However, this will have minimal effect on the overall histograms but implies that the low-frequency channel (e.g., at 20 cycles/picture) will have histograms based on fewer independent samples than the high-frequency channels with smaller receptive fields (e.g., 40 cycles/degree).

4.3 Results. Figure 10A shows the histogram for image 1 with a single condition (spatial frequency bandwidth: 1.4 octave–20° orientation bandwidths). With these filters, the response of any function is as likely to be positive as negative. One can see that the general form of the histogram is much like that shown in the kurtosis plots described previously. Indeed, this pattern has a kurtosis of 6.2. Figure 10B shows the results describing the kurtosis for the original image, the DOG function, and the wavelet when the bandwidth was fixed at 1.4 octaves. These results show that both the DOG function and the oriented wavelet show increased kurtosis. Figure 10C shows the results for 20 $1/f$ noise patterns like those shown in Figure 3. These images have random phase spectra but similar amplitude spectra to natural scenes (and therefore the same principal components).

Figure 11A shows the results describing the kurtosis of the response histograms for the wavelet as a function of the spatial frequency bandwidth. Results are shown for the six images shown in Figure 3. Figure 11B provides a histogram of the bandwidths that produce peak kurtosis for all 55 of our natural scenes. These results show that the bandwidth that produces the maximum kurtosis typically falls in the range of 1.0 to 3.0 octaves. This falls within the range of bandwidths that are most commonly found in the mammalian visual system (e.g., Tolhurst and Thompson 1982).

5 Discussion

The results shown above support the notion that codes that have similar properties to that found in the mammalian visual system are effective at producing a sparse representation of the natural scenes. The results in Figure 10 suggest that as one moves from the retina to the cortex, the kurtosis of the distribution increases. Higher levels appear to be more capable of taking advantage of the redundancy in natural scenes.

The redundancy that is captured by these codes is not due to the amplitude spectra of the images. Figure 10B shows that images with

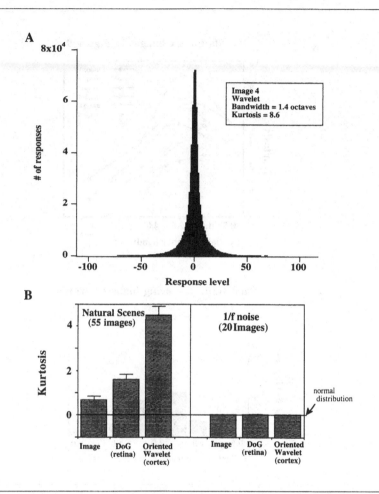

Figure 10: (A) The response histogram for a single image using the wavelet. The histogram is based on the response at four orientations at spatial frequencies of 20 and 40 cycles/picture and two phases (even- and odd-symmetric). (B) The mean kurtosis for the images calculated from the pixels of the original image, after convolution with the difference of gaussians and after convolution with the wavelet. The bottom right shows the same processes with 20 $1/f$ noise patterns that have approximately the same amplitude spectra as that in the natural scenes.

similar amplitude spectra as natural scenes but random phase spectra produce histograms with kurtosis values of 0.0 (normal distributions). Since these images differ only in their phase spectra, it is clear that the

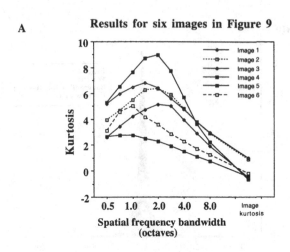

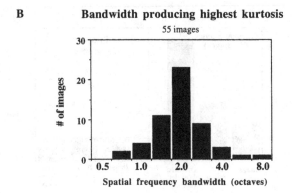

Figure 11: Distribution of peak kurtosis as a function of bandwidth. (A) The kurtosis of the response distributions for the six images shown in Figure 9 as a function of the spatial frequency bandwidth (orientation bandwidth is fixed at 40°). For each of the 55 images, the kurtosis of the response distribution was determined and the bandwidth that produced the highest kurtosis was calculated. (B) The distribution of spatial frequency bandwidths that produced the highest kurtosis.

phase spectra of natural scenes play a major role in determining whether the wavelet transform will produce a sparse output.

5.1 Synthetic Images That Produce High Kurtosis. In Field (1993), it was proposed that self-similar transforms are effective at producing sparse representations with natural scenes because such scenes have sparse, scale-invariant phase spectra. That is, the phases in such scenes are aligned at a relatively small number of locations in space/frequency and the spectral extent of the alignment is proportional to frequency. It is a relatively simple process to synthesize images that have such properties. Figure 12 provides examples of two such images. These particular images were created using the equation:

$$\sum_{m=0}^{a} \sum_{n=1}^{\beta\sigma^2 m} \omega_{nm} g[\tau\sigma^m x - x_{nm}, \tau\sigma^m y - y_{nm}] \tag{5.1}$$

where a is the number of scales in the image, β controls the density of the elements at each scale, σ controls the spectral distance between scales, and τ controls the relative spatial extent of the function at each scale. Figure 12A and B shows two densities where $g(x, y)$ is a gaussian modulated sinusoid. Each of the functions is added with the same average spatial amplitude independent of scale (ω_{nm} has the same average amplitude at all scales). If each function is treated as a vector, then the vector length of each function decreases as the scale increases (proportional to $1/f$). By increasing the number of vectors in proportion to the square of the frequency and adding them in random positions, this technique produces a scale-invariant $1/f$ amplitude spectrum but in which the phases are locally aligned (See Appendix).

Each of these images can be thought of as an "inversion" of the visual code. In a sparse-distributed code, only a subset of the cells is active but each cell has the same probability of activity. The method described in equation 5.1 is roughly equivalent to assigning a low probability to each vector in a wavelet code and summing the sparse set of vectors together. The state space of these images is analogous to the state space shown in Figure 4 but, of course, in higher dimensions. We are currently attempting to provide a better description of the high-dimensional state space and believe that a set of high-dimensional cones of different diameters is a useful analogy. A subset of vectors from the wavelet code can represent this image because it is created by a subset of vectors from the wavelet code. Although these images do not have all the redundancy of natural scenes, they provide a good first approximation and certainly provide a better approximation than the $1/f$ noise patterns shown in Figure 3.[3]

The results in Figure 10 suggest that although the DOG patterns show a significant increase in kurtosis, the oriented wavelet results in higher kurtosis. This suggests, that in natural scenes, when local structure is present (i.e., the phases are aligned), the structure tends to be oriented. This is not mathematically necessary. It is possible to create images

---

[3] As the density approaches 0.5, the images show the same structure as the $1/f$ noise patterns shown earlier in Figure 3.

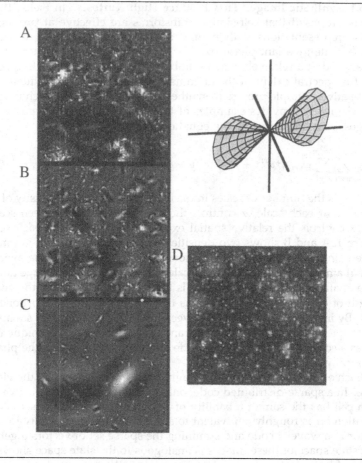

Figure 12: Images that produce high kurtosis can be created by "inverting" the visual code. The top images were created by distributing a set of self-similar functions as described in equation 5.1. The images were created by producing a random sum of the oriented wavelet basis functions. The two images shown were created by assigning a probability of either (A) 0.01, (B) 0.08, or (C) 0.3 to each of the members of the wavelet basis set (e.g., Fig. 8). The lower right image (D) was created using nonoriented difference of gaussians (DOG). It is proposed that images such as these provide a first approximation to the statistical structure of natural scenes. The state space is analogous to the cone (E) with the principal axes aligned with the Fourier vectors.

like that shown in Figure 12 using DOG functions instead of oriented wavelets. Under such circumstances, an oriented wavelet will not produce an increase in kurtosis over the DOG.

It is proposed that because natural scenes have regions where the phases are locally aligned (i.e., the images have local structure), both ganglion cell receptive fields and cortical receptive fields have the shape that they do. The amplitude spectra of natural scenes and the limits in quantal catch may certainly be important in understanding the spatial frequency tuning curves of ganglion cells and the contrast sensitivity function as suggested by Atick and Redlich (1991, 1992). However, it is proposed here that it is the phase spectrum of natural scenes that one must understand to account for the phase spectra of receptive fields in the visual pathway. Indeed, it is likely that many natural phenomena show this self-similar phase structure and may be why the wavelet transform has found so much success in applied mathematics.

5.2 Higher-Order Redundancy in Natural Scenes. Although the images in Figure 12 may provide a good first approximation to the statistics of the environment, these images certainly do not capture all the redundancy that is present in real scenes and do not look that much like real scenes. Consider the analogy of looking at the redundancy in musical symphonies. One might try to find the properties of the typical notes that are played. One might then try to create synthetic symphonies by playing those notes randomly. Although these sounds would be more like symphonies than random noise, they would not sound like symphonies because they would not contain any of the rules of music. Similarly, the images in Figure 12 are more like natural scenes than $1/f$ noise, but they do not contain any of the combinatorial rules found in real scenes.

As previously noted (Field 1993), natural scenes show a significant degree of continuity across space and frequency. Figure 13 shows a simple example of this continuity. A "fractal" edge is split into three frequency bands. Across the different frequency bands and across the length of the edge, the orientation of the edge twists and turns. Locally, the shift in orientation is continuous. The wavelet code does not directly take advantage of this continuity. However, it has recently been proposed (Field et al. 1993) that the visual system may make use of this redundancy by using connections between locally oriented units along the lines of the lateral connections found in the primary visual cortex (e.g., Rockland and Lund 1983; Blasdel et al. 1985; see Gilbert 1992 for a review). Computational studies by Zucker et al. (1989) suggest that such an approach may be an effective strategy in representing continuous features in natural scenes.

It should also be emphasized that the "cells" modeled in this study do not have the spatial nonlinearities that are often found in visual neurons. Such nonlinearities come in various forms. First, in primary visual cortex, "simple cells" do not represent the majority of cells. Both complex and hypercomplex cells certainly represent a major component to visual coding and show highly nonlinear behavior. However, the basic findings described here will at least apply to complex cells. The bandwidths and spatial extents of complex cells are similar to those of simple cells. As noted earlier, one model of complex cells suggests that they detect an

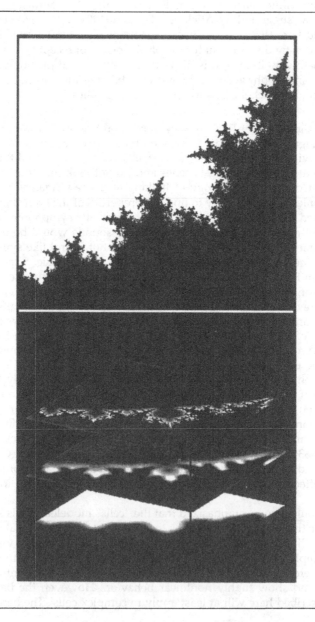

alignment of phases, like simple cells, but do not differentiate the absolute phase of that alignment. Since they are localized in space/frequency in a similar manner to simple cells, it would be expected that complex cells will show a similar sparse representation to the modeled simple cells studied here.

It should also be noted that even classically defined simple cells exhibit a number of important nonlinearities (e.g., end-stopping and cross-orientation inhibition). We currently believe that these nonlinearities may help to increase the "sparseness" of the code by allowing the code to play a local "winner take all" strategy. This is beyond the scope of this paper, but it should be mentioned that the kurtosis values shown in Figures 10 and 11 are likely to be significantly lower than the kurtosis values actually found in the mammalian visual cortex.

It is important to treat the results described in this study with some caution. We have not added the nonlinearities known to exist in the mammalian visual system and we have only searched through a small variety of linear transforms. There may well be linear transforms that produce higher kurtosis than the wavelets tested here and it is quite likely that there exist more effective nonlinear codes. Our main goal in this paper is to demonstrate that the bandpass, localized receptive fields found in the mammalian visual system can take advantage of the redundancy in the environment without compressing the representation (reducing redundancy) and without using the principal components.

5.3 Why Sparse Coding? In this paper, evidence was provided that codes that share properties with the mammalian visual system produce a sparse-distributed output to natural scenes. But the question remains as to why a sensory system would evolve a strategy like sparse coding. As was noted, there are a number of reasons that one might want to produce a compact code. A compact code allows the data to be stored and transmitted with a smaller population of total cells. But what are the advantages of sparse codes?

Under some conditions, it is possible to use the sparse output to produce a compressed image. Techniques such as run-length coding are designed to do just that. There is also a considerable literature on compression techniques with sparse matrices (e.g., Evans 1985; Schendel

---

Figure 13: *Facing page.* Unlike the scenes shown in Figure 12, natural scenes have structures that are continuous across space and frequency. The orientation of the edge shifts across the length of the edge as well as across the different scales. The edge has a well-defined orientation only at a given scale and position along the length of the edge. This oriented structure that is localized in space/frequency makes the wavelet code an effective representation. However, the continuity between scales and across the length of the edge at each scale represents a form of redundancy that is not directly captured by the wavelet and requires more complex processing.

1989). However, it is proposed here that sparse coding serves purposes other than compression. Barlow (1972, 1985) has proposed that codes that minimize the number of active neurons can be useful to the re- sentation and detection of "suspicious coincidences." Zetzsche (1990) has suggested that it is the work on associative memories that provides the most biologically plausible reasons that sensory systems would use sparse coding schemes.

Three interrelated advantages are described below.

Signal-to-Noise. First, a sparse coding scheme can increase the signal-to-noise ratio. As was noted in Field (1987), if most of the variance of a data set is represented by a small subset of cells, then that subset must have a high response relative to the cells that are not part of the subset. The smaller the subset, the higher the response of each member of the subset, given an image with constant variance. If we consider the response of the subset as "the signal" and if all the cells in the population are subject to additive noise, then by increasing the response of the subset of cells relative to the population, it is possible to increase the probability of detecting the correct subset of cells that represent the image. However, it should be emphasized that arguments of this form depend critically on the properties of the noise (e.g., correlated versus uncorrelated) and the location of the noise (e.g., photon versus neural transduction noise).

Correspondence and Feature Detection. Although signal-to-noise consid- erations may be important, it is proposed that the main reason for sparse coding is that it assists in the process of recognition and generalization. In an ideal sparse code, the activity of any particular basis function has a low probability. Because the response of each cell is relatively rare, tasks that require matching of features should be more successful. Con- sider the problem of identifying a corresponding structure (e.g., an edge) across two frames of a movie or across two images of a stereo-pair. If the probability of a cell's response has probability p and there are n com- parable cells of that type within some region of the visual field then, assuming independent probability of response, the probability of detect- ing the correct correspondence depends on the probability that only the corresponding cell responds, which is

$$P(\text{only corresponding cell responds}) = (1 - p)^n$$

The lower the probability p (i.e., the more sparse the code), the more likely a correct correspondence. As noted above, we would not expect cortical cells to be completely independent of their neighbors. Nonetheless, the general rule should still hold. As a code becomes more sparse, the proba- bility of detecting a correct correspondence increases. This suggests that a sparse code should be of assistance in tasks requiring solutions to a correspondence problem and can be related to what Barlow calls a sus- picious coincidence (e.g., Barlow 1989). If the probability that any cell responds is low ($p \ll 0.5$), then the probability of two cells responding is p^2 ($p \ll 0.25$) assuming response independence. Higher-order relations (pairwise, triad, etc.) become increasingly rare and therefore more informative when they are present in the stimulus.

This implies that the unique pattern of activity found with sparse codes may also be of assistance with the general problem of recognition. If relations among units are used to recognize a particular view of an object (e.g., a face), then with a sparse code, any particular high-order relation is relatively rare. In a compact code, a few cells have relatively high probability of response. Therefore, any particular high-order relation among this group is relatively common. Overall, in a compact code different objects are represented in terms of the differential firing of the same subset of cells. With a sparse-distributed code, a large population has a relatively low probability of response. Different objects are represented by a unique subset of cells. That is, different objects are represented by which cells are active rather than how much they are active.

The primary difficulty with this line of thinking is that implementing a process that detects sparse structure in neural architecture may not be so straightforward. Higher-order relations may be relatively rare in a sparse code, but detecting all possible nth-order relations among m cells requires m^n detectors. It is likely that the visual system looks only for "probable" relations by looking at combinations only within local regions and looking only for probable structure (e.g., continuity). This is certainly an interesting problem, but further study of the higher-order structure of natural scenes would be required to determine whether the visual system is using an effective strategy.

Storage and Retrieval with Associative Memory. The third advantage of sparse coding comes from work on networks with associative memories and is related to the above discussion. Several authors have noted that when the inputs to the networks are sparse, the networks can store more memories and provide more effective retrieval with partial information (Palm 1980; Baum *et al.* 1988). Baum *et al.* (1988) suggest that the advantages of sparsity for cell efficiency are "so great that it can be useful to artificially 'sparsify' data or responses which are not sparse to begin with." Indeed, it is not surprising that many types of networks will solve problems more efficiently if the inputs are first "sparsified." Since the sparse representation will have fewer higher-order relations, learning to classify or discriminate inputs should require less computation. Therefore, "sparsifying" the input should help to simplify many of the problems that the network is designed to face. This work with associative memory will hopefully lead to a better understanding of the advantages of sparse codes and help us to understand whether transforming the data to create a sparse input is generally a useful strategy to help networks solve problems.

In this study, there is no attempt to provide a complete description of the possible uses of sparse codes. Rather, the goal is to demonstrate that sparse coding represents one important method for taking advantage of redundancy and that sensory systems show evidence that they make use of this method.

5.4 Factorial Codes and Projection Pursuit. A gaussian distribution has the lowest redundancy (highest entropy) of any distribution given a fixed variance. Thus, a distribution with high kurtosis has a lower entropy than a gaussian distribution. The results shown in Figure 10 show that the visual code has relatively redundant first-order histograms. A sparse-distributed code converts high-order redundancy (relations between units) into first-order redundancy (the response distributions of the basis vectors). Therefore, a transform that produces highly redundant histograms has decreased the higher-order redundancy.

Is it possible to find a code that completely removes higher-order redundancy? In such a case, the responses of the vectors would be independent of one another. For example, if the responses of two vectors are independent then

$$P(V_i \cap V_j) = P(V_i) \cdot P(V_j)$$

and

$$P(V_i \mid V_j) = P(V_i)$$

and in general, if all the vectors are independent then the probability of any given image can be determined by multiplying the probabilities of each of the vectors.

$$P(\text{image}) = \prod P(V_i)$$

In this case, the image is described as having a "factorial code" (Barlow *et al.* 1989; Barlow 1987; Schmidhuber 1992; Atick *et al.* 1993).

A population of images like those shown in Figure 12 can have nearly factorial codes since these were actually generated by combining nearly orthogonal vectors with independent probabilities. That is, the probability that any function was added to the image did not depend on the probability that any other function was added to the image. The differences between the images in Figures 12 and 13 point out the importance of sources of redundancy that remain after coding by the wavelet. Indeed, the fact that the natural scenes do not look like the images in Figure 12 demonstrates that after natural scenes are coded by the wavelet, the responses of wavelet basis functions will not be independent. Thus the individual probabilities of units are unlikely to predict the probability of a particular natural scene. Whether one is searching for a sparse code or a factorial code, the goal is to find a set of units that are as independent from each other as possible. However, the sparse coding approach provides a guide for achieving this goal. By maximizing the kurtosis (i.e., the redundancy) of the response histograms, one effectively minimizes statistical dependencies between units (Field 1987).

In this paper, there has been no discussion of how one might find the optimal sparse code for a given data set. An effective sparse code must have two properties. It must span the space of inputs (i.e., preserve information) and show high kurtosis in the response histograms. At this time, there do not appear to be any learning rules that can achieve these goals. There is a problem related to this, described as "projection pursuit" (e.g., Friedman 1987; Huber 1985; Intrator 1992, 1993). In many domains, where one must deal with high-dimensional data, one is interested in finding interesting projections of the data. The "projections" refer to the response histograms of the vectors describing the data. Intrator (1992, 1993) has noted that one should look for projections (histograms) that are as far from gaussian as possible. Indeed, in line with the above discussion, the more non-gaussian the histogram, the more independent the units should be. High kurtosis represents just one way to deviate from a gaussian distribution. It is not clear whether natural scenes have redundancy that will allow other forms of non-gaussian behavior in the response histograms. It is also not clear that the visual system can take advantage of other forms of non-gaussian behavior. In this paper, it is noted only that the visual system appears to have found one type of non-gaussian distribution (high kurtosis) and this particular distribution results in a sparse representation.

However, at this time, there is no known technique for finding the optimal sparse code. Techniques such as those of Intrator (1992, 1993), Foldiak (1990), Schmidhuber (1992), and Linsker (1993) may ultimately provide insights into this problem, but their work demonstrates that the solution may not be a simple one.

6 Summary

In this paper, we have compared two approaches to sensory coding: compact and sparse-distributed coding. When the statistics of the inputs are stationary, it was noted that compact coding depends primarily on the amplitude spectra of the data (i.e., the correlations). When effective dimensionality reduction is possible, compact coding provides a good first step. Indeed, some aspects of sensory coding (e.g., trichromacy) require a consideration of the efficiency achieved by dimensionality reduction. However, many redundant data sets do not allow effective compression. Furthermore, even if compact coding is possible, there will be a variety of codes that will produce equal compression.

If the goal of a code is to assist higher level processing (e.g., recognition), then other coding strategies and other forms of redundancy must

be considered. To account for the primary receptive field properties of
cells found in the mammalian visual system (i.e., localized, bandpass,
self-similar), it was proposed that one must consider a sparse-distributed
representation of natural scenes. It was noted that when the statistics of
the data are stationary, sparse coding depends primarily on the phase
spectra of the data. In this paper, we have concentrated on the visual
system and the statistics of natural scenes. However, the main ideas
presented here can be applied to any sensory system. Natural sounds,
for example, are likely to have local structure similar to that found in
natural scenes. We are currently working on the question of whether the
sparse coding approach to natural sounds can provide an account of the
frequency selectivity found in auditory neurons.

It is proposed that the evidence for this selectivity will be found in the
kurtosis of the response distribution. If a sensory system is designed for
sparse coding, then we would expect cells in that sensory system to show
high kurtosis in the presence of the typical sensory environment. If the
general goal of sensory coding is to produce a sparse representation of
the environment, then we would expect that recording from any sensory
neuron in any animal will produce a histogram with high kurtosis—as
long as the recording is performed in an awake, behaving animal in its
natural environment. This is a general claim that is left for future work
to answer.

Appendix

An image consisting of the appropriate functions distributed across the
image in the appropriate manner will result in an image that is scale
invariant in both contrast and structure. As noted previously (Field 1987),
a two-dimensional image that is scale invariant in contrast will have an
amplitude spectrum that falls with frequency as $1/f$. In this appendix, it
is demonstrated that images that obey the rules described in equation 5.1
will be scale-invariant in their contrast (have $1/f$ amplitude spectra) and
also have a scale-invariant structure. Consider a simple function localized
in space and assigned a scale k. In equation 5.1, the scale $k = \sigma^m$. By the
scaling theorem, it follows that

$$g(kx, ky) \leftrightarrow G(u/k, v/k)/k^2$$

Now consider a sum of scaled functions that are placed in random positions relative to one another. Functions that are in random position will,
on average, have phases that are orthogonal. In line with the sum of
intensities in incoherent optics, the power spectrum (square of the am-

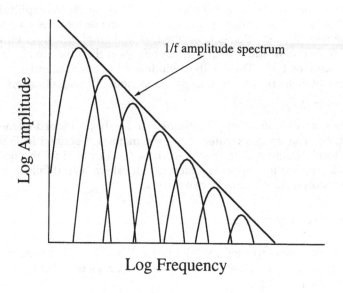

Figure 14: See text.

plitude spectrum) is equal to the sum of the power spectra of each of the functions, thus

$$\begin{array}{cc} \text{Space} & \text{Amplitude spectra} \end{array}$$

$$\sum_i^n g(kx + x_i, ky + y_i) \quad \leftrightarrow \quad \sqrt{n[G(u/k, v/k)k^2]^2}$$
$$= \sqrt{n}|G(u/k, v/k)|/k^2$$

In equation 5.1, the images are created by summing $\beta \cdot k^2$ functions at each scale where $k \propto \sigma^m$. Thus at each scale, the spectrum is proportional to

$$\begin{aligned} G(u, v, k) &= \sqrt{k^2} G(u/k, v/k)/k^2 \\ &= G(u/k, v/k)/k \end{aligned}$$

Thus at each scale, the peak of the spectrum falls by a factor of $1/k$. Figure 14 shows an example of the spectra at different scales. The spacing in the frequency domain is proportional to σ^m ($m = 1, 2, 3, \ldots$). On a log frequency axis, the spacing is

$$\log(\sigma^m) \propto m \quad (m = 1, 2, 3, \ldots)$$

With this sum of scaled functions, the amplitude spectra of the synthetic image will fall as $1/f$, that is, the contrast is scale-invariant. The local structure is also scale invariant. At each scale k (i.e., within each frequency band), the image consists of $\beta \cdot k^2$ elements of amplitude w_{nm} and size $1/\tau k$. If we magnify the image by some factor r then we shift to a scale with $\beta \cdot (r \cdot k)^2$ elements of size $1/\tau k$ and amplitude w_{nm}. However, if we scale our window with the magnification then the area is reduced by a factor of $1/r^2$. Thus with a window of constant angular size, the number of elements at any scale is independent of magnification.

$$\beta \cdot (r \cdot k)^2/r^2 = \beta \cdot k^2$$

Thus, at all scales there remain βk^2 randomly positioned elements of size $1/\tau k$. The images created using the method described in Figure 12 have local structure that is scale-invariant. As noted in the text, this provides a good first approximation to natural scenes but fails to capture combinatorial rules found in real scenes.

Acknowledgments

This work was supported by NIH Grant R29MR50588. I would like to thank Peter Foldiak, Nuala Brady, and the six reviewers for their helpful comments.

References

Adelson, E. H., Simoncelli, E., and Hingorani, R. 1987. Orthogonal pyramid transforms for image coding. *SPIE Visual Commun. Image Process.* II, 845.

Atick, J. J., and Redlich, A. N. 1990. Towards a theory of early visual processing. *Neural Comp.* **4**, 196–210.

Atick, J. J. 1992. Could information theory provide an ecological theory of sensory processing? *Network* **3**, 213–251.

Atick, J. J., and Redlich, A. N. 1992. What does the retina know about natural scenes? *Neural Comp.* **4**, 449–572.

Atick, J. J., Li, Zhaoping, and Redlich, N. 1993. What does post-adaptation color appearance reveal about cortical color coding? *Vision Res.* **33**, 123–129.

Baddeley, R. J., and Hancock, P. J. 1991. A statistical analysis of natural images matches psychophysically derived orientation tuning curves. *Proc. Roy. Soc. London B* **246**, 219–223.

Barlow, H. B. 1961. The coding of sensory messages. *Current Problems in Animal Behavior.* Cambridge, Cambridge University Press.

Barlow, H. B. 1972. Single units and sensation: A neuron doctrine for perceptual psychology? *Perception* **1**, 371–394.

Barlow, H. B. 1985. The Twelfth Bartlett Memorial Lecture: The role of single neurons in the psychology of perception. *Q. J. Exp. Psychol.* **37A**, 121–145.

Barlow, H. B. 1989. Unsupervised learning. *Neural Comp.* **1**, 295–311.

Barlow, H. B., and Foldiak, P. 1989. Adaptation and decorrelation in the cortex. In *The Computing Neuron*, R. Durbin, C. Miall, and G. Mitchison, eds., pp. 54–72. Addison-Wesley, Reading, MA.

Barlow, H. B., Kaushal, T. P., and Mitchison, G. J. 1989. Finding minimum entropy codes. *Neural Comp.* **1**, 412–423.

Baum, E. B., Moody, J., and Wilczek, F. 1988. Internal representations for associative memory. *Biol. Cybern.* **59**, 217–228.

Bialek, W., Ruderman, D. L., and Zee, A. 1991. Optimal sampling of natural images: A design principle for the visual system? In *Advances in Neural Information Processing 3*, R. Lippmann, J. Moody, and D. Touretzky, eds., pp. 363–369. Morgan Kaufmann, San Mateo, CA.

Blasdel, G. G., Lund, J. S., and Fitzpatrick, D. 1985. Intrinsic connections of macaque striate cortex: Axonal projections of cells outside lamina 4C. *J. Neurosci.* **5**, 3350–3369.

Bossomaier, T., and Snyder, A. W. 1986. Why spatial frequency processing in the visual cortex? *Vision Res.* **26**, 1307–1309.

Brady, N., and Field, D. J. 1993. What's constant in contrast constancy?: A vector length model of suprathreshold sensitivity. *Vision Res.*, submitted.

Buchsbaum, G., and Gottschalk, A. 1983. Trichromacy, opponent colors coding and optimum color information transmission in the retina. *Proc. Roy. Soc. London B* **220**, 89–113.

Burt, P. J., and Adelson, E. H. 1983. The Laplacian pyramid as a compact image code. *IEEE Transactions on Communications* **31**, 532–540.

Burton, G. J., and Moorhead, I. R. 1987. Color and spatial structure in natural scenes. *Appl. Opt.* **26**, 157–170.

Churchland, P. S., and Sejnowski, T. J. 1992. *The Computational Brain.* MIT Press, Cambridge, MA.

Daubechies, I. 1988. Orthonormal bases of compactly supported wavelets. *Comm. Pure Appl. Math.* **41**, 909–996.

Daugman, J. 1985. Uncertainty relation for resolution in space, spatial frequency, and orientation optimized by two-dimensional visual cortical filters. *J. Opt. Soc. Amer.* **2(7)**, 1160–1169.

Daugman, J. G. 1988. Complete discrete 2-D Gabor transforms by neural networks for image analysis and compression. *IEEE Transact. Acoustics, Speech Signal Process.* **36(7)**, 1169–1179.

Daugman, J. G. 1991. Self-similar oriented wavelet pyramids: Conjectures about neural non-orthogonality. In A. Gorea, ed., *Representations of Vision.* Cambridge University Press, Cambridge.

Derrico, J. B., and Buchsbaum, G. 1991. A computational model of spatiochromatic coding in early vision. *J. Visual Commun. Image Process.* **2**, 31–38.

DeValois, R. L., Albrecht, D. G., and Thorell, L. G. 1982. Spatial frequency selectivity of cells in macaque visual cortex. *Vision Res.* **22**, 545–559.

Eckert, M. P., and Buchsbaum, G. 1993. Efficient coding of natural time varying images in the early visual system. *Phil. Trans. R. Soc. London B* **339**, 385–395.

Evans, D. 1985. *Sparsity and Its Applications.* Cambridge University Press, Cambridge.

Farge, M., Hunt, J., and Vassilicos, J. C., eds. 1992. *Wavelets, Fractals and Fourier Transforms: New Developments and New Applications.* Oxford University Press, Oxford.

Field, D. J. 1987. Relations between the statistics of natural images and the response properties of cortical cells. *J. Opt. Soc. Amer.* **4**, 2379–2394.

Field, D. J. 1989. What the statistics of natural images tell us about visual coding. *Proc. SPIE* **1077**, 269–276.

Field, D. J. 1993. Scale-invariance and self-similar 'wavelet' transforms: An analysis of natural scenes and mammalian visual systems. In *Wavelets, Fractals and Fourier Transforms*, M. Farge, J. Hunt, and J. C. Vassilicos, eds. Oxford University Press, Oxford.

Field, D. J., and Tolhurst, D. J. 1986. The structure and symmetry of simple-cell receptive field profiles in the cat's visual cortex. *Proc. Roy. Soc. London B* **228**, 379–400.

Field, D. J., Hayes, A., and Hess, R. F. 1993. Contour integration by the human visual system: Evidence for a local "association field." *Vision Res.* **33**, 173–193.

Foldiak, P. 1989. Adaptive network for optimal linear feature extraction. In *Proceedings of the IEEE/INNS International Joint Conference on Neural Networks*, Vol. 1, pp. 401–405. IEEE Press, New York.

Foldiak, P. 1990. Forming sparse representations by local anti-Hebbian learning. *Biol. Cybern.* **64**, 165–170.

Friedman, J. H. 1987. Exploratory projection pursuit. *J. Amer. Statist. Assoc.* **82**, 249–266.

Gabor, D. 1946. Theory of Communication. *J. IEE London* **93**(III), 429–457.

Gilbert, C. D. 1992. Horizontal integration and cortical dynamics. *Neuron* **9**, 1–13.

Hancock, P. J., Baddeley, R. J., and Smith, L. S. 1992. The principal components of natural images. *Network* **3**, 61–70.

Huber, P. J. 1985. Projection pursuit. *Ann. Statist.* **13**, 435–475.

Intrator, N. 1992. Feature extraction using an unsupervised neural network. *Neural Comp.* **4**, 98–107.

Intrator, N. 1993. Combining exploratory projection pursuit and projection pursuit regression with application to neural networks. *Neural Comp.* **5**, 443–455.

Jones, J., and Palmer, L. 1987. An evaluation of the two-dimensional Gabor filter model of simple receptive fields in cat striate cortex. *J. Neurophysiol.* **58**(6), 1233–1258.

Kersten, D. 1987. Predictability and redundancy of natural images. *J. Opt. Soc. Amer.* **4**, 2395–2400.

Klein, S. A., and Levi, D. M. 1985. Hyperacuity thresholds of 1 sec: Theoretical predictions and empirical validation. *J. Opt. Soc. Amer.* **2**(7), 1170–1190.

Kulikowski, J. J., Marcelja, S., and Bishop, P. O. 1982. Theory of spatial position and spatial frequency relations in the receptive fields of simple cells in the visual cortex. *Biol. Cybern.* **43**, 187–198.

Lehky, S. R., and Sejnowski, T. J. 1990. Network model of shape-from-shading: Neural function arises from both receptive and projective receptive fields. *Nature (London)* **333**, 452–454.

Linsker, R. 1988. Self-organization in a perceptual network. *Computer* **21**, 105–117.

Linsker, R. 1993. Deriving receptive fields using an optimal encoding criterion. In *Advances in Neural Information Processing Systems 5*, S. J. Hanson, J. D. Cowan, and C. L. Giles, eds., pp. 953–960. Morgan Kaufmann, San Mateo, CA.

MacKay, D. J., and Miller, K. D. 1990. Analysis of Linsker's simulation of Hebbian rules. *Neural Comp.* **1**, 173–187.

Mallat, S. G. 1989. A theory for multiresolution signal decomposition: The wavelet representation. *IEEE Transact. Pattern Anal. Machine Intelligence* **11**(7), 674–693.

Maloney, L. T. 1986. Evaluation of linear models of surface spectral reflectance with small numbers of parameters. *J. Opt. Soc. Amer. A* **3**, 1673–1683.

Morrone, M. C., and Burr, D. C. 1988. Feature detection in human vision: A phase-dependent energy model. *Proc. Roy. Soc. London B* **235**, 221–245.

Oja, E. 1982. A simplified neuron model as a principal component analyzer. *J. Math. Biol.* **15**, 267–273.

Palm, G. 1980. On associative memory. *Biol. Cybern.* **36**, 19–31.

Pratt, W. K. 1978. *Digital Image Processing*. Wiley, New York.

Rockland, K., and Lund, J. S. 1983. Intrinsic laminar lattice connections in primary visual cortex. *J. Comp. Neurol.* **216**, 303–318.

Sanger, T. D. 1989. Optimal unsupervised learning in a single layer network. *Neural Networks* **2**, 459–473.

Schendel, U. 1989. *Sparse Matrices*. Wiley, New York.

Schmidhuber, J. 1992. Learning factorial codes by predictability minimization. *Neural Comp.* **4**, 863–879.

Shapley, R. M., and Lennie, P. 1985. Spatial frequency analysis in the visual system. *Annu. Rev. Neurosci.* **8**, 547–583.

Tolhurst, D. J., and Thompson, I. D. 1982. On the variety of spatial frequency selectivities shown by neurons in area 17 of the cat. *Proc. Roy. Soc. London Ser. B* **213**, 183–199.

Tolhurst, D. J., Tadmor, Y., and Tang Chao 1992. The amplitude spectra of natural images. *Ophthal. Physiol. Opt.* **12**, 229–232.

van Hateren, J. H. 1992. Real and optimal neural images in early vision. *Nature (London)* **360**, 68–69.

Webber, C. J. St. C. 1991. Competitive learning, natural images and cortical cells. *Network* **2**, 169–187.

Watson, A. B. 1983. Detection and recognition of simple spatial forms. In *Physical and Biological Processing of Images*, O. J. Braddick and A. C. Slade, eds. Springer-Verlag, Berlin.

Webster, M. A., and DeValois, R. L. 1985. Relationship between spatial-frequency and orientation tuning of striate-cortex cells. *J. Opt. Soc. Amer.* **2**(2), 1124–1132.

Zetzsche, C. 1990. Sparse coding: The link between low level vision and associative memory. In *Parallel Processing in Neural Systems and Computers*, R. Eckmiller, G. Hartmann, and G. Hauske, eds. North-Holland, Amsterdam.

Zucker, S. W., Dobbins, A., Iverson, L. 1989. Two stages of curve detection suggest two styles of visual computation. *Neural Comp.* **1**, 68–81.

8

An Information-Maximization Approach to Blind Separation and Blind Deconvolution

Anthony J. Bell
Terrence J. Sejnowski
Howard Hughes Medical Institute,
Computational Neurobiology Laboratory, The Salk Institute,
10010 N. Torrey Pines Road, La Jolla, CA 92037 USA and
Department of Biology, University of California, San Diego, La Jolla, CA 92093 USA

We derive a new self-organizing learning algorithm that maximizes the information transferred in a network of nonlinear units. The algorithm does not assume any knowledge of the input distributions, and is defined here for the zero-noise limit. Under these conditions, information maximization has extra properties not found in the linear case (Linsker 1989). The nonlinearities in the transfer function are able to pick up higher-order moments of the input distributions and perform something akin to true redundancy reduction between units in the output representation. This enables the network to separate statistically independent components in the inputs: a higher-order generalization of principal components analysis. We apply the network to the source separation (or cocktail party) problem, successfully separating unknown mixtures of up to 10 speakers. We also show that a variant on the network architecture is able to perform blind deconvolution (cancellation of unknown echoes and reverberation in a speech signal). Finally, we derive dependencies of information transfer on time delays. We suggest that information maximization provides a unifying framework for problems in "blind" signal processing.

1 Introduction

This paper presents a convergence of two lines of research. The first, the development of information-theoretic unsupervised learning rules for neural networks, has been pioneered by Linsker (1992), Becker and Hinton (1992), Atick and Redlich (1993), Plumbley and Fallside (1988), and others. The second is the use, in signal processing, of higher-order statistics for separating out mixtures of independent sources (blind separation) or reversing the effect of an unknown filter (blind deconvolution). Methods exist for solving these problems, but it is fair to say that many of them are ad hoc. The literature displays a diversity of approaches and justifications—for historical reviews see Comon (1994) and Haykin (1994a).

In this paper, we supply a common theoretical framework for these problems through the use of information-theoretic objective functions applied to neural networks with nonlinear units. The resulting learning rules have enabled a principled approach to the signal processing problems, and opened a new application area for information-theoretic unsupervised learning.

Blind separation techniques can be used in any domain where an array of N receivers picks up linear mixtures of N source signals. Examples include speech separation (the "cocktail party problem"), processing of arrays of radar or sonar signals, and processing of multisensor biomedical recordings. A previous approach has been implemented in analog VLSI circuitry for real-time source separation (Vittoz and Arreguit 1989; Cohen and Andreou 1992). The application areas of blind deconvolution techniques include the cancellation of acoustic reverberations (for example, the "barrel effect" observed when using speaker phones), the processing of geophysical data (seismic deconvolution), and the restoration of images.

The approach we take to these problems is a generalization of Linsker's *infomax* principle to nonlinear units with arbitrarily distributed inputs uncorrupted by any *known* noise sources. The principle is that described by Laughlin (1981) (see Figure 1a): when inputs are to be passed through a sigmoid function, maximum information transmission can be achieved when the sloping part of the sigmoid is optimally lined up with the high-density parts of the inputs. As we show, this can be achieved in an adaptive manner, using a stochastic gradient ascent rule. The generalization of this rule to multiple units leads to a system that, in maximizing information transfer, also reduces the redundancy between the units in the output layer. It is this latter process, also called independent component analysis (ICA), that enables the network to solve the blind separation task.

The paper is organized as follows. Section 2 describes the new information maximization learning algorithm, applied, respectively to a single input, an $N \rightarrow N$ mapping, a causal filter, a system with time delays, and a "flexible" nonlinearity. Section 3 describes the blind separation and blind deconvolution problems. Section 4 discusses the conditions under which the information maximization process can find factorial codes (perform ICA), and therefore solve the separation and deconvolution problems. Section 5 presents results on the separation and deconvolution of speech signals. Section 6 attempts to place the theory and results in the context of previous work and mentions the limitations of the approach.

A brief report of this research appears in Bell and Sejnowski (1995).

2 Information Maximization

The basic problem tackled here is how to maximize the mutual information that the output Y of a neural network processor contains about its input X. This is defined as

$$I(Y, X) = H(Y) - H(Y \mid X) \tag{2.1}$$

where $H(Y)$ is the entropy of the output, while $H(Y \mid X)$ is whatever entropy the output has that did not come from the input. In the case that we have no noise (or rather, we do not know what is noise and what is signal in the input), the mapping between X and Y is deterministic, and $H(Y \mid X)$ has its lowest possible value: it diverges to $-\infty$. This divergence is one of the consequences of the generalization of information theory to continuous variables. What we call $H(Y)$ is really the "differential" entropy of Y with respect to some reference, such as the noise level or the accuracy of our discretization of the variables in X and Y.[1] To avoid such complexities, we consider here only the *gradient* of information-theoretic quantities with respect to some parameter, w, in our network. Such gradients are as well behaved as discrete-variable entropies, because the reference terms involved in the definition of differential entropies disappear. The above equation can be differentiated as follows, with respect to a parameter, w, involved in the mapping from X to Y:

$$\frac{\partial}{\partial w} I(Y, X) = \frac{\partial}{\partial w} H(Y) \tag{2.2}$$

because $H(Y \mid X)$ does not depend on w. This can be seen by considering a system that avoids infinities: $Y = G(X) + N$, where G is some invertible transformation and N is additive noise on the outputs. In this case, $H(Y \mid X) = H(N)$ (Nadal and Parga 1995). Whatever the level of this additive noise, maximization of the mutual information, $I(Y, X)$, is equivalent to the maximization of the output entropy, $H(Y)$, because $(\partial/\partial w)H(N) = 0$. There is nothing mysterious about the deterministic case, despite the fact that $H(Y \mid X)$ tends to minus infinity as the noise variance goes to zero.

Thus for invertible continuous deterministic mappings, the mutual information between inputs and outputs can be maximized by maximizing the entropy of the outputs alone.

2.1 For One Input and One Output. When we pass a single input x through a transforming function $g(x)$ to give an output variable y, both $I(y, x)$ and $H(y)$ are maximized when we align high density parts of the *probability density function* (pdf) of x with highly sloping parts of the function $g(x)$. This is the idea of "matching a neuron's input–output function to the expected distribution of signals" that we find in (Laughlin 1981). See Figure 1a for an illustration.

When $g(x)$ is monotonically increasing or decreasing (i.e., has a unique inverse), the pdf of the output, $f_y(y)$, can be written as a function of the

---

[1] See the discussion in Haykin (1994b, chap. 11), and in Cover and Thomas (1991, chap. 9).

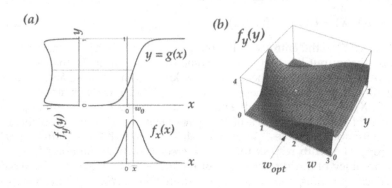

Figure 1: Optimal information flow in sigmoidal neurons. (a) Input x having density function $f_x(x)$, in this case a gaussian, is passed through a nonlinear function $g(x)$. The information in the resulting density, $f_y(y)$ depends on matching the mean and variance of x to the threshold, w_0, and slope, w, of $g(x)$ (see Schraudolph *et al.* 1991). (b) $f_y(y)$ is plotted for different values of the weight w. The optimal weight, w_{opt}, transmits most information.

pdf of the input, $f_x(x)$, (Papoulis 1984, equation 5-5):

$$f_y(y) = \frac{f_x(x)}{|\partial y/\partial x|} \tag{2.3}$$

where the bars denote absolute value. The entropy of the output, $H(y)$, is given by

$$H(y) = -E\left[\ln f_y(y)\right] = -\int_{-\infty}^{\infty} f_y(y) \ln f_y(y)\, dy \tag{2.4}$$

where $E[\cdot]$ denotes expected value. Substituting 2.3 into 2.4 gives

$$H(y) = E\left[\ln \left|\frac{\partial y}{\partial x}\right|\right] - E\left[\ln f_x(x)\right] \tag{2.5}$$

The second term on the right (the entropy of x) may be considered to be unaffected by alterations in a parameter w determining $g(x)$. Therefore in order to maximize the entropy of y by changing w, we need only concentrate on maximizing the first term, which is the average log of how the input affects the output. This can be done by considering the "training set" of x's to approximate the density $f_x(x)$, and deriving an "online," stochastic gradient ascent learning rule:

$$\Delta w \propto \frac{\partial H}{\partial w} = \frac{\partial}{\partial w}\left(\ln \left|\frac{\partial y}{\partial x}\right|\right) = \left(\frac{\partial y}{\partial x}\right)^{-1}\frac{\partial}{\partial w}\left(\frac{\partial y}{\partial x}\right) \tag{2.6}$$

In the case of the logistic transfer function:

$$y = \frac{1}{1 + e^{-u}}, \quad u = wx + w_0 \tag{2.7}$$

in which the input is multiplied by a weight w and added to a bias-weight w_0, the terms above evaluate as

$$\frac{\partial y}{\partial x} = wy(1 - y) \tag{2.8}$$

$$\frac{\partial}{\partial w}\left(\frac{\partial y}{\partial x}\right) = y(1 - y)[1 + wx(1 - 2y)] \tag{2.9}$$

Dividing 2.9 by 2.8 gives the learning rule for the logistic function, as calculated from the general rule of 2.6:

$$\Delta w \propto \frac{1}{w} + x(1 - 2y) \tag{2.10}$$

Similar reasoning leads to the rule for the bias-weight:

$$\Delta w_0 \propto 1 - 2y \tag{2.11}$$

The effect of these two rules can be seen in Figure 1a. For example, if the input pdf $f_x(x)$ were gaussian, then the Δw_0-rule would center the steepest part of the sigmoid curve on the peak of $f_x(x)$, matching input density to output slope, in a manner suggested intuitively by 2.3. The Δw-rule would then scale the slope of the sigmoid curve to match the variance of $f_x(x)$. For example, narrow pdf's would lead to sharply sloping sigmoids. The Δw-rule is *anti-Hebbian*,[2] with an *anti-decay* term. The anti-Hebbian term keeps y away from one uninformative situation: that of y being saturated at 0 or 1. But an anti-Hebbian rule alone makes weights go to zero, so the anti-decay term $(1/w)$ keeps y away from the other uninformative situation: when w is so small that y stays around 0.5.

The effect of these two balanced forces is to produce an output pdf, $f_y(y)$, that is close to the flat unit distribution; that is, the maximum entropy distribution for a variable bounded between 0 and 1. Figure 1b shows a family of these distributions, with the most informative one occurring at w_{opt}.

A rule that maximizes information for one input and one output may be suggestive for structures such as synapses and photoreceptors that must position the gain of their nonlinearity at a level appropriate to the average value and size of the input fluctuations (Laughlin 1981). However, to see the advantages of this approach in artificial neural networks, we now analyze the case of multidimensional inputs and outputs.

---

[2]If $y = \tanh(wx + w_0)$ then $\Delta w \propto (1/w) - 2xy$.

2.2 For an $N \to N$ Network. Consider a network with an input vector
x, a weight matrix **W**, a bias vector $\mathbf{w}_0$, and a monotonically transformed
output vector $\mathbf{y} = g(\mathbf{Wx} + \mathbf{w}_0)$. Analogously to 2.3, the multivariate
probability density function of **y** can be written (Papoulis 1984, equation
6-63):

$$f_\mathbf{y}(\mathbf{y}) = \frac{f_\mathbf{x}(\mathbf{x})}{|J|} \tag{2.12}$$

where $|J|$ is the absolute value of the Jacobian of the transformation. The
Jacobian is the determinant of the matrix of partial derivatives:

$$J = \det \begin{bmatrix} \frac{\partial y_1}{\partial x_1} & \cdots & \frac{\partial y_1}{\partial x_n} \\ \vdots & & \vdots \\ \frac{\partial y_n}{\partial x_1} & \cdots & \frac{\partial y_n}{\partial x_n} \end{bmatrix} \tag{2.13}$$

The derivation proceeds as in the previous section except instead of maxi-
mizing $\ln |\partial y/\partial x|$, now we maximize $\ln |J|$. This latter quantity represents
the log of the volume of space in **y** into which points in **x** are mapped. By
maximizing it, we attempt to spread our training set of **x**-points evenly
in **y**.

For sigmoidal units, $\mathbf{y} = g(\mathbf{u})$, $\mathbf{u} = \mathbf{Wx} + \mathbf{w}_0$, with g being the logistic
function: $g(u) = (1 + e^{-u})^{-1}$, the resulting learning rules are familiar in
form (proof given in the Appendix):

$$\Delta\mathbf{W} \propto \left[\mathbf{W}^T\right]^{-1} + (\mathbf{1} - 2\mathbf{y})\mathbf{x}^T \tag{2.14}$$

$$\Delta\mathbf{w}_0 \propto \mathbf{1} - 2\mathbf{y} \tag{2.15}$$

except that now x, y, $\mathbf{w}_0$, and **1** are vectors (**1** is a vector of ones), **W** is
a matrix, and the anti-Hebbian term has become an outer product. The
anti-decay term has generalized to an *anti-redundancy* term: the inverse
of the transpose of the weight matrix. For an individual weight, w_{ij}, this
rule amounts to

$$\Delta w_{ij} \propto \frac{\text{cof } w_{ij}}{\det \mathbf{W}} + x_j(1 - 2y_i) \tag{2.16}$$

where cof w_{ij}, the *cofactor* of w_{ij}, is $(-1)^{i+j}$ times the determinant of the
matrix obtained by removing the ith row and the jth column from **W**.

This rule is the same as the one for the single unit mapping, except
that instead of $w = 0$ being an unstable point of the dynamics, now any
degenerate weight matrix is unstable, since $\det \mathbf{W} = 0$ if **W** is degenerate.
This fact enables different output units y_i to learn to represent different
things in the input. When the weight vectors entering two output units
become too similar, $\det \mathbf{W}$ becomes small and the natural dynamic of
learning causes these weight vectors to diverge from each other. This
effect is mediated by the numerator, cof w_{ij}. When this cofactor becomes

small, it indicates that there is a degeneracy in the weight matrix of the *rest* of the layer (i.e., those weights not associated with input x_j or output y_i). In this case, any degeneracy in **W** has less to do with the specific weight w_{ij} that we are adjusting. Further discussion of the convergence conditions of this rule (in terms of higher-order moments) is deferred to Section 6.2.

The utility of this rule for performing blind separation is demonstrated in Section 5.1.

2.3 For a Causal Filter. It is not necessary to restrict our architecture to weight *matrices*. Consider the top part of Figure 3b, in which a time series $x(t)$, of length M, is convolved with a causal filter $w_1, \ldots, w_L$ of impulse response $w(t)$, to give an output time series $u(t)$, which is then passed through a nonlinear function, g, to give $y(t)$. We can write this system either as a convolution or as a matrix equation:

$$y(t) = g[u(t)] = g[w(t) * x(t)] \tag{2.17}$$

$$Y = g(U) = g(WX) \tag{2.18}$$

in which Y, X, and U are vectors of the whole time series, and W is an $M \times M$ matrix. When the filtering is causal, W will be lower triangular:

$$W = \begin{bmatrix} w_L & 0 & \cdots & 0 & 0 \\ w_{L-1} & w_L & 0 & \cdots & 0 \\ \vdots & & & & \vdots \\ w_1 & \cdots & w_L & \cdots & 0 \\ \vdots & & & & \vdots \\ 0 & \cdots & w_1 & \cdots & w_L \end{bmatrix} \tag{2.19}$$

At this point, we take the liberty of imagining there is an ensemble of such time series, so that we can write,

$$f_Y(Y) = \frac{f_X(X)}{|J|} \tag{2.20}$$

where again, $|J|$ is the Jacobian of the transformation. We can "create" this ensemble from a single time series by chopping it into bits (of length L for example, making W in 2.19 an $L \times L$ matrix). The Jacobian in 2.20 is written as follows:

$$J = \det \left[\frac{\partial y(t_i)}{\partial x(t_j)} \right]_{ij} = (\det W) \prod_{t=1}^{M} y'(t) \tag{2.21}$$

and may be decomposed into the determinant of the weight matrix 2.19, and the product of the slopes of the squashing function, $y'(t) = \partial y(t)/\partial u(t)$, for all times t (see Appendix A.6). Because W is lower-triangular, its determinant is simply the product of its diagonal values, that is w_L^M. As in the previous section, we maximize the joint entropy

$H(Y)$ by maximizing $\ln |J|$, which can then be simply written as

$$\ln |J| = \ln |w_L^M| + \sum_{t=1}^{M} \ln |y'(t)| \tag{2.22}$$

If we assume that our nonlinear function g is the hyperbolic tangent (tanh), then differentiation with respect to the weights in our filter $w(t)$, gives two simple[3] rules:

$$\Delta w_L \propto \sum_{t=1}^{M} \left(\frac{1}{w_L} - 2x_t\, y_t \right) \tag{2.23}$$

$$\Delta w_{L-j} \propto \sum_{t=j}^{M} \left(-2x_{t-j}\, y_t \right) \tag{2.24}$$

Here, w_L is the 'leading' weight, and the w_{L-j}, where $j > 0$, are tapped delay lines linking x_{t-j} to y_t. The leading weight thus adjusts just as would a weight connected to a neuron with only that one input (see Section 2.1). The delay weights attempt to decorrelate the past input from the present output. Thus the filter is kept from "shrinking" by its leading weight.

The utility of this rule for performing blind deconvolution is demonstrated in Section 5.2.

2.4 For Weights with Time Delays. Consider a weight, w, with a time delay, d, and a sigmoidal nonlinearity, g, so that

$$y(t) = g[wx(t - d)] \tag{2.25}$$

We can maximize the entropy of y with respect to the time delay, again by maximizing the log slope of y (as in 2.6):

$$\Delta d \propto \frac{\partial H}{\partial d} = \frac{\partial}{\partial d} \left(\ln |y'| \right) \tag{2.26}$$

The crucial step in this derivation is to realize that

$$\frac{\partial}{\partial d} x(t - d) = -\frac{\partial}{\partial t} x(t - d) \tag{2.27}$$

Calling this quantity simply $-\dot{x}$, we may then write

$$\frac{\partial y}{\partial d} = -w\dot{x}y' \tag{2.28}$$

Our general rule is therefore given as follows:

$$\frac{\partial}{\partial d} \left(\ln |y'| \right) = \frac{1}{y'} \frac{\partial y'}{\partial y} \frac{\partial y}{\partial d} = -w\dot{x} \frac{\partial y'}{\partial y} \tag{2.29}$$

---

[3]The corresponding rules for *noncausal* filters are substantially more complex.

When g is the tanh function, for example, this yields the following rule for adapting the time delay:

$$\Delta d \propto 2w\dot{x}y \tag{2.30}$$

This rule holds regardless of the architecture in which the network is embedded, and it is local, unlike the Δw rule in 2.16. It bears a resemblance to the rule proposed by Platt and Faggin (1992) for adjustable time delays in the network architecture of Jutten and Herault (1991).

The rule has an intuitive interpretation. First, if $w = 0$, there is no reason to adjust the delay. Second, the rule maximizes the delivered *power* of the inputs, stabilizing when $\langle \dot{x}y \rangle = 0$. As an example, if y received several sinusoidal inputs of the same frequency, ω, and different phase, each with its own adjustable time delay, then the time delays would adjust until the phases of the time-delayed inputs were all the same. Then, for each input, $\langle \dot{x}y \rangle$ would be proportional to $\langle \cos \omega t \cdot \tanh(\sin \omega t) \rangle$, which would be zero.

In adjusting delays, therefore, the rule will attempt to line up similar signals in time, and cancel time delays caused by the same signal taking alternate paths.

We hope to explore, in future work, the usefulness of this rule for adjusting time delays and tap-spacing in blind separation and blind deconvolution tasks.

2.5 For a Generalized Sigmoid Function. In Section 4, we will show how it is sometimes necessary not only to train the weights of the network, but also to select the form of the nonlinearity, so that it can "match" input pdf's. In other words, if the input to a neuron is u, with a pdf of $f_u(u)$, then our sigmoid should approximate, as closely as possible, the cumulative distribution of this input:

$$y = g(u) \simeq \int_{-\infty}^{u} f_u(v)\,dv \tag{2.31}$$

One way to do this is to define a "flexible" sigmoid that can be altered to *fit* the data, in the sense of 2.31. An example of such a function is the asymmetric generalized logistic function (see also Baram and Roth 1994) described by the differential equation:

$$y' = \frac{dy}{du} = y^p(1-y)^r \tag{2.32}$$

where p and r are positive real numbers. Numerical integration of this equation produces sigmoids suitable for very peaked (as $p, r > 1$, see Fig. 2b) and flat, unit-like (as $p, r < 1$, see Fig. 2c) input distributions. So by varying these coefficients, we can mold the sigmoid so that its slope fits unimodal distributions of varying kurtosis. By having $p \neq r$,

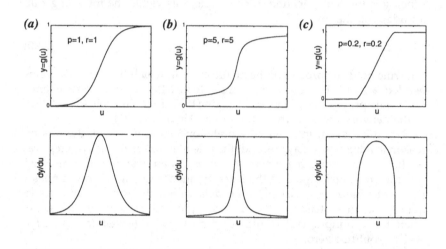

Figure 2: The generalized logistic sigmoid (top row) of 2.32, and its slope, y' (bottom row), for (a) $p = r = 1$, (b) $p = r = 5$ and (c) $p = r = 0.2$. Compare the slope of (b) with the pdf in Figure 5a: it provides a good match for natural speech signals.

we can also account for some skew in the distributions. When we have chosen values for p and r, perhaps by some optimization process, the rules for changing a single input–output weight, w, and a bias, w_0, are subtly altered from 2.14 and 2.11, but clearly the same when $p = r = 1$:

$$\Delta w \;\propto\; \frac{1}{w} + x[p(1-y) - ry] \tag{2.33}$$

$$\Delta w_0 \;\propto\; p(1-y) - ry \tag{2.34}$$

The importance of being able to train a general function of this type will be explained in Section 4.

3 Background to Blind Separation and Blind Deconvolution

Blind separation and blind deconvolution are related problems in signal processing. In *blind separation*, as introduced by Herault and Jutten (1986), and illustrated in Figure 3a, a set of sources, $s_1(t), \ldots, s_N(t)$, (different people speaking, music, etc.) is mixed together linearly by a matrix **A**. We do not know anything about the sources, or the mixing process. All

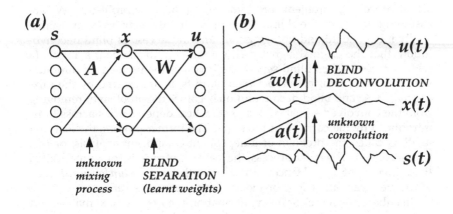

Figure 3: Network architectures for (a) blind separation of five mixed signals, and (b) blind deconvolution of a single signal.

we receive are the N superpositions of them, $x_1(t), \ldots, x_N(t)$. The task is to recover the original sources by finding a square matrix, $\mathbf{W}$, which is a permutation and rescaling of the inverse of the unknown matrix, $\mathbf{A}$. The problem has also been called the "cocktail-party" problem.[4]

In *blind deconvolution*, described in Haykin (1991, 1994a) and illustrated in Figure 3b, a single unknown signal $s(t)$ is convolved with an unknown tapped delay-line filter $a_1, \ldots, a_K$, giving a corrupted signal $x(t) = a(t)*s(t)$ where $a(t)$ is the impulse response of the filter. The task is to recover $s(t)$ by convolving $x(t)$ with a learnt filter $w_1, \ldots, w_L$, which reverses the effect of the filter $a(t)$.

There are many similarities between the two problems. In one, sources are corrupted by the superposition of other sources. In the other, a source is corrupted by time-delayed versions of itself. In both cases, unsupervised learning must be used because no error signals are available. In both cases, second-order statistics are inadequate to solve the problem.

For example, for blind separation, a second-order decorrelation technique such as that of Barlow and Földiák (1989) would find uncorrelated, or linearly independent, projections, $\mathbf{y}$, of the input data, $\mathbf{x}$. But it could only find a symmetric decorrelation matrix, that would not suffice if the mixing matrix, $\mathbf{A}$, were asymmetric (Jutten and Herault 1991). Similarly, for blind deconvolution, second-order techniques based on the autocorrelation function, such as prediction-error filters, are *phase-blind*. They do not have sufficient information to estimate the phase of the corrupting filter, $a(t)$, only its amplitude (Haykin 1994a).

---

[4]Though for now, we ignore the problem of signal propagation delays.

The reason why second-order techniques fail is that these two "blind" signal processing problems are information-theoretic problems. We are assuming, in the case of blind separation, that the sources, s, are statistically independent and non-gaussian, and in the case of blind deconvolution, that the original signal, $s(t)$, consists of independent symbols (a white process). Then blind separation becomes the problem of minimizing the mutual information between outputs, u_i, introduced by the mixing matrix A; and blind deconvolution becomes the problem of removing from the convolved signal, $x(t)$, any statistical dependencies across time, introduced by the corrupting filter $a(t)$. The former process, the learning of W, is called the problem of independent component analysis, or *ICA* (Comon 1994). The latter process, the learning of $w(t)$, is sometimes called the *whitening* of $x(t)$. Henceforth, we use the term *redundancy reduction* when we mean either ICA or the whitening of a time series.

In either case, it is clear in an information-theoretic context that second-order statistics are inadequate for reducing redundancy, because the mutual information between two variables involves statistics of all orders, except in the special case that the variables are jointly gaussian.

In the various approaches in the literature, the higher-order statistics required for redundancy reduction have been accessed in two main ways. The first way is the explicit estimation of cumulants and polyspectra. See Comon (1994) and Hatzinakos and Nikias (1994) for the application of this approach to separation and deconvolution, respectively. The drawbacks of such direct techniques are that they can sometimes be computationally intensive, and may be inaccurate when cumulants higher than fourth order are ignored, as they usually are. It is currently not clear why direct approaches can be surprisingly successful despite errors in the estimation of the cumulants, and in the usage of these cumulants to estimate mutual information.

The second main way of accessing higher-order statistics is through the use of static nonlinear functions. The Taylor series expansions of these nonlinearities yield higher-order terms. The hope, in general, is that learning rules containing such terms will be sensitive to the right higher-order statistics necessary to perform ICA or whitening. Such reasoning has been used to justify both the Herault-Jutten (or H-J) approach to blind separation (Comon *et al.* 1991) and the so-called "Bussgang" approaches to blind deconvolution (Bellini 1994). The drawback here is that there is no guarantee that the higher-order statistics yielded by the nonlinearities are weighted in a way relating to the calculation of statistical dependency. For the H-J algorithm, the standard approach is to try different nonlinearities on different problems to see if they work.

Clearly, it would be of benefit to have some method of rigorously linking our choice of a static nonlinearity to a learning rule performing gradient ascent in some quantity relating to statistical dependency. Because of the infinite number of higher-order statistics involved in statistical dependency, this has generally been thought to be impossible. As we now show, this belief is incorrect.

4 When Does Information Maximization Reduce Statistical Dependence?

In this section, we consider under what conditions the information *maximization* algorithm presented in Section 2 *minimizes* the mutual information between outputs (or time points) and therefore performs redundancy reduction.

Consider a system with two outputs, y_1 and y_2 (two output channels in the case of separation, or two time points in the case of deconvolution). The joint entropy of these two variables may be written as (Papoulis 1984, equation 15-93):

$$H(y_1, y_2) = H(y_1) + H(y_2) - I(y_1, y_2) \tag{4.1}$$

Maximizing this joint entropy consists of maximizing the individual entropies while minimizing the mutual information, $I(y_1, y_2)$, shared between the two. When this latter quantity is zero, the two variables are statistically independent, and the pdf can be factored: $f_{y_1 y_2}(y_1, y_2) = f_{y_1}(y_1) f_{y_2}(y_2)$. Both ICA and the "whitening" approach to deconvolution are examples of minimizing $I(y_1, y_2)$ for all pairs y_1 and y_2. This process is variously known as factorial code learning (Barlow 1989), predictability minimization (Schmidhuber 1992), as well as independent component analysis (Comon 1994) and redundancy reduction (Barlow 1961; Atick 1992).

The algorithm presented in Section 2 is a stochastic gradient ascent algorithm that maximizes the joint entropy in 4.1. In doing so, it will, in general, reduce $I(y_1, y_2)$, reducing the statistical dependence of the two outputs.

However, it is not guaranteed to reach the absolute minimum of $I(y_1, y_2)$, because of interference from the other terms, the $H(y_i)$. Figure 4 shows one pathological situation where a "diagonal" projection (Fig. 4c) of two independent, uniformly distributed variables x_1 and x_2 is preferred over an "independent" projection (Fig. 4b). This is because of a "mismatch" between the input pdf's and the slope of the sigmoid nonlinearity. The learning procedure is able to achieve higher values in Figure 4c for the individual output entropies, $H(y_1)$ and $H(y_2)$, because the pdf's of $x_1 + x_2$ and $x_1 - x_2$ are triangular, more closely matching the slope of the sigmoid. This interferes with the minimization of $I(y_1, y_2)$.

In many practical situations, however, such interference will have minimal effect. We conjecture that only when the pdf's of the inputs are *sub-gaussian* (meaning their kurtosis, or fourth-order standardized cumulant, is less than 0), may unwanted higher entropy solutions for logistic

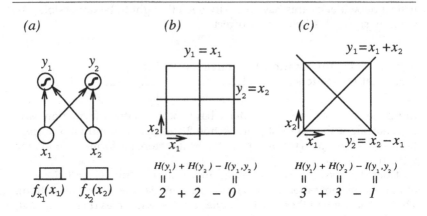

Figure 4: An example of when joint entropy maximization fails to yield statistically independent components. (a) Two independent input variables, x_1 and x_2, having uniform (flat) pdf's, are input into an entropy maximization network with sigmoidal outputs. Because the input pdf's are not well matched to the nonlinearity, the "diagonal" solution (c) has higher joint entropy than the "independent-component" solution (b), despite its having nonzero mutual information between the outputs. The values given are for illustration purposes only.

sigmoid networks be found by combining inputs in the way shown in Figure 4c (Kenji Doya, personal communication). Many real-world analog signals, including the speech signals we used, are super-gaussian. They have longer tails and are more sharply peaked than gaussians (see Fig. 5). For such signals, in our experience, maximizing the joint entropy in simple logistic sigmoidal networks always minimizes the mutual information between the outputs (see the results in Section 5).

We can tailor conditions so that the mutual information between outputs *is* minimized, by constructing our nonlinear function, $g(u)$, so that it matches, in the sense of 2.31, the known pdf's of the independent variables. When this is the case, $H(y)$ will be maximized [meaning $f_y(y)$ will be the flat unit distribution] only when u carries one single independent variable. Any linear combination of the variables will produce a "more gaussian" $f_u(u)$ (due to central limit tendencies) and a resulting suboptimal (nonflat) $f_y(y)$.

We have presented, in Section 2.5, one possible "flexible" nonlinearity. This suggests a two-stage algorithm for performing independent component analysis. First, a nonlinearity such as that defined by 2.32 is optimized to approximate the cumulative distributions, 2.31, of known independent components (sources). Then networks using this nonlinear-

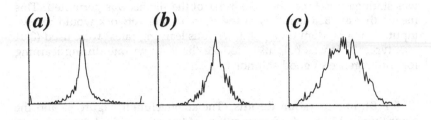

Figure 5: Typical probability density functions for (a) speech, (b) rock music, and (c) gaussian white noise. The kurtosis of pdf's (a) and (b) was greater than 0, and they would be classified as super-gaussian.

ity are trained using the full weight matrix and bias vector generalization of 2.33 and 2.34:

$$\Delta \mathbf{W} \propto \left[\mathbf{W}^T \right]^{-1} + [p(\mathbf{1} - \mathbf{y}) - r\mathbf{y}]\mathbf{x}^T \tag{4.2}$$

$$\Delta \mathbf{w}_0 \propto p(\mathbf{1} - \mathbf{y}) - r\mathbf{y} \tag{4.3}$$

This way, we can be sure that the problem of maximizing the mutual information between the inputs and outputs, and the problem of minimizing the mutual information between the outputs, have the same solution.

This argument is well supported by the analysis of Nadal and Parga (1995), who independently reached the conclusion that in the low-noise limit, information maximization yields factorial codes when both the non-linear function, $g(u)$, and the weights, w, can be optimized. Here, we provide a practical optimization method for the weights and a framework for optimizing the nonlinear function. Having discussed these caveats, we now present results for blind separation and blind deconvolution using the standard logistic function.

5 Methods and Results

The experiments presented here were obtained using 7 second segments of speech recorded from various speakers (only one speaker per recording). All signals were sampled at 8 kHz from the output of the auxiliary microphone of a Sparc-10 workstation. No special postprocessing was performed on the waveforms, other than that of normalizing their amplitudes so they were appropriate for use with our networks (input values roughly between −3 and 3). The method of training was stochastic gradient ascent, but because of the costly matrix inversion in 2.14, weights were usually adjusted based on the summed $\Delta \mathbf{W}$'s of small "batches" of length B, where $5 \leq B \leq 300$. Batch training was made efficient using vectorized code written in MATLAB. To ensure that the input ensemble was stationary in time, the time index of the signals was permuted. This means that at each iteration of the training, the network would receive input from a random time point. Various learning rates[5] were used (0.01 was typical). It was helpful to reduce the learning rate during learning for convergence to good solutions.

5.1 Blind Separation Results. The architecture in Figure 3a and the algorithm in 2.14 and 2.15 were sufficient to perform blind separation. A random mixing matrix, A, was generated with values usually uniformly distributed between -1 and 1. This was used to make the mixed time series, x, from the original sources, s. The matrices s and x, then, were both $N \times M$ matrices (N signals, M timepoints), and x was constructed from s by (1) permuting the time index of s to produce $s^{\dagger}$, and (2) creating the mixtures, x, by multiplying by the mixing matrix: $x = As^{\dagger}$. The unmixing matrix W and the bias vector w_0 were then trained.

An example run with five sources is shown in Figure 6. The mixtures, x, formed an incomprehensible babble. This unmixed solution was reached after around 10^6 time points were presented, equivalent to about 20 passes through the complete time series,[6] though much of the improvement occurred on the first few passes through the data. Any residual interference in u is inaudible. This is reflected in the permutation structure of the matrix WA:

$$WA = \begin{bmatrix} \boxed{-4.09} & 0.13 & 0.09 & -0.07 & -0.01 \\ 0.07 & \boxed{-2.92} & 0.00 & 0.02 & -0.06 \\ 0.02 & -0.02 & -0.06 & -0.08 & \boxed{-2.20} \\ 0.02 & 0.03 & 0.00 & \boxed{1.97} & 0.02 \\ -0.07 & 0.14 & \boxed{-3.50} & -0.01 & 0.04 \end{bmatrix} \quad (5.1)$$

As can be seen, only one substantial entry (boxed) exists in each row and column. The interference was attenuated by between 20 and 70 dB in all cases, and the system was continuing to improve slowly with a learning rate of 0.0001.

In our most ambitious attempt, 10 sources (six speakers, rock music, raucous laughter, a gong, and the Hallelujah chorus) were successfully separated, though the fine tuning of the solution took many hours and required some annealing of the learning rate (lowering it with time). For two sources, convergence is normally achieved in less than one pass through the data (50,000 data points), and on a Sparc-10 on-line learning

---

[5]The learning rate is defined as the proportionality constant in 2.14–2.15 and 2.23–2.24.

[6]This took on the order of 5 min on a Sparc-10. Two hundred data points were presented at a time in a "batch," then the weights were changed with a learning rate of 0.01 based on the sum of the 200 accumulated Δws.

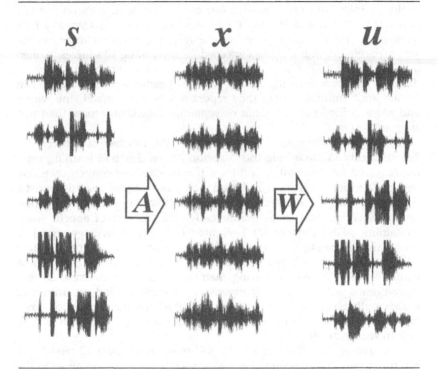

Figure 6: A 5×5 information maximization network performed blind separation, learning the unmixing matrix **W**. The outputs, **u**, are shown here unsquashed by the sigmoid. They can be visually matched to their corresponding sources, **s**, even though their order was different and some (for example u_1) were recovered as negative (upside down).

can occur at twice the speed at which the sounds themselves are played. Real-time separation for more than, say, three sources, may require further work to speed convergence, or special-purpose hardware.

In all our attempts at blind separation, the algorithm has failed under only two conditions:

1. when more than one of the sources were gaussian white noise, and

2. when the mixing matrix **A** was almost singular.

Both are understandable. First, no procedure can separate out independent gaussian sources since the sum of two gaussian variables has itself a gaussian distribution. Second, if **A** is almost singular, then any unmixing **W** must also be almost singular, making the learning in 2.14 quite unstable in the vicinity of a solution.

In contrast with these results, our experience with tests on the H-J network of Jutten and Herault (1991) has been that it occasionally fails to converge for two sources and only rarely converges for three, on the same speech and music signals we used for separating 10 sources. Cohen and Andreou (1992) report separation of up to six sinusoidal signals of different frequencies using analog VLSI H-J networks. In addition, in Cohen and Andreou (1995), they report results with mixed sine waves and noise in 5×5 networks, but no separation results for more than two speakers.

How does convergence time scale with the number of sources, N? The difficulty in answering this question is that different learning rates are required for different N and for different stages of convergence. We expect to address this issue in future work, and employ useful heuristic or explicit second-order techniques (Battiti 1992) to speed convergence. For now, we present rough estimates for the number of epochs (each containing 50,000 data vectors) required to reach an average signal to noise ratio on the ouput channels of 20 dB. At such a level, approximately 80% of each output channel amplitude is devoted to one signal. These results were collected for mixing matrices of unit determinant, so that convergence would not be hampered by having to find an unmixing matrix with especially large entries. Therefore these convergence times may be lower than for randomly generated matrices. The batch size, B, was in each case 20.

The average numbers of epochs to convergence (over 10 trials) and the computer times consumed per epoch (on a Sparc-10) are given in the following table:

No. of sources, N	2	3	4	5	6	7	8	9	10
Learning rate	0.1	0.1	0.1	0.05	0.05	0.025	0.025	0.025	0.0125
Epochs to convergence	< 1	< 1	2.25	5.0	9.0	9.2	13.8	14.9	30.6
Time in secs./epoch	12.1	13.3	14.6	15.6	16.9	18.4	19.9	21.7	23.6

5.2 Blind Deconvolution Results. Speech signals were convolved with various filters and the learning rules in 2.23 and 2.24 were used to perform blind deconvolution. Some results are shown in Figure 7. The convolving filters generally contained some zero values. For example, Figure 7e is the filter [0.8,0,0,0,1]. In addition, the taps were sometimes adjacent to each other (Fig. 7a–d) and sometimes spaced out in time (Fig. 7i–l). The "leading weight" of each filter is the rightmost bar in each histogram.

For each of the three experiments shown in Figure 7, we display the convolving filter, $a(t)$, the truncated inverting filter, $w_{ideal}(t)$, the filter produced by our algorithm, $w(t)$, and the convolution of $w(t)$ and $a(t)$.

task	WHITENING	BARREL EFFECT	MANY ECHOES
no. of taps	15	25	30
tap spacing	1 (= 0.125ms)	10 (= 1.25ms)	100 (= 12.5ms)
convolving filter 'a'	(a)	(e)	(i)
ideal deconvolving filter 'w_{ideal}'	(b)	(f)	(j)
learnt deconvolving filter 'w'	(c)	(g)	(k)
w * a	(d)	(h)	(l)

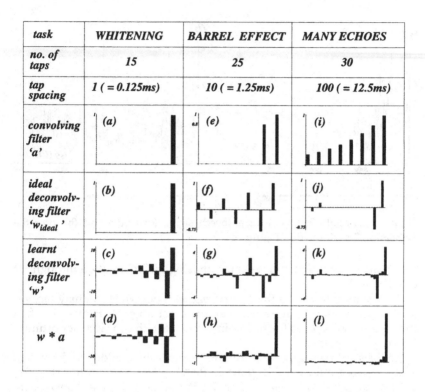

Figure 7: Blind deconvolution results. (a,e,i) Filters used to convolve speech signals, (b,f,j) their inverses, (c,g,k) deconvolving filters learned by the algorithm, and (d,h,l) convolution of the convolving and deconvolving filters. See text for further explanation.

The latter should be a delta-function (i.e., consist of only a single high value, at the position of the leading weight) if $w(t)$ correctly inverts $a(t)$.

The first example, Figure 7a–d, shows what happens when one tries to "deconvolve" a speech signal that has not actually been corrupted [filter $a(t)$ is a delta function]. If the tap spacing is close enough (in this case, as close as the samples), the algorithm learns a whitening filter (Fig. 7c), which flattens the amplitude spectrum of the speech right up to the Nyquist limit, the frequency corresponding to half the sampling rate. The spectra before and after such "deconvolution" are shown in Figure 8. Whitened speech sounds like a clear sharp version of the original signal since the phase structure is preserved. Using all available frequency lev-

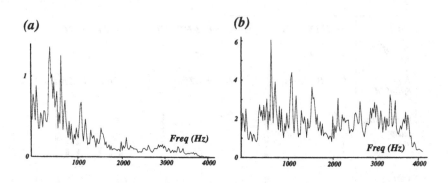

Figure 8: Amplitude spectra of a speech signal (a) before and (b) after the "whitening" performed in Figure 7c.

els equally is another example of maximizing the information throughput of a channel.

This shows that when the original signal is not white, we may recover a whitened version of it, rather than the exact original. However, when the taps are spaced out further, as in Figure 7e–l, there is less opportunity for simple whitening.

In the second example (Fig. 7e) a 6.25-msec echo is added to the signal. This creates a mild audible "barrel effect."[7] Because the filter (Fig. 7e) is finite in length, its inverse (Fig. 7f) is infinite in length, shown here truncated. The inverting filter learned in Figure 7g resembles it, though the resemblance tails off toward the left since we are really learning an optimal filter of finite length, not a truncated infinite filter. The resulting deconvolution (Fig. 7h) is quite good.

The cleanest results, though, come when the ideal deconvolving filter is of finite length, as in our third example. A set of exponentially decaying echoes spread out over 275 msec (Fig. 7i) may be inverted by a two-point filter (Fig. 7j) with a small decaying correction on its left, an artifact of the truncation of the convolving filter (Fig. 7i). As seen in Figure 7k, the learned filter corresponds almost exactly to the ideal one, and the deconvolution in Figure 7l is almost perfect. This result shows the sensitivity of the learning algorithm in cases where the tap-spacing is great enough (12.5 msec) that simple whitening does not interfere noticeably with the deconvolution process. The deconvolution result, in this case, represents an improvement of the signal-to-noise ratio from −23 to 12 dB. In all cases, convergence was relatively rapid, with these solutions being produced after on the order of 70,000 data points were presented,

[7]An example of the barrel effect is the acoustic echoes heard when someone talks into a "speaker-phone."

which amounts to 2 sec training on 8 sec of speech, amounting to four times as fast as real-time on a Sparc-10.

5.3 Combining Separation and Deconvolution. The blind separation rules in 2.14 and 2.15 and the blind deconvolution rules in 2.23 and 2.24 can be easily combined. The objective then becomes the maximization of the log of a Jacobian with *local* lower triangular structure. This yields exactly the learning rule one would expect: the leading weights in the filters follow the blind separation rules and all the others follow a decorrelation rule similar to 2.24 except that now there are tapped weights w_{ikj} between an input $x_j(t - k)$ and an output $y_i(t)$.

We have performed experiments with speech signals in which signals have been simultaneously separated and deconvolved using these rules. We used mixtures of two signals with convolution filters like those in Figure 7e and 7i, and convergence to separated, deconvolved speech was almost perfect.

6 Discussion

We will consider these techniques first in the context of previous information-theoretic approaches within neural networks, and then in the context of related approaches to "blind" signal processing problems.

6.1 Comparison with Previous Work on Information Maximization. Many authors have formulated optimality criteria similar to ours, for both neural networks and sensory systems (Barlow 1989; Atick 1992; Bialek *et al.* 1991). However, our work is most similar to that of Linsker, who in 1989 proposed an "infomax" principle for linear mappings with various forms of noise. Linsker (1992) derived a learning algorithm for maximizing the mutual information between two layers of a network. This "infomax" criterion is the same as ours (see 2.1). However, the problem as formulated here is different in the following respects:

1. There is no noise, or rather, there is no noise *model* in this system.
2. There is no assumption that inputs or outputs have gaussian statistics.
3. The transfer function is in general nonlinear.

These differences lead to quite a different learning rule. Linsker's 1992 rule uses (for input signal X and output Y) a Hebbian term to maximize $H(Y)$ when the network receives both signal and noise, an anti-Hebbian term to minimize $H(Y \mid X)$ when the system receives only noise, and an anti-Hebbian lateral interaction to decorrelate the outputs Y. When the network is deterministic, however, the $H(Y \mid X)$ term does not contribute. A deterministic linear network can increase its information throughput without bound, as the $[\mathbf{W}^T]^{-1}$ term in 2.14 suggests.

However, the information capacity in the networks we have considered *is* bounded, not by noise, but by the saturation of a squashing function. Our network shares with Linsker's the property that this bound gives rise to an anti-Hebbian term in the learning rule. This is true for various squashing functions (see Table 1 in the Appendix).

This nonlinear, non-gaussian, deterministic formulation of the "infomax" problem leads to more powerful algorithms, since, as demonstrated, the nonlinear function enables the network to compute with non-gaussian statistics, and find higher-order forms of redundancy inherent in the inputs. (As emphasized in Section 3, linear approaches are inadequate for solving the problems of blind separation and blind deconvolution.) These observations also apply to the approaches of Atick and Redlich (1993) and Bialek *et al.* 1991).

The problem of information maximization through nonlinear sigmoidal neurons has been considered before without a learning rule actually being proposed. Schraudolph *et al.* (1991), in work that inspired this approach, considered it as a method for initializing weights in a neural network. Before this, Laughlin (1981) used it to characterize as optimal, the exact contrast sensitivity curves of interneurons in the insect's compound eye. Various other authors have considered unsupervised learning rules for nonlinear units, without justifying them in terms of information theory (see Karhunen and Joutsensalo 1994, and references therein).

Several recent papers, however, have touched closely on the work presented in this paper. Deco and Brauer (1995) use cumulant expansions to approximate mutual information between outputs. Parra and Deco (1995) use symplectic transforms to train *nonlinear* information-preserving mappings. Most notably, Baram and Roth (1994) perform substantially the same analysis as ours, but apply their networks to probability density estimation and time series forecasting. None of this work was known to us when we developed our approach.

Finally, another group of information-theoretic algorithms has been proposed by Becker and Hinton (1992). These employ nonlinear networks to *maximize* mutual information between different sets of outputs. This *increasing* of redundancy enables the network to discover invariants in separate groups of inputs (see also Schraudolph and Sejnowski 1992). This is, in a sense, the opposite of our objective, though some way may be found to view the two in the same light.

6.2 Comparison with Previous Work on Blind Separation. As indicated in Section 3, approaches to blind separation and blind deconvolution have divided into those using nonlinear functions (Jutten and Herault 1991; Bellini 1994) and those using explicit calculations of cumulants and polyspectra (Comon 1994; Hatzinakos and Nikias 1994). We have shown that an information maximization approach can provide a theoretical framework for approaches of the former type.

In the case of blind separation, the architecture of our $N \to N$ network, although it is a feedforward network, maps directly onto that of the recurrent Herault–Jutten network. The relationship between our weight matrix, $\mathbf{W}$, and the H-J recurrent weight matrix, $\mathbf{W_{HJ}}$, can be written as $\mathbf{W} = (\mathbf{I} + \mathbf{W_{HJ}})^{-1}$, where $\mathbf{I}$ is the identity matrix. From this we may write

$$\Delta \mathbf{W_{HJ}} = \Delta \left(\mathbf{W}^{-1} \right) = \left(\mathbf{W}^{-1} \right) \Delta \mathbf{W} \left(\mathbf{W}^{-1} \right) \tag{6.1}$$

so that our learning rule, 2.14 forms part of a rule for the recurrent H-J network. Unfortunately, this rule is complex and not obviously related to the nonlinear anti-Hebbian rule proposed for the H-J net:

$$\Delta \mathbf{W_{HJ}} \propto -g(\mathbf{u})h(\mathbf{u})^T \tag{6.2}$$

where g and h are odd nonlinear functions. It remains to conduct a detailed performance comparison between 6.2 and the algorithm presented here. We have performed many simulations in which the H-J net failed to converge, but because there is substantial freedom in the choice of g and h in 6.2, we cannot be sure that our choices were good ones.

We now compare the convergence criteria of the two algorithms to show how they are related. The explanation (Jutten and Herault 1991) for the success of the H-J network is that the Taylor series expansion of $g(\mathbf{u})h(\mathbf{u})^T$ in 6.2 yields odd cross moments, such that the weights stop changing when

$$\sum_{i,j} b_{ijpq} \langle u_i^{2p+1} u_j^{2q+1} \rangle = 0 \tag{6.3}$$

for all output unit pairs $i \neq j$, for $p, q = 0, 1, 2, 3 \ldots$, and for the coefficients b_{ijpq} coming from the Taylor series expansion of g and h. This, they argue, provides an "approximation of an independence test."

This can be compared with the convergence criterion of our algorithm. For the tanh nonlinearity, we derive

$$\Delta \mathbf{W} \propto \left[\mathbf{W}^T \right]^{-1} - 2\mathbf{y}\mathbf{x}^T \tag{6.4}$$

This converges in the mean (ignoring bias weights and assuming $\mathbf{x}$ to be zero mean) when:

$$\left[\mathbf{W}^T \right]^{-1} = 2 \langle \tanh(\mathbf{Wx})\mathbf{x}^T \rangle \tag{6.5}$$

This condition can be readily rewritten (multiplying it by $\mathbf{W}^T$ and using $\mathbf{u} = \mathbf{Wx}$) as

$$\mathbf{I} = 2 \langle \tanh(\mathbf{u})\mathbf{u}^T \rangle \tag{6.6}$$

Since tanh is an odd function, its series expansion is of the form $\tanh(u) = \sum_j b_j u^{2p+1}$, the b_j being coefficients, and thus the convergence criterion 6.6

amounts to the condition

$$\sum_{i,j} b_{ijp} \langle u_i^{2p+1} u_j \rangle = 0 \qquad (6.7)$$

for all output unit pairs $i \neq j$, for $p = 0, 1, 2, 3 \ldots$, and for the coefficients b_{ijp} coming from the Taylor series expansion of the tanh function.

The convergence criterion 6.7 involves fewer cross-moments than that of 6.3 and in this sense may be viewed as a less restrictive condition. More relevant, however, is the fact that the weighting, or relative importance, b_{ijp}, of the moments in 6.7 is determined by the information-theoretic objective function in conjunction with the nonlinear function g, while in 6.3, the b_{ijpq} values are accidents of the particular nonlinear functions, g and h, that we choose. These observations may help to explain the existence of spurious solutions for H-J, as revealed, for example, in the stability analysis of Sorouchyari (1991).

Several other approaches to blind separation exist. Comon (1994) expands the mutual information in terms of cumulants up to order 4, amounting to a truncation of the constraints in 6.7. A similar proposal that combines separation with deconvolution is to be found in Yellin and Weinstein (1994). Such cumulant-based methods seem to work, though they are complex. It is not clear how the truncation of the expansion affects the solution. In addition, Molgedey and Schuster (1994) proposed a novel technique that uses time-delayed correlations to constrain the solution. Finally, Hopfield (1991) has applied a variant of the H-J architecture to odor separation in a model of the olfactory bulb.

6.3 Comparison with Previous Work on Blind Deconvolution. In the case of blind deconvolution, our approach most resembles the "Bussgang" family of techniques (Bellini 1994; Haykin 1991). These algorithms assume some knowledge about the input distributions to sculpt a nonlinearity that may be used in the creation of a memoryless conditional estimator for the input signal. In our notation, the nonlinearly transformed output, y, is exactly this conditional estimator:

$$y = g(u) = E[s \mid u] \qquad (6.8)$$

and the goal of the system is to change weights until u, the actual output, is the same as y, our estimate of s. An error is thus defined, $error = y - u$, and a stochastic weight update rule follows directly from gradient descent in mean-squared error. This gives the blind deconvolution rule for a tapped delay weight at time t [compare with 2.24]:

$$\Delta w_{L-j}(t) \propto x_{t-j}(y_t - u_t) \qquad (6.9)$$

If $g(u) = \tanh(u)$ then this rule is very similar to 2.24. The only difference is that 2.24 contains the term $\tanh(u)$ where 6.9 has the term $u - \tanh(u)$, but as can be easily verified, these terms are of the same sign at all times, so the algorithms should behave similarly.

The theoretical justifications for the Bussgang approaches are, however, a little obscure, and, as with the Herault–Jutten rules, part of their appeal derives from the fact that they have been shown to work in many circumstances. The primary difficulty lies in the consideration, 6.8, of y as a conditional estimator for s. Why, a priori, should we consider a nonlinearly transformed output to be a conditional estimator for the unconvolved input? The answer comes from Bayesian considerations. The output, u, is considered to be a noisy version of the original signal, s. Models of the pdf's of the original signal and this noise are then constructed, and Bayesian reasoning yields a nonlinear conditional estimator of s from u, which can be quite complex (see 20.39 in Haykin 1991). It is not clear, however, that the "noise" introduced by the convolving filter, a, is well modeled as gaussian. Nor will we generally have justifiable estimates of its mean and variance, and how they compare with the means and variances of the input, s.

In short, the selection of a nonlinearity, g, is a black art. Haykin does note, though, that in the limit of high convolutional noise, g can be well approximated by the tanh sigmoid nonlinearity (see 20.44 in Haykin 1991), exactly the nonlinearity we have been using. Could it be that the success of the Bussgang approaches using Bayesian conditional estimators is due less to the exact form of the conditional estimator than to the general goal of squeezing as much information as possible through a sigmoid function? As noted, a similarity exists between the information maximization rule 2.24, derived without any Bayesian modeling, and the Bussgang rule 6.9 when convolutional noise levels are high. This suggests that the higher-order moments and information maximization properties may be the important factors in blind deconvolution, rather than the minimization of a contrived error measure, and its justification in terms of estimation theory.

Finally, we note that the idea of using a variable-slope sigmoid function for blind deconvolution was first described in Haykin (1992).

6.4 Conclusion. In their current forms, the algorithms presented here are limited. First, since only single layer networks are used, the optimal mappings discovered are constrained to be linear, while some multilayer system could be more powerful. With layers of hidden units, the Jacobian in 2.13 becomes more complicated, as do the learning rules derived from it. Second, the networks require, for N inputs, that there be N outputs, which makes them unable to perform the computationally useful tasks of dimensionality reduction or optimal data compression. Third, realistic acoustic environments are characterized by substantial propagation delays. As a result, blind separation techniques without adaptive time delays do not work for speech recorded in a natural environment. An approach to this problem using "beamforming" may be found in Li and Sejnowski (1994). Fourth, no account has yet been given for cases where there is known noise in the inputs. The beginning of such an analysis may be found in Nadal and Parga (1995) and Schuster (1992), and it may be possible to define learning rules for such cases.

Finally, and most seriously from a biological point of view, the learning rule in equation 2.16 is decidedly nonlocal. Each "neuron" must know the cofactors either of all the weights entering it, or all those leaving it. Some architectural trick may be found that enables information maximization to take place using only local information. The existence of local learning rules such as the H-J network suggests that it may be possible to develop local learning rules approximating the nonlocal ones derived here. For now, however, the network learning rule in 2.14 remains unbiological.

Despite these concerns, we believe that the information maximization approach presented here could serve as a unifying framework that brings together several lines of research, and as a guiding principle for further advances. The principles may also be applied to other sensory modalities such as vision, where Field (1994) has recently argued that phase-insensitive information maximization (using only second-order statistics) is unable to predict local (non-Fourier) receptive fields.

Appendix: Proof of Learning Rule (2.14)

Consider a network with an input vector $\mathbf{x}$, a weight matrix $\mathbf{W}$, a bias vector $\mathbf{w}_0$, and a nonlinearly transformed output vector $\mathbf{y} = g(\mathbf{u})$, $\mathbf{u} = \mathbf{W}\mathbf{x} + \mathbf{w}_0$. Providing $\mathbf{W}$ is a square matrix and g is an invertible function, the multivariate probability density function of $\mathbf{y}$ can be written (Papoulis 1984, eq. 6-63):

$$f_y(\mathbf{y}) = \frac{f_x(\mathbf{x})}{|J|} \tag{A.1}$$

where $|J|$ is the absolute value of the Jacobian of the transformation. This simplifies to the product of the determinant of the weight matrix and the derivatives, y'_i, of the outputs, y_i, with respect to their net inputs:

$$J = (\det \mathbf{W}) \prod_{i=1}^{N} y'_i \tag{A.2}$$

For example, in the case where the nonlinearity is the logistic sigmoid,

$$y_i = \frac{1}{1 + e^{-u_i}} \quad \text{and} \quad y'_i = \frac{\partial y_i}{\partial u_i} = y_i(1 - y_i) \tag{A.3}$$

We can perform gradient ascent in the information that the outputs transmit about inputs by noting that the information gradient is the same as the entropy gradient 2.2 for invertible deterministic mappings. The joint entropy of the outputs is

$$\begin{aligned} H(\mathbf{y}) &= -E[\ln f_y(\mathbf{y})] & \tag{A.4} \\ &= E[\ln |J|] - E[\ln f_x(\mathbf{x})] \quad \text{from A.1} & \tag{A.5} \end{aligned}$$

Table 1: Different Nonlinearities, $g(u_i)$, Give Different Slopes and Anti-Hebbian Terms That Appear When Deriving Information Maximization Rules Using equation A.6.

	Function: $y_i = g(u_i)$	Slope: $y_i' = \dfrac{\partial y_i}{\partial u_i}$	Anti-Hebb term: $\dfrac{\partial}{\partial w_{ij}} \ln |y_i'|$
A	$\dfrac{1}{1+e^{-u_i}}$	$y_i(1-y_i)$	$x_j(1-2y_i)$
B	$\tanh(u_i)$	$1-y_i^2$	$-2x_jy_i$
C	$\arctan(u_i)$	$\dfrac{1}{1+u_i^2}$	$-\dfrac{2x_ju_i}{1+u_i^2}$
D	$\text{erf}(u_i)$	$\dfrac{2}{\sqrt{\pi}}e^{-u_i^2}$	$-2x_ju_i$
E	$\int_{-\infty}^{u_i} e^{-|v|^r}\,dv$	$e^{-|u_i|^r}$	$-rx_j|u_i|^{r-1}\text{sgn}(u_i)$
F	$\int_{-\infty}^{u_i}(1-|g(v)|^r)\,dv$	$1-|y_i|^r$	$-rx_j|y_i|^{r-1}\text{sgn}(y_i)$
G	$e^{-u_i^2}$	$-2u_iy_i$	$x_j\dfrac{1+2u_i^2}{u_i}$

Weights can be adjusted to maximize $H(\mathbf{y})$. As before, they only affect the $E[\ln |J|]$ term above, and thus, substituting A.2 into A.5:

$$\Delta\mathbf{W} \propto \frac{\partial H}{\partial \mathbf{W}} = \frac{\partial}{\partial \mathbf{W}}\ln|J| = \frac{\partial}{\partial \mathbf{W}}\ln|\det\mathbf{W}| + \frac{\partial}{\partial \mathbf{W}}\ln\prod_i |y_i'| \qquad (A.6)$$

The first term is the same regardless of the transfer function, and since $\det\mathbf{W} = \sum_j w_{ij}\operatorname{cof} w_{ij}$ for any row i ($\operatorname{cof} w_{ij}$ being the cofactor of w_{ij}), we have, for a single weight:

$$\frac{\partial}{\partial w_{ij}}\ln|\det\mathbf{W}| = \frac{\operatorname{cof} w_{ij}}{\det\mathbf{W}} \qquad (A.7)$$

For the full weight matrix, we use the definition of the inverse of a matrix, and the fact that the *adjoint* matrix, $\operatorname{adj}\mathbf{W}$, is the transpose of the matrix of cofactors. This gives

$$\frac{\partial}{\partial \mathbf{W}}\ln|\det\mathbf{W}| = \frac{(\operatorname{adj}\mathbf{W})^T}{\det\mathbf{W}} = \left[\mathbf{W}^T\right]^{-1} \qquad (A.8)$$

For the second term in A.6, we note that the product, $\ln\prod_i y_i'$, splits up into a sum of log-terms, only one of which depends on a particular w_{ij}. The calculation of this dependency proceeds as in the one-to-one mapping of 2.8 and 2.9. Different squashing functions give different forms of anti-Hebbian terms. Some examples are given in Table 1.

Thus, for units computing weighted sums, the information-maximization rule consists of an *anti-redundancy* term, which always has the form of A.8, and an *anti-Hebb* term, which keeps the unit from saturating. □

Several points are worth noting in Table 1:

1. The logistic (A) and tanh (B) functions produce anti-Hebb terms that use higher-order statistics. The other functions use the net input u_i as their output variable, rather than the actual, nonlinearly transformed output y_i. Tests have shown the erf function (D) to be unsuitable for blind separation problems. In fact, it can be shown to converge in the mean when (compare with 6.6) $I = 2\langle \mathbf{u}\mathbf{u}^T \rangle$, showing clearly that it is just a decorrelator.

2. The generalized cumulative gaussian function (E) has a variable exponent, r. This can be varied between 0 and ∞ to produce squashing functions suitable for symmetrical input distributions with very high or low kurtosis. When r is very large, then $g(u_i)$ is suitable for unit input distributions such as those in Figure 4. When close to zero, it fits high kurtosis input distributions, that are peaked with long tails.

3. Analogously, it is possible to define a generalized "tanh" sigmoid (F), of which the hyperbolic tangent (B) is a special case ($r = 2$). The values of function F can in general only be attained by numerical integration (in both directions) of the differential equation, $g'(u) = 1 - |g(u)|^r$, from a boundary condition of $g(0) = 0$. Once this is done, however, and the values are stored in a look-up table, the slope and anti-Hebb terms are easily evaluated at each presentation. Again, as in Section 2.5, it should be useful for data that may have flat ($r > 2$) or peaky ($r < 2$) pdf's.

4. The learning rule for a gaussian radial basis function node (G) shows the unsuitability of nonmonotonic functions for information maximization learning. The u_i term on the denominator would make such learning unstable when the net input to the unit was zero.

Acknowledgments

This research was supported by a grant from the Office of Naval Research. We are much indebted to Nicol Schraudolph, who not only supplied the original idea in Figure 1 and shared his unpublished calculations (Schraudolph *et al.* 1991), but also provided detailed criticism at every stage of the work. Many helpful observations also came from Paul Viola, Barak Pearlmutter, Kenji Doya, Misha Tsodyks, Alexandre Pouget, Peter Dayan, Olivier Coenen, and Iris Ginzburg.

References

Atick, J. J. 1992. Could information theory provide an ecological theory of sensory processing? *Network* **3**, 213–251.

Atick, J. J., and Redlich, A. N. 1993. Convergent algorithm for sensory receptive field development. *Neural Comp.* **5**, 45–60.

Baram, Y., and Roth, Z. 1994. Multi-dimensional density shaping by sigmoidal networks with application to classification, estimation and forecasting. CIS report No. 9420, October 1994, Centre for Intelligent systems, Dept. of Computer Science, Technion, Israel Institute of Technology, Haifa, submitted for publication.

Barlow, H. B. 1961. Possible principles underlying the transformation of sensory messages. In *Sensory Communication*, W. A. Rosenblith, ed., pp. 217–234. MIT Press, Cambridge, MA.

Barlow, H. B. 1989. Unsupervised learning. *Neural Comp.* **1**, 295–311.

Barlow, H. B., and Földiák, P. 1989. Adaptation and decorrelation in the cortex. In *The Computing Neuron*, R. Durbin et al., eds., pp. 54–72. Addison-Wesley, Reading, MA.

Battiti, R. 1992. First- and second-order methods for learning: Between steepest descent and Newton's method. *Neural Comp.* **4**(2), 141–166.

Becker, S., and Hinton, G. E. 1992. A self-organising neural network that discovers surfaces in random-dot stereograms. *Nature (London)* **355**, 161–163.

Bell, A. J., and Sejnowski, T. J. 1995. A nonlinear information maximization algorithm that performs blind separation. In *Advances in Neural Information Processing Systems 7*, G. Tesauro et al., eds., pp. 467–474. MIT Press, Cambridge, MA.

Bellini, S. 1994. Bussgang techniques for blind deconvolution and equalisation. In *Blind Deconvolution*, S. Haykin, ed. Prentice-Hall, Englewood Cliffs, NJ.

Bialek, W., Ruderman, D. L., and Zee, A. 1991. Optimal sampling of natural images: A design principle for the visual system? In *Advances in Neural Information Processing Systems 3*. R. P. Lippmann et al., eds., pp. 363–369. Morgan Kaufmann, San Mateo, CA.

Burel, G. 1992. Blind separation of sources: A nonlinear neural algorithm. *Neural Networks* **5**, 937–947

Cohen, M. H., and Andreou, A. G. 1992. Current-mode subthreshold MOS implementation of the Herault-Jutten autoadaptive network. *IEEE J. Solid-State Circuits* **27**(5), 714–727.

Cohen, M. H., and Andreou, A. G. 1995. Analog CMOS integration and experimentation with an autoadaptive independent component analyzer. *IEEE Trans. Circuits Systems-II: Analog Digital Signal Process.* **42**(2), 65–77.

Comon, P. 1994. Independent component analysis, a new concept? *Signal Process.* **36**, 287–314.

Comon, P., Jutten, C., and Herault, J. 1991. Blind separation of sources, part II: Problems statement. *Signal Process.* **24**, 11–21.

Cover, T. M., and Thomas, J. A. 1991. *Elements of Information Theory.* John Wiley, New York.

Deco, G., and Brauer, W. 1995. Non-linear higher-order statistical decorrelation by volume-conserving neural architectures. *Neural Networks*, in press.

Field, D. J. 1994. What is the goal of sensory coding? *Neural Comp.* **6**, 559–601.

Hatzinakos, D., and Nikias, C. L. 1994. Blind equalisation based on higher-order statistics. In *Blind Deconvolution*, S. Haykin, ed., pp. 181–258. Prentice-Hall, Englewood Cliffs, NJ.

Haykin, S. 1991. *Adaptive Filter Theory*, 2nd ed. Prentice-Hall, Englewood Cliffs, NJ.

Haykin, S. 1992. Blind equalisation formulated as a self-organized learning process. *Proceedings of the 26th Asilomar Conference on Signals, Systems and Computers*. Pacific Grove, CA.

Haykin, S. (ed.) 1994a. *Blind Deconvolution*. Prentice-Hall, Englewood Cliffs, NJ.

Haykin, S. (ed.) 1994b. *Neural Networks: A Comprehensive Foundation*. Macmillan, New York.

Herault, J., and Jutten, C. 1986. Space or time adaptive signal processing by neural network models. In *Neural Networks for Computing: AIP Conference Proceedings 151*, J. S. Denker, ed. American Institute for Physics, New York.

Hopfield, J. J. 1991. Olfactory computation and object perception. *Proc. Natl. Acad. Sci. U.S.A.* **88**, 6462–6466.

Jutten, C., and Herault, J. 1991. Blind separation of sources, part I: An adaptive algorithm based on neuromimetic architecture. *Signal Process.* **24**, 1–10.

Karhunen, J., and Joutsensalo, J. 1994. Representation and separation of signals using nonlinear PCA type learning. *Neural Networks* **7**(1), 113–127.

Laughlin, S. 1981. A simple coding procedure enhances a neuron's information capacity. *Z. Naturforsch.* **36**, 910–912.

Li, S., and Sejnowski, T. J. 1994. Adaptive separation of mixed broadband sound sources with delays by a beamforming Herault-Jutten network. *IEEE J. Oceanic Eng.* **20**(1), 73–79.

Linsker, R. 1989. An application of the principle of maximum information preservation to linear systems. In *Advances in Neural Information Processing Systems 1*, D. S. Touretzky, ed. Morgan Kaufmann, San Mateo, CA.

Linsker, R. 1992. Local synaptic learning rules suffice to maximize mutual information in a linear network. *Neural Comp.* **4**, 691–702.

Molgedey, L., and Schuster, H. G. 1994. Separation of independent signals using time-delayed correlations. *Phys. Rev. Lett.* **72**(23), 3634–3637.

Nadal, J-P., and Parga, N. 1994. Non-linear neurons in the low noise limit: A factorial code maximizes information transfer. *Network* **5**, 565–581.

Papoulis, A. 1984. *Probability, Random Variables and Stochastic Processes*, 2nd ed. McGraw-Hill, New York.

Parra, L., Deco, G., and Miesbach, S. 1995. Redundancy reduction with information-preserving maps. *Network* **6**, 61–72.

Platt, J. C., and Faggin, F. 1992. Networks for the separation of sources that are superimposed and delayed. In *Advances in Neural Information Processing Systems 4*. J. E. Moody et al., eds., pp. 730–737. Morgan Kaufmann, San Mateo, CA.

Plumbley, M. D., and Fallside, F. 1988. An information-theoretic approach to unsupervised connectionist models. In *Proceedings of the 1988 Connectionist Models Summer School*, 239–245. D. Touretzky, G. Hinton, and T. Sejnowski, eds. Morgan Kaufmann, San Mateo, CA.

Schmidhuber, J. 1992. Learning factorial codes by predictability minimization. *Neural Comp.* **4**(6), 863–887.

Schraudolph, N. N., and Sejnowski, T. J. 1992. Competitive anti-Hebbian learning of invariants. In *Advances in Neural Information Processing Systems 4*, J. E. Moody et al., eds. Morgan Kaufmann, San Mateo, CA.

Schraudolph, N. N., Hart, W. E., and Belew, R. K. 1991. Optimal information flow in sigmoidal neurons. Unpublished manuscript.

Schuster, H. G. 1992. Learning by maximizing the information transfer through nonlinear noisy neurons and "noise breakdown", *Phys. Rev. A* **46**(4), 2131–2138.

Sorouchyari, E. 1991. Blind separation of sources, part III: Stability analysis. *Signal Process.* **24**(1), 11–20.

Vittoz, E. A., and Arreguit, X. 1989. CMOS integration of Herault-Jutten cells for separation of sources. In *Analog VLSI Implementation of Neural Systems*, 57–84. C. Mead and M. Ismail, eds. Kluwer, Boston.

Yellin, D., and Weinstein, E. 1994. Criteria for multichannel signal separation. *IEEE Trans. Signal Process.* **42**(8), 2158–2168.

9

Natural Gradient Works Efficiently in Learning

Shun-ichi Amari
RIKEN Frontier Research Program, Saitama 351-01, Japan

When a parameter space has a certain underlying structure, the ordinary gradient of a function does not represent its steepest direction, but the natural gradient does. Information geometry is used for calculating the natural gradients in the parameter space of perceptrons, the space of matrices (for blind source separation), and the space of linear dynamical systems (for blind source deconvolution). The dynamical behavior of natural gradient online learning is analyzed and is proved to be Fisher efficient, implying that it has asymptotically the same performance as the optimal batch estimation of parameters. This suggests that the plateau phenomenon, which appears in the backpropagation learning algorithm of multilayer perceptrons, might disappear or might not be so serious when the natural gradient is used. An adaptive method of updating the learning rate is proposed and analyzed.

1 Introduction

The stochastic gradient method (Widrow, 1963; Amari, 1967; Tsypkin, 1973; Rumelhart, Hinton, & Williams, 1986) is a popular learning method in the general nonlinear optimization framework. The parameter space is not Euclidean but has a Riemannian metric structure in many cases. In these cases, the ordinary gradient does not give the steepest direction of a target function; rather, the steepest direction is given by the natural (or contravariant) gradient. The Riemannian metric structures are introduced by means of information geometry (Amari, 1985; Murray and Rice, 1993; Amari, 1997a; Amari, Kurata, & Nagoska, 1992). This article gives the natural gradients explicitly in the case of the space of perceptrons for neural learning, the space of matrices for blind source separation, and the space of linear dynamical systems for blind multichannel source deconvolution. This is an extended version of an earlier article (Amari, 1996), including new results.

How good is natural gradient learning compared to conventional gradient learning? The asymptotic behavior of online natural gradient learning is studied for this purpose. Training examples can be used only once in online learning when they appear. Therefore, the asymptotic performance of online learning cannot be better than the optimal batch procedure where all the examples can be reused again and again. However, we prove that natural gradient online learning gives the Fisher-efficient estimator in the sense of asymptotic statistics when the loss function is differentiable, so that it is asymptotically equivalent to the optimal batch procedure (see also Amari, 1995; Opper, 1996). When the loss function is nondifferentiable, the accuracy of asymptotic online learning is worse than batch learning by a factor of 2 (see, for example, Van den Broeck & Reimann, 1996). It was shown in Amari et al. (1992) that the dynamic behavior of natural gradient in the Boltzmann machine is excellent.

It is not easy to calculate the natural gradient explicitly in multilayer perceptrons. However, a preliminary analysis (Yang & Amari, 1997), by using a simple model, shows that the performance of natural gradient learning is remarkably good, and it is sometimes free from being trapped in plateaus, which give rise to slow convergence of the backpropagation learning method (Saad & Solla, 1995). This suggests that the Riemannian structure might eliminate such plateaus or might make them not so serious.

Online learning is flexible, because it can track slow fluctuations of the target. Such online dynamics were first analyzed in Amari (1967) and then by many researchers recently. Sompolinsky, Barkai, and Seung (1995), and Barkai, Seung, and Sompolinsky (1995) proposed an adaptive method of adjusting the learning rate (see also Amari, 1967). We generalize their idea and evaluate its performance based on the Riemannian metric of errors.

The article is organized as follows. The natural gradient is defined in section 2. Section 3 formulates the natural gradient in various problems of stochastic descent learning. Section 4 gives the statistical analysis of efficiency of online learning, and section 5 is devoted to the problem of adaptive changes in the learning rate. Calculations of the Riemannian metric and explicit forms of the natural gradients are given in sections 6, 7, and 8.

2 Natural Gradient

Let $S = \{w \in R^n\}$ be a parameter space on which a function $L(w)$ is defined. When S is a Euclidean space with an orthonormal coordinate system w, the squared length of a small incremental vector dw connecting w and $w + dw$ is given by

$$|dw|^2 = \sum_{i=1}^{n}(dw_i)^2,$$

where dw_i are the components of dw. However, when the coordinate system is nonorthonormal, the squared length is given by the quadratic form

$$|dw|^2 = \sum_{i,j} g_{ij}(w)dw_i dw_j. \tag{2.1}$$

When S is a curved manifold, there is no orthonormal linear coordinates, and the length of dw is always written as in equation 2.1. Such a space is a Riemannian space. We show in later sections that parameter spaces of neural networks have the Riemannian character. The $n \times n$ matrix $G = (g_{ij})$ is called the Riemannian metric tensor, and it depends in general on w. It reduces to

$$g_{ij}(w) = \delta_{ij} = \begin{cases} 1, & i = j, \\ 0, & i \neq j \end{cases}$$

in the Euclidean orthonormal case, so that G is the unit matrix I in this case.

The steepest descent direction of a function $L(w)$ at w is defined by the vector dw that minimizes $L(w + dw)$ where $|dw|$ has a fixed length, that is, under the constraint

$$|dw|^2 = \varepsilon^2 \tag{2.2}$$

for a sufficiently small constant ε.

Theorem 1. *The steepest descent direction of $L(w)$ in a Riemannian space is given by*

$$-\tilde{\nabla}L(w) = -G^{-1}(w)\nabla L(w) \tag{2.3}$$

where $G^{-1} = (g^{ij})$ is the inverse of the metric $G = (g_{ij})$ and ∇L is the conventional gradient,

$$\nabla L(w) = \left(\frac{\partial}{\partial w_1} L(w), \ldots, \frac{\partial}{\partial w_n} L(w) \right)^T,$$

the superscript T denoting the transposition.

Proof.   We put

$$dw = \varepsilon a,$$

and search for the a that minimizes

$$L(w + dw) = L(w) + \varepsilon \nabla L(w)^T a$$

under the constraint

$$|a|^2 = \sum g_{ij} a_i a_j = 1.$$

By the Lagrangean method, we have

$$\frac{\partial}{\partial a_i} \{ \nabla L(w)^T a - \lambda a^T G a \} = 0.$$

This gives

$$\nabla L(w) = 2\lambda Ga$$

or

$$a = \frac{1}{2\lambda} G^{-1} \nabla L(w),$$

where λ is determined from the constraint.

We call

$$\tilde{\nabla} L(w) = G^{-1} \nabla L(w)$$

the natural gradient of L in the Riemannian space. Thus, $-\tilde{\nabla} L$ represents the steepest descent direction of L. (If we use the tensorial notation, this is nothing but the contravariant form of $-\nabla L$.) When the space is Euclidean and the coordinate system is orthonormal, we have

$$\tilde{\nabla} L = \nabla L. \tag{2.4}$$

This suggests the natural gradient descent algorithm of the form

$$w_{t+1} = w_t - \eta_t \tilde{\nabla} L(w_t), \tag{2.5}$$

where η_t is the learning rate that determines the step size.

3 Natural Gradient Learning

Let us consider an information source that generates a sequence of independent random variables $z_1, z_2, \ldots, z_t, \ldots$, subject to the same probability distribution $q(z)$. The random signals z_t are processed by a processor (like a neural network) that has a set of adjustable parameters w. Let $l(z, w)$ be a loss function when signal z is processed by the processor whose parameter is w. Then the risk function or the average loss is

$$L(w) = E[l(z, w)], \tag{3.1}$$

where E denotes the expectation with respect to z. Learning is a procedure to search for the optimal w^* that minimizes $L(w)$.

The stochastic gradient descent learning method can be formulated in general as

$$w_{t+1} = w_t - \eta_t C(w_t) \nabla l(z_t, w_t), \tag{3.2}$$

where η_t is a learning rate that may depend on t and $C(w)$ is a suitably chosen positive definite matrix (see Amari, 1967). In the natural gradient online learning method, it is proposed to put $C(w)$ equal to $G^{-1}(w)$ when the Riemannian structure is defined. We give a number of examples to be studied in more detail.

3.1 Statistical Estimation of Probability Density Function. In the case of statistical estimation, we assume a statistical model $\{p(z, w)\}$, and the problem is to obtain the probability distribution $p(z, \hat{w})$ that approximates the unknown density function $q(z)$ in the best way—that is, to estimate the true w or to obtain the optimal approximation w from the observed data. A typical loss function is

$$l(z, w) = -\log p(z, w). \tag{3.3}$$

The expected loss is then given by

$$\begin{aligned} L(w) &= -E[\log p(z, w)] \\ &= E_q\left[\log \frac{q(z)}{p(z, w)}\right] + H_Z, \end{aligned}$$

where H_Z is the entropy of $q(z)$ not depending on w. Hence, minimizing L is equivalent to minimizing the Kullback-Leibler divergence

$$D[q(z) : p(z, w)] = \int q(z) \log \frac{q(z)}{p(z, w)} dz \tag{3.4}$$

of two probability distributions $q(z)$ and $p(z, w)$. When the true distribution $q(z)$ is written as $q(z) = p(z, w^*)$, this is equivalent to obtain the maximum likelihood estimator $\hat{w}$.

The Riemannian structure of the parameter space of a statistical model is defined by the Fisher information (Rao, 1945; Amari, 1985)

$$g_{ij}(w) = E\left[\frac{\partial \log p(x, w)}{\partial w_i} \frac{\partial \log p(x, w)}{\partial w_j}\right] \tag{3.5}$$

in the component form. This is the only invariant metric to be given to the statistical model (Chentsov, 1972; Campbell, 1985; Amari, 1985). The learning equation (see equation 3.2) gives a sequential estimator $\hat{w}_t$.

3.2 Multilayer Neural Network. Let us consider a multilayer feedforward neural network specified by a vector parameter $w = (w_1, \ldots, w_n)^T \in R^n$. The parameter w is composed of modifiable connection weights and thresholds. When input x is applied, the network processes it and calculates the outputs $f(x, w)$. The input x is subject to an unknown probability distribution $q(x)$. Let us consider a teacher network that, by receiving x, generates the corresponding output y subject to a conditional probability distribution $q(y \mid x)$. The task is to obtain the optimal w^* from examples such that the student network approximates the behavior of the teacher.

Let us denote by $l(x, w)$ a loss when input signal x is processed by a network having parameter w. A typical loss is given,

$$l(x, y, w) = \frac{1}{2}|y - f(x, w)|^2, \tag{3.6}$$

where y is the output given by the teacher.

Let us consider a statistical model of neural networks such that its output y is given by a noisy version of $f(x, w)$,

$$y = f(x, w) + n, \tag{3.7}$$

where n is a multivariate gaussian noise with zero mean and unit covariance matrix I. By putting $z = (x, y)$, which is an input-output pair, the model specifies the probability density of z as

$$p(z, w) = cq(x) \exp\left\{-\frac{1}{2}|y - f(x, w)|^2\right\}, \tag{3.8}$$

where c is a normalizing constant and the loss function (see equation 3.6) is rewritten as

$$l(z, w) = \text{const} + \log q(x) - \log p(z, w). \tag{3.9}$$

Given a sequence of examples $(x_1, y_1), \ldots, (x_t, y_t), \ldots$, the natural gradient online learning algorithm is written as

$$w_{t+1} = w_t - \eta_t \tilde{\nabla} l(x_t, y_t, w_t). \tag{3.10}$$

Information geometry (Amari, 1985) shows that the Riemannian structure is given to the parameter space of multilayer networks by the Fisher information matrix,

$$g_{ij}(w) = E\left[\frac{\partial \log p(x, y; w)}{\partial w_i} \frac{\partial p(x, y; w)}{\partial w_j}\right]. \tag{3.11}$$

We will show how to calculate $G = (g_{ij})$ and its inverse in a later section.

3.3 Blind Separation of Sources. Let us consider m signal sources that produce m independent signals $s_i(t)$, $i = 1, \ldots, m$, at discrete times $t = 1, 2, \ldots$. We assume that $s_i(t)$ are independent at different times and that the expectations of s_i are 0. Let $r(s)$ be the joint probability density function of s. Then it is written in the product form

$$r(s) = \prod_{i=1}^{m} r_1(s_1). \tag{3.12}$$

Consider the case where we cannot have direct access to the source signals $s(t)$ but we can observe their m instantaneous mixtures $x(t)$,

$$x(t) = As(t) \tag{3.13}$$

or

$$x_i(t) = \sum_{j=1}^{m} A_{ij}s_j(t),$$

where $A = (A_{ij})$ is an $m \times m$ nonsingular mixing matrix that does not depend on t, and $x = (x_1, \ldots, x_m)^T$ is the observed mixtures.

Blind source separation is the problem of recovering the original signals $s(t)$, $t = 1, 2, \ldots$ from the observed signals $x(t)$, $t = 1, 2, \ldots$ (Jutten & Hérault, 1991). If we know A, this is trivial, because we have

$$s(t) = A^{-1}x(t).$$

The "blind" implies that we do not know the mixing matrix A and the probability distribution densities $r_i(s_i)$.

A typical algorithm to solve the problem is to transform $x(t)$ into

$$y(t) = W_t x(t), \tag{3.14}$$

where W_t is an estimate of A^{-1}. It is modified by the following learning equation:

$$W_{t+1} = W_t - \eta_t F(x_t, W_t). \tag{3.15}$$

Here, $F(x, W)$ is a special matrix function satisfying

$$E[F(x, W)] = 0 \tag{3.16}$$

for any density functions $r(s)$ in equation 3.12 when $W = A^{-1}$. For W_t of equation 3.15 to converge to A^{-1}, equation 3.16 is necessary but not sufficient, because the stability of the equilibrium is not considered here.

Let $K(W)$ be an operator that maps a matrix to a matrix. Then

$$\tilde{F}(x, W) = K(W)F(x, W)$$

satisfies equation 3.16 when F does. The equilibrium of F and $\tilde{F}$ is the same, but their stability can be different. However, the natural gradient does not alter the stability of an equilibrium, because G^{-1} is positive-definite.

Let $l(x, W)$ be a loss function whose expectation

$$L(W) = E[l(x, W)]$$

is the target function minimized at $W = A^{-1}$. A typical function F is obtained by the gradient of l with respect to W,

$$F(x, W) = \nabla l(x, W). \tag{3.17}$$

Such an F is also obtained by heuristic arguments. Amari and Cardoso (in press) gave the complete family of F satisfying equation 3.16 and elucidated the statistical efficiency of related algorithms.

From the statistical point of view, the problem is to estimate $W = A^{-1}$ from observed data $x(1), \ldots, x(t)$. However, the probability density function of x is written as

$$p_X(x; W, r) = |W|r(Wx), \tag{3.18}$$

which is specified not only by W to be estimated but also by an unknown function r of the form 3.12. Such a statistical model is said to be semiparametric and is a difficult problem to solve (Bickel, Klassen, Ritov, & Wellner, 1993), because it includes an unknown function of infinite degrees of freedom. However, we can apply the information-geometrical theory of estimating functions (Amari & Kawanabe, 1997) to this problem.

When F is given by the gradient of a loss function (see equation 3.17), where ∇ is the gradient $\partial/\partial W$ with respect to a matrix, the natural gradient is given by

$$\tilde{\nabla} l = G^{-1} \circ \nabla l. \tag{3.19}$$

Here, G is an operator transforming a matrix to a matrix so that it is an $m^2 \times m^2$ matrix. G is the metric given to the space $Gl(m)$ of all the nonsingular $m \times m$ matrices. We give its explicit form in a later section based on the Lie group structure. The inverse of G is also given explicitly. Another important problem is the stability of the equilibrium of the learning dynamics. This has recently been solved by using the Riemannian structure (Amari, Chen, & Chichocki, in press; see also Cardoso & Laheld, 1996). The superefficiency of some algorithms has been also proved in Amari (1997b) under certain conditions.

3.4 Blind Source Deconvolution. When the original signals $s(t)$ are mixed not only instantaneously but also with past signals as well, the problem is called blind source deconvolution or equalization. By introducing the time delay operator z^{-1},

$$z^{-1}s(t) = s(t-1), \tag{3.20}$$

we have a mixing matrix filter A denoted by

$$A(z) = \sum_{k=0}^{\infty} A_k z^{-k}, \tag{3.21}$$

where A_k are $m \times m$ matrices. The observed mixtures are

$$x(t) = A(z)s(t) = \sum_k A_k s(t-k). \tag{3.22}$$

To recover the original independent sources, we use the finite impulse response model

$$W(z) = \sum_{k=0}^{d} W_k z^{-1} \tag{3.23}$$

of degree d. The original signals are recovered by

$$y(t) = W_t(z)x(t), \tag{3.24}$$

where W_t is adaptively modified by

$$W_{t+1}(z) = W_t(z) - \eta_t \nabla l\{x_t, x_{t-1}, \dots, W_t(z)\}. \tag{3.25}$$

Here, $l(x_t, x_{t-1}, \dots, W)$ is a loss function that includes some past signals. We can summarize the past signals into a current state variable in the on-line learning algorithm. Such a loss function is obtained by the maximum entropy method (Bell & Sejnowski, 1995), independent component analysis (Comon, 1994), or the statistical likelihood method.

In order to obtain the natural gradient learning algorithm

$$W_{t+1}(z) = W_t(z) - \eta_t \tilde{\nabla} l(x_t, x_{t-1}, \dots, W_t),$$

we need to define the Riemannian metric in the space of all the matrix filters (multiterminal linear systems). Such a study was initiated by Amari (1987). It is possible to define G and to obtain G^{-1} explicitly (see section 8). A preliminary investigation into the performance of the natural gradient learning algorithm has been undertaken by Douglas, Chichocki, and Amari (1996) and Amari et al. (1997).

4 Natural Gradient Gives Fisher-Efficient Online Learning Algorithms

This section studies the accuracy of natural gradient learning from the statistical point of view. A statistical estimator that gives asymptotically the best result is said to be Fisher efficient. We prove that natural gradient learning attains Fisher efficiency.

Let us consider multilayer perceptrons as an example. We study the case of a realizable teacher, that is, the behavior of the teacher is given by $q(y \mid x) = p(y \mid x, w^*)$. Let $D_T = \{(x_1, y_1), \ldots, (x_T, y_T)\}$ be T-independent input-output examples generated by the teacher network having parameter w^*. Then, minimizing the log loss,

$$l(x, y; w) = -\log p(x, y; w),$$

over the training data D_T is to obtain $\hat{w}_T$ that minimizes the training error

$$L_{\text{train}}(w) = \frac{1}{T} \sum_{t=1}^{T} l(x_t, y_t; w). \qquad (4.1)$$

This is equivalent to maximizing the likelihood $\prod_{t=1}^{T} p(x_t, y_t; w)$. Hence, $\hat{w}_T$ is the maximum likelihood estimator. The Cramér-Rao theorem states that the expected squared error of an unbiased estimator satisfies

$$E[(\hat{w}_T - w^*)(\hat{w}_T - w^*)^T] \geq \frac{1}{T} G^{-1}, \qquad (4.2)$$

where the inequality holds in the sense of positive definiteness of matrices. An estimator is said to be efficient or Fisher efficient when it satisfies equation 4.2 with equality for large T. The maximum likelihood estimator is Fisher efficient, implying that it is the best estimator attaining the Cramér-Rao bound asymptotically,

$$\lim_{T \to \infty} T E[(\hat{w}_T - w^*)(\hat{w}_T - w^*)^T] = G^{-1}, \qquad (4.3)$$

where G^{-1} is the inverse of the Fisher information matrix $G = (g_{ij})$ defined by equation 3.11.

Examples (x_1, y_1), $(x_2, y_2) \ldots$ are given one at a time in the case of online learning. Let $\tilde{w}_t$ be an online estimator at time t. At the next time, $t + 1$, the estimator $\tilde{w}_t$ is modified to give a new estimator $\tilde{w}_{t+1}$ based on the current observation (x_t, y_t). The old observations $(x_1, y_1), \ldots, (x_{t-1}, y_{t-1})$ cannot be reused to obtain $\tilde{w}_{t+1}$, so the learning rule is written as

$$\tilde{w}_{t+1} = m(x_t, y_t, \tilde{w}_t).$$

The process $\{\tilde{w}_t\}$ is Markovian. Whatever learning rule m is chosen, the behavior of the estimator $\tilde{w}_t$ is never better than that of the optimal batch estimator $\hat{w}_t$ because of this restriction. The gradient online learning rule

$$\tilde{w}_{t+1} = \tilde{w}_t - \eta_t C \frac{\partial l(x_t, y_t; \tilde{w}_t)}{\partial w},$$

was proposed where C is a positive-definite matrix, and its dynamical behavior was studied by Amari (1967) when the learning constant $\eta_t = \eta$ is fixed. Heskes and Kappen (1991) obtained similar results, which ignited research into online learning. When η_t satisfies some condition, say, $\eta_t = c/t$, for a positive constant c, the stochastic approximation guarantees that $\tilde{w}_t$ is a consistent estimator converging to w^*. However, it is not Fisher efficient in general.

There arises a question of whether there exists a learning rule that gives an efficient estimator. If it exists, the asymptotic behavior of online learning is equivalent to that of the best batch estimation method. This article answers the question affirmatively, by giving an efficient online learning rule (see Amari, 1995; see also Opper, 1996).

Let us consider the natural gradient learning rule,

$$\tilde{w}_{t+1} = \tilde{w}_t - \frac{1}{t}\tilde{\nabla} l(x_t, y_t, \tilde{w}_t). \tag{4.4}$$

Theorem 2. *Under the learning rule (see equation 4.4), the natural gradient online estimator $\tilde{w}_t$ is Fisher efficient.*

Proof. Let us denote the covariance matrix of estimator $\tilde{w}_t$ by

$$\tilde{V}_{t+1} = E[(\tilde{w}_{t+1} - w^*)(\tilde{w}_{t+1} - w^*)^T]. \tag{4.5}$$

This shows the expectation of the squared error. We expand

$$\frac{\partial l(x_t, y_t; \tilde{w}_t)}{\partial w} = \frac{\partial l(x_t, y_t; w^*)}{\partial w} + \frac{\partial^2 l(x_t, y_t; w^*)}{\partial w \partial w}(\tilde{w}_t - w^*)$$
$$+ O(|\tilde{w}_t - w^*|^2).$$

By subtracting w^* from the both sides of equation 4.4 and taking the expectation of the square of the both sides, we have

$$\tilde{V}_{t+1} = \tilde{V}_t - \frac{2}{t}\tilde{V}_t + \frac{1}{t^2}G^{-1} + O\left(\frac{1}{t^3}\right), \tag{4.6}$$

where we used

$$E\left[\frac{\partial l(x_t, y_t; w^*)}{\partial w}\right] = 0, \tag{4.7}$$

$$E\left[\frac{\partial^2 l(x_t, y_t; w^*)}{\partial w \partial w}\right] = G(w^*), \tag{4.8}$$

$$G(\tilde{w}_t) = G(w^*) + O\left(\frac{1}{t}\right),$$

because $\tilde{w}_t$ converges to w^* as guaranteed by stochastic approximation under certain conditions (see Kushner & Clark, 1978). The solution of equation 4.6 is written asymptotically as

$$\tilde{V}_t = \frac{1}{t}G^{-1} + O\left(\frac{1}{t^2}\right),$$

proving the theorem.

The theory can be extended to be applicable to the unrealizable teacher case, where

$$K(w) = E\left[\frac{\partial^2}{\partial w \partial w} l(x, y; w)\right] \tag{4.9}$$

should be used instead of $G(w)$ in order to obtain the same efficient result as the optimal batch procedure. This is locally equivalent to the Newton-Raphson method. The results can be stated in terms of the generalization error instead of the covariance of the estimator, and we can obtain more universal results (see Amari, 1993; Amari & Murata, 1993).

Remark. In the cases of blind source separation and deconvolution, the models are semiparametric, including the unknown function r (see equation 3.18). In such cases, the Cramér-Rao bound does not necessarily hold. Therefore, Theorem 2 does not hold in these cases. It holds when we can estimate the true r of the source probability density functions and use it to define the loss function $l(x, W)$. Otherwise equation 4.8 does not hold. The stability of the true solution is not necessarily guaranteed either. Amari, Chen, & Cichocki (in press) have analyzed this situation and proposed a universal method of attaining the stability of the equilibrium solution.

5 Adaptive Learning Constant

The dynamical behavior of the learning rule (see equation 3.2) was studied in Amari (1967) when η_t is a small constant η. In this case, w_t fluctuates around the (local) optimal value w^* for large t. The expected value and variance of w_t was studied, and the trade-off between the convergence speed and accuracy of convergence was demonstrated.

When the current w_t is far from the optimal w^*, it is desirable to use a relatively large η to accelerate the convergence. When it is close to w^*, a small η is preferred in order to eliminate fluctuations. An idea of an adaptive change of η was discussed in Amari (1967) and was called "learning of learning rules."

Sompolinsky et al. (1995) (see also Barkai et al., 1995) proposed a rule of adaptive change of η_t, which is applicable to the pattern classification problem where the expected loss $L(w)$ is not differentiable at w^*. This article generalizes their idea to a more general case where $L(w)$ is differentiable and analyzes its behavior by using the Riemannian structure.

We propose the following learning scheme:

$$w_{t+1} = w_t - \eta_t \tilde{\nabla} l(x_t, y_t; \hat{w}_t) \tag{5.1}$$

$$\eta_{t+1} = \eta_t \exp\{\alpha[\beta l(x_t, y_t; \hat{w}_t) - \eta_t]\}, \tag{5.2}$$

where α and β are constants. We also assume that the training data are generated by a realizable deterministic teacher and that $L(w^*) = 0$ holds at the optimal value. (See Murata, Müller, Ziehe, and Amari (1996) for a more general case.) We try to analyze the dynamical behavior of learning by using the continuous version of the algorithm for the sake of simplicity,

$$\frac{d}{dt} w_t = -\eta_t G^{-1}(w_t) \frac{\partial}{\partial w} l(x_t, y_t; w_t), \tag{5.3}$$

$$\frac{d}{dt} \eta_t = \alpha \eta_t [\beta l(x_t, z_t; w_t) - \eta_t]. \tag{5.4}$$

In order to show the dynamical behavior of (w_t, η_t), we use the averaged version of equations 5.3 and 5.4 with respect to the current input-output pair (x_t, y_t). The averaged learning equation (Amari, 1967, 1977) is written as

$$\frac{d}{dt} w_t = -\eta_t G^{-1}(w_t) \left\langle \frac{\partial}{\partial w} l(x, y; w_t) \right\rangle, \tag{5.5}$$

$$\frac{d}{dt} \eta_t = \alpha \eta_t \{\beta \langle l(x, y; w_t) \rangle - \eta_t\}, \tag{5.6}$$

where $\langle \ \rangle$ denotes the average over the current (x, y). We also use the asymptotic evaluations

$$\left\langle \frac{\partial}{\partial w} l(x, y; w_t) \right\rangle = \left\langle \frac{\partial}{\partial w} l(x, y; w^*) \right\rangle + \left\langle \frac{\partial^2}{\partial w \partial w} l(x, y; w^*)(w_t - w^*) \right\rangle$$

$$= G^*(w_t - w^*),$$

$$\langle l(x, y; w_t) \rangle = \frac{1}{2}(w_t - w^*)^T G^*(w_t - w^*),$$

where $G^* = G(w^*)$ and we used $L(w^*) = 0$. We then have

$$\frac{d}{dt} w_t = -\eta_t(w_t - w^*), \tag{5.7}$$

$$\frac{d}{dt}\eta_t = \alpha\eta_t \left\{ \frac{\beta}{2}(w_t - w^*)^T G^*(w_t - w^*) - \eta_t \right\}. \tag{5.8}$$

Now we introduce the squared error variable,

$$e_t = \frac{1}{2}(w_t - w^*)^T G^*(w_t - w^*), \tag{5.9}$$

where e_t is the Riemannian magnitude of $w_t - w^*$. It is easy to show

$$\frac{d}{dt}e_t = -2\eta_t e_t, \tag{5.10}$$

$$\frac{d}{dt}\eta_t = \alpha\beta\eta_t e_t - \alpha\eta_t^2. \tag{5.11}$$

The behavior of equations 5.10 and 5.11 is interesting. The origin $(0, 0)$ is its attractor. However, the basin of attraction has a boundary of fractal structure. Anyway, starting from an adequate initial value, it has the solution of the form

$$e_t = \frac{a}{t},$$

$$\eta_t = \frac{b}{t}.$$

The coefficients a and b are determined from

$$a = 2ab$$
$$b = -\alpha\beta ab + \alpha b^2.$$

This gives

$$b = \frac{1}{2},$$

$$a = \frac{1}{\beta}\left(\frac{1}{2} - \frac{1}{\alpha}\right), \qquad \alpha > 2.$$

This proves the $1/t$ convergence rate of the generalization error, that is, the optimal order for any estimator $\hat{w}_t$ converging to w^*. The adaptive η_t shows a nice characteristic when the target teacher is slowly fluctuating or changes suddenly.

6 Natural Gradient in the Space of Perceptrons

The Riemannian metric and its inverse are calculated in this section to obtain the natural gradient explicitly. We begin with an analog simple perceptron whose input-output behavior is given by

$$y = f(w \cdot x) + n, \tag{6.1}$$

where n is a gaussian noise subject to $N(0, \sigma^2)$ and

$$f(u) = \frac{1 - e^{-u}}{1 + e^{-u}}. \tag{6.2}$$

The conditional probability density of y when x is applied is

$$p(y \mid x; w) = \frac{1}{\sqrt{2\pi}\sigma} \exp\left\{ -\frac{1}{2\sigma^2}[y - f(w \cdot x)]^2 \right\}. \tag{6.3}$$

The distribution $q(x)$ of inputs x is assumed to be the normal distribution $N(0, I)$. The joint distribution of (x, y) is

$$p(y, x; w) = q(x)p(y \mid x; w).$$

In order to calculate the metric G of equation 3.11 explicitly, let us put

$$w^2 = |w|^2 = \sum w_i^2 \tag{6.4}$$

where $|w|$ is the Euclidean norm. We then have the following theorem.

Theorem 3.   *The Fisher information metric is*

$$G(w) = w^2 c_1(w)I + \{c_2(w) - c_1(w)\}ww^T, \tag{6.5}$$

where $c_1(w)$ and $c_2(w)$ are given by

$$c_1(w) = \frac{1}{4\sqrt{2\pi}\sigma^2 w^2} \int \{f^2(w\varepsilon) - 1\}^2 \exp\left\{ -\frac{1}{2}\varepsilon^2 \right\} d\varepsilon,$$

$$c_2(w) = \frac{1}{4\sqrt{2\pi}\sigma^2 w^2} \int \{f^2(w\varepsilon) - 1\}^2 \varepsilon^2 \exp\left\{ -\frac{1}{2}\varepsilon^2 \right\} d\varepsilon.$$

Proof.   We have

$$\log p(y, x; w) = \log q(x) - \log(\sqrt{2\pi}\sigma) - \frac{1}{2\sigma^2}[y - f(w \cdot x)]^2.$$

Hence,

$$\frac{\partial}{\partial w_i} \log p(y, x; w) = \frac{1}{\sigma^2}\{y - f(w \cdot x)\}f'(w \cdot x)x_i$$

$$= \frac{1}{\sigma^2}nf'(w \cdot x)x_i.$$

The Fisher information matrix is given by

$$g_{ij}(w) = E\left[\frac{\partial}{\partial w_i}\log p\frac{\partial}{\partial w_j}\log p\right]$$

$$= \frac{1}{\sigma^2}E[\{f'(w \cdot x)\}^2 x_i x_j],$$

where $E[n^2] = \sigma^2$ is taken into account. This can be written, in the vector-matrix form, as

$$G(w) = \frac{1}{\sigma^2}E[(f')^2 x x^T].$$

In order to show equation 6.5, we calculate the quadratic form $r^T G(w)r$ for arbitrary r. When $r = w$,

$$w^T G w = \frac{1}{\sigma^2}E[\{f'(w \cdot x)\}^2(w \cdot x)^2].$$

Since $u = w \cdot x$ is subject to $N(0, w^2)$, we put $u = w\varepsilon$, where ε is subject to $N(0, 1)$. Noting that

$$f'(u) = \frac{1}{2}\{1 - f^2(u)\},$$

we have,

$$w^T G(w)w = \frac{w^2}{4\sqrt{2\pi}\sigma^2}\int \varepsilon^2\{f^2(w\varepsilon) - 1\}^2 \exp\left\{-\frac{\varepsilon^2}{2}\right\}d\varepsilon,$$

which confirms equation 6.5 when $r = w$. We next put $r = v$, where v is an arbitrary unit vector orthogonal to w (in the Euclidean sense). We then have

$$v^T G(w)v = \frac{1}{4\sigma^2}E[\{f^2(w \cdot x) - 1\}^2(v \cdot x)^2].$$

Since $u = w \cdot x$ and $v = v \cdot x$ are independent, and v is subject to $N(0, 1)$, we have

$$v^T G(w)v = \frac{1}{4\sigma^2}E[(v \cdot x)^2]E[(f^2\{w \cdot x\} - 1\}^2]$$

$$= \frac{1}{4\sqrt{2\pi}\sigma^2}\int\{f^2(w\varepsilon) - 1\}^2 \exp\left\{-\frac{\varepsilon^2}{2}\right\}d\varepsilon.$$

Since $G(w)$ in equation 6.5 is determined by the quadratic forms for n-independent w and v's, this proves equation 6.5.

To obtain the natural gradient, it is necessary to have an explicit form of G^{-1}. We can calculate $G^{-1}(w)$ explicitly in the perceptron case.

Theorem 4.　The inverse of the Fisher information metric is

$$G^{-1}(w) = \frac{1}{w^2 c_1(w)} I + \frac{1}{w^4} \left(\frac{1}{c_2(w)} - \frac{1}{c_1(w)} \right) ww^T. \tag{6.6}$$

This can easily be proved by direct calculation of GG^{-1}. The natural gradient learning equation (3.10) is then given by

$$w_{t+1} = w_t + \eta_t \{y_t - f(w_t \cdot x_t)\} f'(w_t \cdot x_t)$$
$$\left[\frac{1}{w_t^2 c_1(w_t)} x_t + \frac{1}{w_t^4} \left(\frac{1}{c_2(w_t)} - \frac{1}{c_1(w_t)} \right) (w_t \cdot x_t) w_t \right]. \tag{6.7}$$

We now show some other geometrical characteristics of the parameter space of perceptrons. The volume V_n of the manifold of simple perceptrons is measured by

$$V_n = \int \sqrt{|G(w)|} dw \tag{6.8}$$

where $|G(w)|$ is the determinant of $G = (g_{ij})$, which represents the volume density by the Riemannian metric. It is interesting to see that the manifold of perceptrons has a finite volume.

Bayesian statistics considers that w is randomly chosen subject to a prior distribution $\pi(w)$. A choice of $\pi(w)$ is the Jeffrey prior or noninformative prior given by

$$\pi(w) = \frac{1}{V_n} \sqrt{|G(w)|}. \tag{6.9}$$

The Jeffrey prior is calculated as follows.

Theorem 5.　*The Jeffrey prior and the volume of the manifold are given, respectively, by*

$$\sqrt{|G(w)|} = \frac{w}{V_n} \sqrt{c_2(w)\{c_1(w)\}^{n-1}}, \tag{6.10}$$

$$V_n = a_{n-1} \int \sqrt{c_2(w)\{c_1(w)\}^{n-1}} w^n dw, \tag{6.11}$$

respectively, where a_{n-1} is the area of the unit $(n-1)$-sphere.

The Fisher metric G can also be calculated for multilayer perceptrons. Let us consider a multilayer perceptron having m hidden units with sigmoidal activation functions and a linear output unit. The input-output relation is

$$y = \sum v_i f(w_i \cdot x) + n,$$

or the conditional probability is

$$p(y \mid x; v, w_1, \ldots, w_m) = c \exp\left[-\frac{1}{2}\{y - \sum v_i f(w_i \cdot x)\}^2\right]. \qquad (6.12)$$

The total parameter w consist of $\{v, w_1, \ldots, w_m\}$. Let us calculate the Fisher information matrix G. It consists of $m+1$ blocks corresponding to these w_i's and v.

From

$$\frac{\partial}{\partial w_i} \log p(y \mid x; w) = n v_i f'(w_i \cdot x)x,$$

we easily obtain the block submatrix corresponding to w_i as

$$E\left[\frac{\partial}{\partial w_i} \log p \frac{\partial}{\partial w_i} \log p\right] = \frac{1}{\sigma^4} E[n^2] v_i^2 E[\{f'(w_i \cdot x)\}^2 xx^T]$$

$$= \frac{1}{\sigma^2} v_i^2 E[\{f'(w_i \cdot x)\}^2 xx^T].$$

This is exactly the same as the simple perceptron case except for a factor of $(v_i)^2$. For the off-diagonal block, we have

$$E\left[\frac{\partial}{\partial w_i} \log p \frac{\partial}{\partial w_j} \log p\right] = \frac{1}{\sigma^2} v_i v_j E[f'(w_i \cdot x) f'(w_j \cdot x) xx^T].$$

In this case, we have the following form,

$$G_{w_i w_j} = c_{ij} I + d_{ii} w_i w_i^T + d_{ij} w_i w_j^T + d_{ji} w_j w_i^T + d_{jj} w_j w_j^T, \qquad (6.13)$$

where the coefficients c_{ij} and d_{ij}'s are calculated explicitly by similar methods.

The v block and v and w_i block are also calculated similarly. However, the inversion of G is not easy except for simple cases. It requires inversion of a $2(m + 1)$ dimensional matrix. However, this is much better than the direct inversion of the original $(n + 1)m$-dimensional matrix of G. Yang and Amari (1997) performed a preliminary study on the performance of the natural gradient learning algorithm for a simple multilayer perceptron. The result shows that natural gradient learning might be free from the plateau phenomenon. Once the learning trajectory is trapped in a plateau, it takes a long time to get out of it.

7 Natural Gradient in the Space of Matrices and Blind Source Separation _____

We now define a Riemannian structure to the space of all the $m \times m$ nonsingular matrices, which forms a Lie group denoted by $Gl(m)$, for the purpose of introducing the natural gradient learning rule to the blind source separation problem. Let dW be a small deviation of a matrix from W to $W + dW$. The tangent space T_W of $Gl(m)$ at W is a linear space spanned by all such small deviations dW_{ij}'s and is called the Lie algebra.

We need to introduce an inner product at W by defining the squared norm of dW

$$ds^2 = \langle dW, dW \rangle_W = \| dW \|^2 .$$

By multiplying W^{-1} from the right, W is mapped to $WW^{-1} = I$, the unit matrix, and $W + dW$ is mapped to $(W + dW)W^{-1} = I + dX$, where

$$dX = dWW^{-1}. \tag{7.1}$$

This shows that a deviation dW at W is equivalent to the deviation dX at I by the correspondence given by multiplication of W^{-1}. The Lie group invariance requires that the metric is kept invariant under this correspondence, that is, the inner product of dW at W is equal to the inner product of dWY at WY for any Y,

$$\langle dW, dW \rangle_W = \langle dWY, dWY \rangle_{WY}. \tag{7.2}$$

When $Y = W^{-1}$, $WY = I$. This principle was used to derive the natural gradient in Amari, Cichocki, and Yang (1996); see also Yang and Amari (1997) for detail. Here we give its analysis by using dX.

We define the inner product at I by

$$\langle dX, dX \rangle_I = \sum_{i,j} (dX_{ij})^2 = \text{tr}(dX^T dX). \tag{7.3}$$

We then have the Riemannian metric structure at W as

$$\langle dW, dW \rangle_W = \text{tr}\{(W^{-1})^T dW^T dW W^{-1}\}. \tag{7.4}$$

We can write the metric tensor G in the component form. It is a quantity having four indices $G_{ij.kl}(W)$ such that

$$ds^2 = \sum G_{ij.kl}(W) dW_{ij} dW_{kl},$$
$$G_{ij.kl}(W) = \sum_m \delta_{ik} W_{jm}^{-1} W_{lm}^{-1}, \tag{7.5}$$

where W_{jm}^{-1} are the components of W^{-1}. While it may not appear to be straightforward to obtain the explicit form of G^{-1} and natural gradient $\tilde{\nabla}L$, in fact it can be calculated as shown below.

Theorem 6.   *The natural gradient in the matrix space is given by*

$$\tilde{\nabla}L = (\nabla L)W^T W. \tag{7.6}$$

Proof.   The metric is Euclidean at I, so that both $G(I)$ and its inverse, $G^{-1}(I)$, are the identity. Therefore, by mapping dW at W to dX at I, the natural gradient learning rule in terms of dX is written as

$$\frac{dX}{dt} = -\eta_t G^{-1}(I)\frac{\partial L}{\partial X} = -\eta_t \frac{\partial L}{\partial X}, \tag{7.7}$$

where the continuous time version is used. We have from equation 7.1

$$\frac{dX}{dt} = \frac{dW}{dt}W^{-1}. \tag{7.8}$$

The gradient $\partial L/\partial X$ is calculated as

$$\frac{\partial L}{\partial X} = \frac{\partial L(W)}{\partial W}\left(\frac{\partial W^T}{\partial X}\right) = \frac{\partial L}{\partial W}W^T.$$

Therefore, the natural gradient learning rule is

$$\frac{dW}{dt} = -\eta_t \frac{\partial L}{\partial W}W^T W,$$

which proves equation 7.6.

   The $dX = dWW^{-1}$ forms a basis of the tangent space at W, but this is not integrable; that is, we cannot find any matrix function $X = X(W)$ that satisfies equation 7.1. Such a basis is called a nonholonomic basis. This is a locally defined basis but is convenient for our purpose. Let us calculate the natural gradient explicitly. To this end, we put

$$l(x, W) = -\log\det|W| - \sum_{i-1}^{n}\log f_i(y_i), \tag{7.9}$$

where $y = Wx$ and $f_i(y_i)$ is an adequate probability distribution. The expected loss is

$$L(W) = E[l(x, W)],$$

which represents the entropy of the output y after a componentwise non-linear transformation (Nadal & Parga, 1994; Bell & Sejnowski, 1995). The independent component analysis or the mutual information criterion also gives a similar loss function (Comon, 1994; Amari et al., 1996; see also Oja & Karhunen, 1995). When f_i is the true probability density function of the ith source, $l(x, W)$ is the negative of the log likelihood.

The natural gradient of l is calculated as follows. We calculate the differential

$$dl = l(x, W + dW) - l(x, W) = -d \log \det |W| - \sum d \log f_i(y_i)$$

due to change dW. Then,

$$\begin{aligned} d \log \det |W| &= \log \det |W + dW| - \log \det |W| \\ &= \log \det |(W + dW)W^{-1}| = \log(\det |I + dX|) \\ &= \mathrm{tr}\, dX. \end{aligned}$$

Similarly, from $dy = dWx$,

$$\begin{aligned} \sum d \log f_i(y_i) &= -\varphi(y)^T dWx \\ &= -\varphi(y)^T dXy, \end{aligned}$$

where $\varphi(y)$ is the column vector

$$\varphi(y) = [\varphi_1(y_1), \ldots, \varphi_m(y_m)],$$
$$\varphi_i(y_i) = -\frac{d}{dy} \log f_i(y_i). \tag{7.10}$$

This gives $\partial L / \partial X$, and the natural gradient learning equation is

$$\frac{dW}{dt} = \eta_t (I - \varphi(y)^T y)W. \tag{7.11}$$

The efficiency of this equation is studied from the statistical and information geometrical point of view (Amari & Kawanabe, 1997; Amari & Cardoso, in press). We further calculate the Hessian by using the natural frame dX,

$$d^2 l = y^T dX^T \dot{\varphi}(y) dXy + \varphi(y)^T dX dXy, \tag{7.12}$$

where $\dot{\varphi}(y)$ is the diagonal matrix with diagonal entries $d\varphi_i(y_i)/dy_i$. Its expectation can be explicitly calculated (Amari et al., in press). The Hessian is decomposed into diagonal elements and two-by-two diagonal blocks (see also Cardoso & Laheld, 1996). Hence, the stability of the above learning rule is easily checked. Thus, in terms of dX, we can solve the two fundamental problems: the efficiency and the stability of learning algorithms of blind source separation (Amari & Cardoso, in press; Amari et al., in press).

8 Natural Gradient in Systems Space

The problem is how to define the Riemannian structure in the parameter space $\{W(z)\}$ of systems, where z is the time-shift operator. This was given in Amari (1987) from the point of view of information geometry (Amari, 1985, 1997a; Murray & Rice, 1993). We show here only ideas (see Douglas et al., 1996; Amari, Douglas, Cichocki, & Yang, 1997, for preliminary studies).

In the case of multiterminal deconvolution, a typical loss function l is given by

$$l = -\log \det |W_0| - \sum_i \int p\{y_i; W(z)\} \log f_i(y_i) dy_i, \tag{8.1}$$

where $p\{y_i; W(z)\}$ is the marginal distribution of $y(t)$ which is derived from the past sequence of $x(t)$ by matrix convolution $W(z)$ of equation 3.24. This type of loss function is obtained from maximization of entropy, independent component analysis, or maximum likelihood.

The gradient of l is given by

$$\nabla_m l = -(W_0^{-1})^T \delta_{0m} + \varphi(y_t) x^T (t - m), \tag{8.2}$$

where

$$\nabla_m = \frac{\partial}{\partial W_m},$$

and

$$\nabla l = \sum_{m=0}^{d} (\nabla_m l) z^{-m}. \tag{8.3}$$

In order to calculate the natural gradient, we need to define the Riemannian metric G in the manifold of linear systems. The geometrical theory of the manifold of linear systems by Amari (1987) defines the Riemannian metric and a pair of dual affine connections in the space of linear systems.

Let

$$dW(z) = \sum_m dW_m z^{-m} \tag{8.4}$$

be a small deviation of $W(z)$. We postulate that the inner product $\langle dW(z), dW(z) \rangle$ is invariant under the operation of any matrix filter $Y(z)$,

$$\langle dW(z), dW(z) \rangle_{W(z)} = \langle dW(z)Y(z), dW(z)Y(z) \rangle_{WY}. \tag{8.5}$$

where $Y(z)$ is any system matrix. If we put

$$Y(z) = \{W(z)\}^{-1},$$

which is a general system not necessarily belonging to FIR,

$$W(z)\{W(z)\}^{-1} = I(z),$$

which is the identity system

$$I(z) = I$$

not including any z^{-m} terms. The tangent vector $dW(z)$ is mapped to

$$dX(z) = dW(z)\{W(z)\}^{-1}. \tag{8.6}$$

The inner product at I is defined by

$$\langle dX(z), dX(z)\rangle_I = \sum_{m.ij}(dX_{m.ij})^2, \tag{8.7}$$

where $dX_{m.ij}$ are the elements of matrix dX_m.
    The natural gradient

$$\tilde{\nabla}l = G^{-1} \circ \nabla l$$

of the manifold of systems is given as follows.

Theorem 7.   *The natural gradient of the manifold of systems is given by*

$$\tilde{\nabla}l = \nabla l(z)W^T(z^{-1})W(z), \tag{8.8}$$

where operator z^{-1} should be operated adequately.

   The proof is omitted. It should be remarked that $\tilde{\nabla}l$ does not belong to the class of FIR systems, nor does it satisfy the causality condition either. Hence, in order to obtain an online learning algorithm, we need to introduce time delay to map it to the space of causal FIR systems. This article shows only the principles involved; details will published in a separate article by Amari, Douglas, and Cichocki.

9 Conclusions

This article introduces the Riemannian structures to the parameter spaces of multilayer perceptrons, blind source separation, and blind source deconvolution by means of information geometry. The natural gradient learning method is then introduced and is shown to be statistically efficient. This implies that optimal online learning is as efficient as optimal batch learning when the Fisher information matrix exists. It is also suggested that natural gradient learning might be easier to get out of plateaus than conventional stochastic gradient learning.

Acknowledgments

I thank A. Cichocki, A. Back, and H. Yang at RIKEN Frontier Research Program for their discussions.

References

Amari, S. (1967). Theory of adaptive pattern classifiers. *IEEE Trans., EC-16*(3), 299–307.

Amari, S. (1977). Neural theory of association and concept-formation. *Biological Cybernetics, 26,* 175–185.

Amari, S. (1985). *Differential-geometrical methods in statistics.* Lecture Notes in Statistics 28. New York: Springer-Verlag.

Amari, S. (1987). Differential geometry of a parametric family of invertible linear systems—Riemannian metric, dual affine connections and divergence. *Mathematical Systems Theory, 20,* 53–82.

Amari, S. (1993). Universal theorem on learning curves. *Neural Networks, 6,* 161–166.

Amari, S. (1995). Learning and statistical inference. In M. A. Arbib (Ed.), *Handbook of brain theory and neural networks* (pp. 522–526). Cambridge, MA: MIT Press.

Amari, S. (1996). Neural learning in structured parameter spaces—Natural Riemannian gradient. In M. C. Mozer, M. I. Jordan, & Th. Petsche (Eds.), *Advances in neural processing systems, 9.* Cambridge, MA: MIT Press.

Amari, S. (1997a). Information geometry. *Contemporary Mathematics, 203,* 81–95.

Amari, S. (1997b). *Superefficiency in blind source separation.* Unpublished manuscript.

Amari, S., & Cardoso, J. F. (In press). Blind source separation—Semi-parametric statistical approach. *IEEE Trans. on Signal Processing.*

Amari, S., Chen, T.-P., & Cichocki, A. (In press). Stability analysis of learning algorithms for blind source separation. *Neural Networks.*

Amari, S., Cichocki, A., & Yang, H. H. (1996). A new learning algorithm for blind signal separation, in *NIPS'95,* vol. 8, Cambridge, MA: MIT Press.

Amari, S., Douglas, S. C., Cichocki, A., & Yang, H. H. (1997). Multichannel blind deconvolution and equalization using the natural gradient. *Signal Processing*

Advance in Wireless Communication Workshop, Paris.

Amari, S., & Kawanabe, M. (1997). Information geometry of estimating functions in semiparametric statistical models, *Bernoulli, 3*, 29–54.

Amari, S., Kurata, K., & Nagaoka, H. (1992). Information geometry of Boltzmann machines. *IEEE Trans. on Neural Networks, 3*, 260–271.

Amari, S., & Murata, N. (1993). Statistical theory of learning curves under entropic loss criterion. *Neural Computation, 5*, 140–153.

Barkai, N., Seung, H. S., & Sompolinsky, H. (1995). Local and global convergence of on-line learning. *Phys. Rev. Lett., 75*, 1415–1418.

Bell, A. J., & Sejnowski, T. J. (1995). An information-maximization approach to blind separation and blind deconvolution. *Neural Computation, 7*, 1129–1159.

Bickel, P. J., Klassen, C. A. J., Ritov, Y., & Wellner, J. A. (1993). *Efficient and adaptive estimation for semiparametric models.* Baltimore: Johns Hopkins University Press.

Campbell, L. L. (1985). The relation between information theory and the differential-geometric approach to statistics. *Information Sciences, 35*, 199–210.

Cardoso, J. F., & Laheld, B. (1996). Equivariant adaptive source separation. *IEEE Trans. on Signal Processing, 44*, 3017–3030.

Chentsov, N. N. (1972). *Statistical decision rules and optimal inference* (in Russian). Moscow: Nauka [translated in English (1982), Rhode Island: AMS].

Comon, P. (1994). Independent component analysis, a new concept? *Signal Processing, 36*, 287–314.

Douglas, S. C., Cichocki, A., & Amari, S. (1996). Fast convergence filtered regressor algorithms for blind equalization. *Electronics Letters, 32*, 2114–2115.

Heskes, T., & Kappen, B. (1991). Learning process in neural networks. *Physical Review, A44*, 2718–2762.

Jutten, C., & Hérault, J. (1991). Blind separation of sources, an adaptive algorithm based on neuromimetic architecture. *Signal Processing, 24*(1), 1–31.

Kushner, H. J., & Clark, D. S. (1978). *Stochastic approximation methods for constrained and unconstrained systems.* Berlin: Springer-Verlag.

Murata, N., & Müller, K. R., Ziehe, A., & Amari, S. (1996). Adaptive on-line learning in changing environments. In M. C. Mozer, M. I. Jordan, & Th. Petsche (Eds.), *Advaces in neural processing systems, 9.* Cambridge, MA: MIT Press.

Murray, M. K., & Rice, J. W. (1993). *Differential geometry and statistics.* New York: Chapman & Hall.

Nadal, J. P. & Parga, N. (1994). Nonlinear neurons in the low noise limit—A factorial code maximizes information transfer. *Network, 5*, 561–581.

Oja, E., & Karhunen, J. (1995). Signal separation by nonlinear Hebbian learning. In M. Palaniswami et al. (Eds.), *Computational intelligence—A dynamic systems perspective* (pp. 83–97). New York: IEEE Press.

Opper, M. (1996). Online versus offline learning from random examples: General results. *Phys. Rev. Lett., 77*, 4671–4674.

Rao, C. R. (1945). Information and accuracy attainable in the estimation of statistical parameters. *Bulletin of the Calcutta Mathematical Society, 37*, 81–91.

Rumelhart, D. E., Hinton, G. E., & Williams, R. J. (1986). Learning internal representations by error propagation. *Parallel Distributed Processing* (Vol. 1, pp. 318–362). Cambridge, MA: MIT Press.

Saad, D., & Solla, S. A. (1995). On-line learning in soft committee machines. *Phys. Rev. E, 52,* 4225–4243.

Sompolinsky, H., Barkai, N., & Seung, H. S. (1995). On-line learning of dichotomies: Algorithms and learning curves. In J.-H. Oh et al. (Eds.), *Neural networks: The statistical mechanics perspective* (pp. 105–130). Proceedings of the CTP-PBSRI Joint Workshop on Theoretical Physics. Singapore: World Scientific.

Tsypkin, Ya. Z. (1973). *Foundation of the theory of learning systems.* New York: Academic Press.

Van den Broeck, C., & Reimann, P. (1996). Unsupervised learning by examples: On-line versus off-line. *Phys. Rev. Lett., 76,* 2188–2191.

Widrow, B. (1963). *A statistical theory of adaptation.* Oxford: Pergamon Press.

Yang, H. H., & Amari, S. (1997). *Application of natural gradient in training multilayer perceptrons.* Unpublished manuscript.

Yang, H. H., & Amari, S. (In press). Adaptive on-line learning algorithms for blind separation—Maximum entropy and minimal mutual information. *Neural Computation.*

10

A Fast Fixed-Point Algorithm for Independent Component Analysis

Aapo Hyvärinen
Erkki Oja
Helsinki University of Technology, Laboratory of Computer and Information Science, Espoo, Finland

We introduce a novel fast algorithm for independent component analysis, which can be used for blind source separation and feature extraction. We show how a neural network learning rule can be transformed into a fixed-point iteration, which provides an algorithm that is very simple, does not depend on any user-defined parameters, and is fast to converge to the most accurate solution allowed by the data. The algorithm finds, one at a time, all nongaussian independent components, regardless of their probability distributions. The computations can be performed in either batch mode or a semiadaptive manner. The convergence of the algorithm is rigorously proved, and the convergence speed is shown to be cubic. Some comparisons to gradient-based algorithms are made, showing that the new algorithm is usually 10 to 100 times faster, sometimes giving the solution in just a few iterations.

1 Introduction

Independent component analysis (ICA) (Comon, 1994; Jutten & Herault, 1991) is a signal processing technique whose goal is to express a set of random variables as linear combinations of statistically independent component variables. Two interesting applications of ICA are blind source separation and feature extraction. In the simplest form of ICA (Comon, 1994), we observe m scalar random variables $v_1, v_2, \ldots, v_m$, which are assumed to be linear combinations of n unknown independent components $s_1, s_2, \ldots, s_n$ that are mutually statistically independent and zeromean. In addition, we must assume $n \leq m$. Let us arrange the observed variables v_i into a vector $\mathbf{v} = (v_1, v_2, \ldots, v_m)^T$ and the component variables s_i into a vector $\mathbf{s}$, respectively; then the linear relationship is given by

$$\mathbf{v} = \mathbf{As}. \tag{1.1}$$

Here, $\mathbf{A}$ is an unknown $m \times n$ matrix of full rank, called the mixing matrix. The basic problem of ICA is then to estimate the original components s_i from the mixtures v_j or, equivalently, to estimate the mixing matrix $\mathbf{A}$.

The fundamental restriction of the model is that we can estimate only non-gaussian independent components (except if just one of the independent components is gaussian). Moreover, neither the energies nor the signs of the independent components can be estimated, because any constant multiplying an independent component in equation 1.1 could be cancelled by dividing the corresponding column of the mixing matrix A by the same constant. For mathematical convenience, we define here that the independent components s_i have unit variance. This makes the (nongaussian) independent components unique, up to their signs. Note that no order is defined between the independent components.

In blind source separation (Cardoso, 1990; Jutten & Herault, 1991), the observed values of v correspond to a realization of an m-dimensional discrete-time signal $v(t)$, $t = 1, 2, \ldots$ Then the components $s_i(t)$ are called source signals, which are usually original, uncorrupted signals or noise sources.

Another possible application of ICA is feature extraction (Bell & Sejnowski, 1996, in press; Hurri, Hyvärinen, Karhunen, & Oja, 1996). Then the columns of A represent features, and s_i signals the presence and the amplitude of the ith feature in the observed data v.

The problem of estimating the matrix A in equation 1.1 can be somewhat simplified by performing a preliminary sphering or prewhitening of the data v (Cardoso, 1990; Comon, 1994; Oja & Karhunen, 1995). The observed vector v is linearly transformed to a vector $x = Mv$ such that its elements x_i are mutually uncorrelated, and all have unit variance. Thus the correlation matrix of x equals unity: $E\{xx^T\} = I$. This transformation is always possible and can be accomplished by classical principal component analysis. At the same time, the dimensionality of the data should be reduced so that the dimension of the transformed data vector x equals n, the number of independent components. This also has the effect of reducing noise. After the transformation we have

$$x = Mv = MAs = Bs, \tag{1.2}$$

where $B = MA$ is an orthogonal matrix due to our assumptions on the components s_i: it holds $E\{xx^T\} = BE\{ss^T\}B^T = BB^T = I$. Thus we have reduced the problem of finding an arbitrary full-rank matrix A to the simpler problem of finding an orthogonal matrix B, which then gives $s = B^Tx$. If the ith column of B is denoted b_i, then the ith independent component can be computed from the observed x as $s_i = (b_i)^Tx$.

The current algorithms for ICA can be roughly divided into two categories. The algorithms in the first category (Cardoso, 1992; Comon, 1994) rely on batch computations minimizing or maximizing some relevant criterion functions. The problem with these algorithms is that they require very complex matrix or tensorial operations. The second category contains adaptive algorithms often based on stochastic gradient methods, which may have implementations in neural networks (Amari, Cichocki, & Yang, 1996;

Bell & Sejnowski, 1995; Delfosse & Loubaton, 1995; Hyvärinen & Oja, 1996; Jutten & Herault, 1991; Moreau & Macchi, 1993; Oja & Karhunen, 1995). The main problem with this category is the slow convergence and the fact that the convergence depends crucially on the correct choice of the learning rate parameters.

In this article we introduce a novel approach for performing the computations needed in ICA.[1] We introduce an algorithm using a very simple yet highly efficient fixed-point iteration scheme for finding the local extrema of the kurtosis of a linear combination of the observed variables. It is well known (Delfosse & Loubaton, 1995) that finding the local extrema of kurtosis is equivalent to estimating the nongaussian independent components. However, the convergence of our algorithm will be proved independent of these well-known results. The computations can be performed either in batch mode or semiadaptively.

The new algorithm is introduced and analyzed in section 3, after presenting in section 2 a short review of kurtosis minimization-maximization and its relation to neural network type learning rules.

2 ICA by Kurtosis Minimization and Maximization

Most suggested solutions to the ICA problem use the fourth-order cumulant or kurtosis of the signals, defined for a zero-mean random variable v as

$$\text{kurt}(v) = E\{v^4\} - 3(E\{v^2\})^2. \tag{2.1}$$

For a gaussian random variable, kurtosis is zero; for densities peaked at zero, it is positive, and for flatter densities, negative. Note that for two independent random variables v_1 and v_2 and for a scalar α, it holds $\text{kurt}(v_1 + v_2) = \text{kurt}(v_1) + \text{kurt}(v_2)$ and $\text{kurt}(\alpha v_1) = \alpha^4 \text{kurt}(v_1)$.

Let us search for a linear combination of the sphered observations x_i, say, $\mathbf{w}^T\mathbf{x}$, such that it has maximal or minimal kurtosis. Obviously, this is meaningful only if the norm of $\mathbf{w}$ is somehow bounded; let us assume $\|\mathbf{w}\| = 1$. Using the orthogonal mixing matrix $\mathbf{B}$, let us define $\mathbf{z} = \mathbf{B}^T\mathbf{w}$. Then also $\|\mathbf{z}\| = 1$. Using equation 1.2 and the properties of the kurtosis, we have

$$\text{kurt}(\mathbf{w}^T\mathbf{x}) = \text{kurt}(\mathbf{w}^T\mathbf{B}\mathbf{s}) = \text{kurt}(\mathbf{z}^T\mathbf{s}) = \sum_{i=1}^{n} z_i^4 \, \text{kurt}(s_i). \tag{2.2}$$

Under the constraint $\|\mathbf{w}\| = \|\mathbf{z}\| = 1$, the function in equation 2.2 has a number of local minima and maxima. For simplicity, let us assume for the moment that the mixture contains at least one independent component

---

[1] It was brought to our attention that a similar algorithm for blind deconvolution was proposed by Shalvi and Weinstein (1993).

whose kurtosis is negative and at least one whose kurtosis is positive. Then, as was shown by Delfosse and Loubaton (1995), the extremal points of equation 2.2 are the canonical base vectors $z = \pm e_j$, that is, vectors whose components are all zero except one component that equals ± 1. The corresponding weight vectors are $w = Bz = Be_j = b_j$ (perhaps with a minus sign), i.e., the columns of the orthogonal mixing matrix B. So by minimizing or maximizing the kurtosis in equation 2.2 under the given constraint, the columns of the mixing matrix are obtained as solutions for w, and the linear combination itself will be one of the independent components: $w^T x = (b_i)^T x = s_i$. Equation 2.2 also shows that gaussian components cannot be estimated by this way, because for them kurt(s_i) is zero.

To minimize or maximize kurt($w^T x$), a neural algorithm based on gradient descent or ascent can be used (Delfosse & Loubaton, 1995; Hyvärinen & Oja, 1996). Then w is interpreted as the weight vector of a neuron with input vector x. The objective function can be simplified because the inputs have been sphered. It holds

$$\text{kurt}(w^T x) = E\{(w^T x)^4\} - 3[E\{(w^T x)^2\}]^2 = E\{(w^T x)^4\} - 3\|w\|^4. \quad (2.3)$$

Also the constraint $\|w\| = 1$ must be taken into account, for example, by a penalty term (Hyvärinen & Oja, 1996). Then the final objective function is

$$J(w) = E\{(w^T x)^4\} - 3\|w\|^4 + F(\|w\|^2), \quad (2.4)$$

where F is a penalty term due to the constraint. Several forms for the penalty term have been suggested by Hyvärinen and Oja (1996).[2] In the following, the exact form of F is not important. Denoting by $x(t)$ the sequence of observations, by $\mu(t)$ the learning rate sequence, and by f the derivative of $F/2$, the online learning algorithm then has the form

$$w(t+1) = w(t)$$
$$\pm \mu(t)[x(t)(w(t)^T x(t))^3 - 3\|w(t)\|^2 w(t) + f(\|w(t)\|^2)w(t)]. \quad (2.5)$$

The first two terms in brackets are obtained from the gradient of kurt($w^T x$) when instantaneous values are used instead of the expectation. The third term in brackets is obtained from the gradient of $F(\|w\|^2)$; as long as this is a function of $\|w\|^2$ only, its gradient has the form *scalar* $\times w$. A positive sign before the brackets means finding the local maxima; a negative sign corresponds to local minima.

The convergence of this kind of algorithm can be proved using the principles of stochastic approximation. The advantage of such neural learning

---

[2] Note that in Hyvärinen and Oja (1996), the second term in J was also included in the penalty term.

rules is that the inputs $x(t)$ can be used in the algorithm at once, thus enabling fast adaptation in a nonstationary environment. A resulting trade-off is that the convergence is slow and depends on a good choice of the learning rate sequence $\mu(t)$. A bad choice of the learning rate can, in practice, destroy convergence. Therefore, some ways to make the learning radically faster and more reliable may be needed. The fixed-point iteration algorithms are such an alternative.

The fixed points $\mathbf{w}$ of the learning rule (see equation 2.5) are obtained by taking the expectations and equating the change in the weight to 0:

$$E\{\mathbf{x}(\mathbf{w}^T\mathbf{x})^3\} - 3\|\mathbf{w}\|^2\mathbf{w} + f(\|\mathbf{w}\|^2)\mathbf{w} = 0. \tag{2.6}$$

The time index t has been dropped. A deterministic iteration could be formed from equation 2.6 by a number of ways, for example, by standard numerical algorithms for solving such equations. A very fast iteration is obtained, as shown in the next section, if we write equation 2.6 in the form

$$\mathbf{w} = scalar \times (E\{\mathbf{x}(\mathbf{w}^T\mathbf{x})^3\} - 3\|\mathbf{w}\|^2\mathbf{w}). \tag{2.7}$$

Actually, because the norm of $\mathbf{w}$ is irrelevant, it is the direction of the right-hand side that is important. Therefore the *scalar* in equation 2.7 is not significant, and its effect can be replaced by explicit normalization, or the projection of $\mathbf{w}$ onto the unit sphere.

3 Fixed-Point Algorithm

3.1 The Algorithm. *3.1.1 Estimating One Independent Component.* Assume that we have collected a sample of the sphered (or prewhitened) random vector $\mathbf{x}$, which in the case of blind source separation is a collection of linear mixtures of independent source signals according to equation 1.2. Using the derivation of the preceding section, we get the following fixed-point algorithm for ICA:

1. Take a random initial vector $\mathbf{w}(0)$ of norm 1. Let $k = 1$.

2. Let $\mathbf{w}(k) = E\{\mathbf{x}(\mathbf{w}(k-1)^T\mathbf{x})^3\} - 3\mathbf{w}(k-1)$. The expectation can be estimated using a large sample of $\mathbf{x}$ vectors (say, 1000 points).

3. Divide $\mathbf{w}(k)$ by its norm.

4. If $|\mathbf{w}(k)^T\mathbf{w}(k-1)|$ is not close enough to 1, let $k = k + 1$, and go back to step 2. Otherwise, output the vector $\mathbf{w}(k)$.

The final vector $\mathbf{w}(k)$ given by the algorithm equals one of the columns of the (orthogonal) mixing matrix $\mathbf{B}$. In the case of blind source separation, this means that $\mathbf{w}(k)$ separates one of the nongaussian source signals in the sense that $\mathbf{w}(k)^T\mathbf{x}(t), t = 1, 2, \ldots$ equals one of the source signals.

A remarkable property of our algorithm is that a very small number of iterations, usually 5 to 10, seems to be enough to obtain the maximal accuracy allowed by the sample data. This is due to the cubic convergence shown below.

3.1.2 Estimating Several Independent Components. To estimate n independent components, we run this algorithm n times. To ensure that we estimate each time a different independent component, we need only to add a simple orthogonalizing projection inside the loop. Recall that the columns of the mixing matrix $\mathbf{B}$ are orthonormal because of the sphering. Thus we can estimate the independent components one by one by projecting the current solution $\mathbf{w}(k)$ on the space orthogonal to the columns of the mixing matrix $\mathbf{B}$ previously found. Define the matrix $\overline{\mathbf{B}}$ as a matrix whose columns are the previously found columns of $\mathbf{B}$. Then add the projection operation in the beginning of step 3:

Let $\mathbf{w}(k) = \mathbf{w}(k) - \overline{\mathbf{B}}\,\overline{\mathbf{B}}^T \mathbf{w}(k)$. Divide $\mathbf{w}(k)$ by its norm.

Also the initial random vector should be projected this way before starting the iterations. To prevent estimation errors in $\overline{\mathbf{B}}$ from deteriorating the estimate $\mathbf{w}(k)$, this projection step can be omitted after the first few iterations. Once the solution $\mathbf{w}(k)$ has entered the basin of attraction of one of the fixed points, it will stay there and converge to that fixed point.

In addition to the hierarchical (or sequential) orthogonalization described above, any other method of orthogonalizing the weight vectors could also be used. In some applications, a symmetric orthogonalization might be useful. This means that the fixed-point step is first performed for all the n weight vectors, and then the matrix $\mathbf{W}(k) = (\mathbf{w}_1(k), \ldots, \mathbf{w}_n(k))$ of the weight vectors is orthogonalized, for example, using the well-known formula,

$$\mathbf{W}(k) = \mathbf{W}(k)(\mathbf{W}(k)^T\mathbf{W}(k))^{-1/2}, \tag{3.1}$$

where $(\mathbf{W}(k)^T\mathbf{W}(k))^{-1/2}$ is obtained from the eigenvalue decomposition of $\mathbf{W}(k)^T\mathbf{W}(k) = \mathbf{E}\mathbf{D}\mathbf{E}^T$ as $(\mathbf{W}(k)^T\mathbf{W}(k))^{-1/2} = \mathbf{E}\mathbf{D}^{-1/2}\mathbf{E}^T$. However, the convergence proof below applies only to the hierarchical orthogonalization.

3.1.3 A Semiadaptive Version. A disadvantage of many batch algorithms is that large amounts of data must be stored simultaneously in working memory. Our fixed-point algorithm, however, can be used in a semiadaptive manner so as to avoid this problem. This can be accomplished simply by computing the expectation $E\{\mathbf{x}(\mathbf{w}(k-1)^T\mathbf{x})^3\}$ by an online algorithm for N consecutive sample points, keeping $\mathbf{w}(k-1)$ fixed, and updating the vector $\mathbf{w}(k)$ after the average over all the N sample points has been computed.

This semiadaptive version also makes adaptation to nonstationary data possible. Thus, the semiadaptive algorithm combines many of the advantages usually attributed to either online or batch algorithms.

3.2 Convergence Proof. Now we prove the convergence of our algorithm. To begin, make the change of variables $\mathbf{z}(k) = \mathbf{B}^T\mathbf{w}(k)$. Note that the effect of the projection step is to set to zero all components $z_i(k)$ of $\mathbf{z}(k)$ such that the ith column of $\mathbf{B}$ has already been estimated. Therefore, we can simply consider in the following the algorithm without the projection step, taking into account that the $z_i(k)$ corresponding to the independent components previously estimated are zero.

First, using equation 2.2, we get the following form for step 2 of the algorithm:

$$\mathbf{z}(k) = E\{\mathbf{s}(\mathbf{z}(k-1)^T\mathbf{s})^3\} - 3\mathbf{z}(k-1). \tag{3.2}$$

Expanding the first term, we can calculate explicitly the expectation, and obtain for the ith component of the vector $\mathbf{z}(k)$,

$$z_i(k) = E\{s_i^4\}z_i(k-1)^3 + 3\sum_{j\neq i} z_j(k-1)^2 z_i(k-1) - 3z_i(k-1), \tag{3.3}$$

where we have used the fact that by the statistical independence of the s_i, we have $E\{s_i^2 s_j^2\} = 1$, and $E\{s_i^3 s_j\} = E\{s_i^2 s_j s_l\} = E\{s_i s_j s_l s_m\} = 0$ for four different indices $i, j, l,$ and m. Using $\|\mathbf{z}(k)\| = \|\mathbf{w}(k)\| = 1$, equation 3.3 simplifies to

$$z_i(k) = \text{kurt}(s_i)\, z_i(k-1)^3, \tag{3.4}$$

where $\text{kurt}(s_i) = E\{s_i^4\} - 3$ is the kurtosis of the ith independent component. Note that the subtraction of $3\mathbf{w}(k-1)$ from the right side cancelled the term due to the cross-variances, enabling direct access to the fourth-order cumulants. Choosing j so that $\text{kurt}(s_j) \neq 0$ and $z_j(k-1) \neq 0$, we further obtain,

$$\frac{|z_i(k)|}{|z_j(k)|} = \frac{|\,\text{kurt}(s_i)|}{|\,\text{kurt}(s_j)|}\left(\frac{|z_i(k-1)|}{|z_j(k-1)|}\right)^3. \tag{3.5}$$

Note that the assumption $z_j(k-1) \neq 0$ implies that the jth column of $\mathbf{B}$ is not among those already found. Next note that $|z_i(k)|/|z_j(k)|$ is not changed by the normalization step 3. It is therefore possible to solve explicitly $|z_i(k)|/|z_j(k)|$ from this recursive formula, which yields

$$\frac{|z_i(k)|}{|z_j(k)|} = \frac{\sqrt{|\,\text{kurt}(s_j)|}}{\sqrt{|\,\text{kurt}(s_i)|}}\left(\frac{\sqrt{|\,\text{kurt}(s_i)|}\,|z_i(0)|}{\sqrt{|\,\text{kurt}(s_j)|}\,|z_j(0)|}\right)^{3^k} \tag{3.6}$$

for all $k > 0$. For $j = \arg\max_p \sqrt{|\,\text{kurt}(s_p)|}\,|z_p(0)|$, we see that all the other components $z_i(k)$, $i \neq j$ quickly become small compared to $z_j(k)$. Taking the normalization $\|\mathbf{z}(k)\| = \|\mathbf{w}(k)\| = 1$ into account, this means that $z_j(k) \to 1$

and $z_i(k) \rightarrow 0$ for all $i \neq j$. This implies that $\mathbf{w}(k) = \mathbf{B}\mathbf{z}(k)$ converges to the column $\mathbf{b}_j$ of the mixing matrix $\mathbf{B}$, for which the kurtosis of the corresponding independent component s_j is not zero and which has not yet been found. This proves the convergence of our algorithm.

4 Simulation Results

The fixed-point algorithm was applied to blind separation of four source signals from four observed mixtures. Two of the source signals had a uniform distribution, and the other two were obtained as cubes of gaussian variables. Thus, the source signals included both subgaussian and supergaussian signals. Using different random mixing matrices and initial values $\mathbf{w}(0)$, five iterations were usually sufficient for estimation of one column of the orthogonal mixing matrix to an accuracy of four decimal places.

Next, the convergence speed of our algorithm was compared with the speed of the corresponding neural stochastic gradient algorithm. In the neural algorithm, an empirically optimized learning rate sequence was used. The computational overhead of the fixed-point algorithm was optimized by initially using a small sample size (200 points) in step 2 of the algorithm, and increasing it at every iteration for greater accuracy. The number of floating-point operations was calculated for both methods.

The fixed-point algorithm needed only 10 percent of the floating-point operations required by the neural algorithm. This result was achieved with an empirically optimized learning rate. If we had been obliged to choose the learning rate without preliminary testing, the speed-up factor would have been of the order of 100. In fact, the neural stochastic gradient algorithm might not have converged at all.

These simulation results confirm the theoretical implications of very fast convergence.

5 Discussion

We introduced a batch version of a neural learning algorithm for ICA. This algorithm, which is based on the fixed-point method, has several advantages as compared to other suggested ICA methods.

1. Equation 3.6 shows that the convergence of our algorithm is cubic. This means very fast convergence and is rather unique among the ICA algorithms. It is also in contrast to other similar fixed-point algorithms, like the power method, which often have only linear convergence. In fact, our algorithm can be considered a higher-order generalization of the power method for tensors.

2. Contrary to gradient-based algorithms, there is no learning rate or other adjustable parameters in the algorithm, which makes it easy to use and more reliable.

3. The algorithm, in its hierarchical version, finds the independent components one at a time instead of working in parallel like most of the suggested ICA algorithms that solve the entire mixing matrix. This makes it possible to estimate only certain desired independent components, provided we have sufficient prior information of the weight matrices corresponding to those components. For example, if the initial weight vector of the algorithm is the first principal component, the algorithm finds probably the most important independent component, such that the norm of the corresponding column in the original mixing matrix $\mathbf{A}$ is the largest.

4. Components of both negative kurtosis (i.e., subgaussian components) and positive kurtosis (i.e., supergaussian components) can be found by starting the algorithm from different initial points and possibly removing the effect of the already found independent components by a projection onto an orthogonal subspace. If just one of the independent components is gaussian (or otherwise has zero kurtosis), it can be estimated as the residual that is left over after extracting all other independent components. Recall that more than one gaussian independent component cannot be estimated in the ICA model.

5. Although the algorithm was motivated as a short-cut method to make neural learning for kurtosis minimization and maximization faster, its convergence was proved independent of the neural algorithm and the well-known results on the connection between ICA and kurtosis. Indeed, our proof is based on principles different from those used so far in ICA and thus opens new lines for research.

Recent developments of the theory presented in this article can be found in Hyvärinen (1997a,b).

References

Amari, S., Cichocki, A., & Yang, H. (1996). A new learning algorithm for blind source separation. In *Advances in Neural Information Processing 8 (Proc. NIPS'95)*. Cambridge, MA: MIT Press.

Bell, A., & Sejnowski, T. (1995). An information-maximization approach to blind separation and blind deconvolution. *Neural Computation, 7*, 1129–1159.

Bell, A., & Sejnowski, T. (1996). Learning higher-order structure of a natural sound. *Network, 7*, 261–266.

Bell, A., & Sejnowski, T. (in press). The "independent components" of natural scenes are edge filters. *Vision Research*.

Cardoso, J.-F. (1990). Eigen-structure of the fourth-order cumulant tensor with application to the blind source separation problem. In *Proc. IEEE Int. Conf. on Acoustics, Speech, and Signal Processing* (pp. 2655–2658). Albuquerque, NM.

Cardoso, J.-F. (1992). Iterative techniques for blind source separation using only fourth-order cumulants. In *Proc. EUSIPCO* (pp. 739–742). Brussels.

Comon, P. (1994). Independent component analysis—a new concept? *Signal Processing, 36,* 287–314.

Delfosse, N., & Loubaton, P. (1995). Adaptive blind separation of independent sources: A deflation approach. *Signal Processing, 45,* 59–83.

Hurri, J., Hyvärinen, A., Karhunen, J., & Oja, E. (1996). Image feature extraction using independent component analysis. In *Proc. NORSIG'96.* Espoo, Finland.

Hyvärinen, A. (1997a). A family of fixed-point algorithms for independent component analysis. In *Proc. IEEE Int. Conf. on Acoustics, Speech, and Signal Processing (ICASSP '97)* (pp. 3917–3920). Munich, Germany.

Hyvärinen, A. (1997b). *Independent component analysis by minimization of mutual information* (Technical Report). Helsinki: Helsinki University of Technology, Laboratory of Computer and Information Science.

Hyvärinen, A., & Oja, E. (1996). A neuron that learns to separate one independent component from linear mixtures. In *Proc. IEEE Int. Conf. on Neural Networks* (pp. 62–67). Washington, D.C.

Jutten, C., & Herault, J. (1991). Blind separation of sources, part I: An adaptive algorithm based on neuromimetic architecture. *Signal Processing, 24,* 1–10.

Moreau, E., & Macchi, O. (1993). New self-adaptive algorithms for source separation based on contrast functions. In *Proc. IEEE Signal Processing Workshop on Higher Order Statistics* (pp. 215–219). Lake Tahoe, NV.

Oja, E., & Karhunen, J. (1995). Signal separation by nonlinear Hebbian learning. In M. Palaniswami, Y. Attikiouzel, R. Marks, D. Fogel, & T. Fukuda (Eds.), *Computational intelligence—a dynamic system perspective* (pp. 83–97). New York: IEEE Press.

Shalvi, O., & Weinstein, E. (1993). Super-exponential methods for blind deconvolution. *IEEE Trans. on Information Theory, 39*(2), 504–519.

11

Feature Extraction Using an Unsupervised Neural Network

Nathan Intrator
Center for Neural Science, Brown University
Providence, RI 02912 USA

A novel unsupervised neural network for dimensionality reduction that seeks directions emphasizing multimodality is presented, and its connection to exploratory projection pursuit methods is discussed. This leads to a new statistical insight into the synaptic modification equations governing learning in Bienenstock, Cooper, and Munro (BCM) neurons (1982). The importance of a dimensionality reduction principle based solely on distinguishing features is demonstrated using a phoneme recognition experiment. The extracted features are compared with features extracted using a backpropagation network.

1 Introduction

When a classification of high-dimensional vectors is sought, the *curse of dimensionality* (Bellman 1961) becomes the main factor affecting the classification performance. The curse of dimensionality is due to the inherent sparsity of high-dimensional spaces, implying that, in the absence of simplifying assumptions, the amount of training data needed to get reasonably low variance estimators is ridiculously high. This has led many researchers in recent years to construct methods that specifically avoid this problem (see Geman *et al.* 1991 for review in the context of neural networks). One approach is to assume that important structure in the data actually lies in a much smaller dimensional space, and therefore try to reduce the dimensionality before attempting the classification. This approach can be successful if the dimensionality reduction/feature extraction method loses as little relevant information as possible in the transformation from the high-dimensional space to the low-dimensional one.

Performing supervised feature extraction using the class labels is sensitive to the dimensionality in a similar manner to a high-dimensional classifier, and may result in a strong bias to the training data leading to poor generalization properties of the resulting classifier (Barron and Barron 1988).

A general class of unsupervised dimensionality reduction methods, called exploratory projection pursuit, is based on seeking *interesting* projections of high-dimensional data points (Kruskal 1972; Friedman and

Tukey 1974; Friedman 1987; Huber 1985, for review). The notion of interesting projections is motivated by an observation made by Diaconis and Freedman (1984) that for most high-dimensional clouds, most low-dimensional projections are approximately normal. This finding suggests that important information in the data is conveyed in those directions whose single-dimensional projected distribution is far from gaussian. Various projection indices differ on the assumptions about the nature of deviation from normality, and in their computational efficiency. Friedman (1987) argues that the most computationally efficient measures are based on polynomial moments. However, polynomial moments heavily emphasize departure from normality in the tails of the distribution (Huber 1985). Moreover, although many synaptic plasticity models are based on second-order statistics and lead to extraction of the principal components (Sejnowski 1977; von der Malsburg 1973; Oja 1982; Miller 1988; Linsker 1988), second-order polynomials are not sufficient to characterize the important features of a distribution (see examples in Duda and Hart 1973, p. 212). This suggests that in order to use polynomials for measuring deviation from normality, higher order polynomials are required, and care should be taken to avoid their oversensitivity to outliers. In this paper, the observation that high-dimensional clusters translate to multimodal low-dimensional projections is used for defining a measure of multimodality for seeking interesting projections. In some special cases, where the data are known in advance to be bimodal, it is relatively straightforward to define a good projection index (Hinton and Nowlan 1990), however, when the structure is not known in advance, defining a general multimodal measure of the projected data is not straightforward, and will be discussed in this paper.

There are cases in which it is desirable to make the projection index invariant under certain transformations, and maybe even remove second-order structure (see Huber 1985 for desirable invariant properties of projection indices). In those cases it is possible to make such transformations beforehand (Friedman 1987), and then assume that the data possess these invariant properties.

2 Feature Extraction Using ANN

In this section, the intuitive idea presented above is used to form a statistically plausible objective function whose minimization will find those projections having a single-dimensional projected distribution that is far from gaussian. This is done using a loss function that has an expected value that leads to the desired projection index. Mathematical details are given in Intrator (1990).

Before presenting our version of the loss function, we review some necessary notation and assumptions. Consider a neuron with input vector $x = (x_1, \ldots, x_N)$, synaptic weight vector $m = (m_1, \ldots, m_N)$, both in

R^N, and activity (in the linear region) $c = x \cdot m$. Define the threshold $\Theta_m = E[(x \cdot m)^2]$, and the functions $\hat{\phi}(c, \Theta_m) = c^2 - (2/3)c\Theta_m$, $\phi(c, \Theta_m) = c^2 - (4/3)c\Theta_m$. The ϕ function has been suggested as a biologically plausible synaptic modification function to explain visual cortical plasticity (Bienenstock *et al.* 1982). Θ_m is a dynamic threshold that will be shown later to have an effect on the sign of the synaptic modification. The input x, which is a stochastic process, is assumed to be of Type II φ mixing,[1] bounded, and piecewise constant. These assumptions are plausible, since they represent the closest continuous approximation to the usual training algorithms, in which training patterns are presented at random. The φ mixing property allows for some time dependency in the presentation of the training patterns. These assumptions are needed for the approximation of the resulting deterministic gradient descent by a stochastic one (Intrator and Cooper 1991). For this reason we use a *learning rate* μ that has to decay in time so that this approximation is valid.

We want to base the projection index on polynomial moments of low order, and to use the fact that a projection that leads to a bimodal distribution is already interesting, and any additional mode in the projected distribution should make the projection even more interesting. With this in mind, consider the following family of loss functions that depends on the synaptic weight vector m and on the input x;

$$L_m(x) = -\mu \int_0^{(x \cdot m)} \hat{\phi}(s, \Theta_m)\, ds = -\frac{\mu}{3}\{(x \cdot m)^3 - E[(x \cdot m)^2](x \cdot m)^2\}$$

The motivation for this loss function can be seen in Figure 1, which represents the $\hat{\phi}$ function and the associated loss function $L_m(c)$. For simplicity the loss for a fixed threshold Θ_m and synaptic vector m can be written as $L_m(c) = -(\mu/3)c^2(c - \Theta_m)$, where $c = (x \cdot m)$.

The graph of the loss function shows that for any fixed m and Θ_m, the loss is small for a given input x, when either $c = x \cdot m$ is close to zero, or when $x \cdot m$ is larger than Θ_m. Moreover, the loss function remains negative for $(x \cdot m) > \Theta_m$, therefore any kind of distribution at the right-hand side of Θ_m is possible, and the preferred ones are those that are concentrated further from Θ_m.

It remains to be shown why it is not possible that a minimizer of the average loss will be such that all the mass of the distribution will be concentrated on one side of Θ_m. This can not happen because the threshold Θ_m is dynamic and depends on the projections in a nonlinear way, namely, $\Theta_m = E(x \cdot m)^2$. This implies that Θ_m will always move itself to a position such that the distribution will never be concentrated at only one of its sides.

The risk (expected value of the loss) is given by

$$R_m = -\frac{\mu}{3}\left\{E[(x \cdot m)^3] - E^2[(x \cdot m)^2]\right\}$$

---

[1] The φ mixing property specifies the dependency of the future of the process on its past.

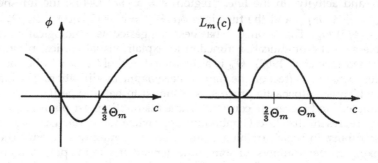

Figure 1: The function ϕ and the loss functions for a fixed m and Θ_m.

Since the risk is continuously differentiable, its minimization can be achieved via a gradient descent method with respect to m, namely

$$\frac{dm_i}{dt} = -\frac{\partial}{\partial m_i} R_m = \mu \, E[\phi(x \cdot m, \Theta_m) x_i]$$

The resulting differential equations give a modified version of the law governing synaptic weight modification in the BCM theory for learning and memory (Bienenstock *et al.* 1982). This theory was presented to account for various experimental results in visual cortical plasticity. The modification lies in the way the threshold Θ_m is calculated. In the original form this threshold was $\Theta_m = E^p(c)$ for $p > 1$, while in the current form $\Theta_m = E(c^p)$ for $p > 1$. The latter takes into account the variance of the activity (for $p = 2$) and therefore is always positive; this ensures stability even when the average of the inputs is zero. The biological relevance of the theory has been extensively studied (Bear *et al.* 1987; Bear and Cooper 1988) and it was shown that the theory is in agreement with the classical deprivation experiments (Clothiaux *et al.* 1991).

The fact that the distribution has part of its mass on both sides of Θ_m makes this loss a plausible projection index that seeks multimodalities. However, we still need to reduce the sensitivity of the projection index to outliers, and for full generality, allow any projected distribution to be shifted so that the part of the distribution that satisfies $c < \Theta_m$ will have its mode at zero. The oversensitivity to outliers is addressed by considering a nonlinear neuron in which the neuron's activity is defined to be $c = \sigma(x \cdot m)$, where σ usually represents a smooth sigmoidal function. A more general definition that would allow symmetry breaking of the projected distributions, as well as provide a solution to the second problem raised above, and will still be consistent with the statistical formulation, is $c = \sigma(x \cdot m - \alpha)$, for an arbitrary threshold α. The threshold α can be found by using gradient descent as well. For the nonlinear neuron, Θ_m is defined to be $\Theta_m = E[\sigma^2(x \cdot m)]$. The loss function is given by

$$L_m(x) = -\mu \int_0^{\sigma(x \cdot m)} \hat{\phi}(s, \Theta_m) ds = -\frac{\mu}{3} \{\sigma^3(x \cdot m) - E[\sigma^2(x \cdot m)]\sigma^2(x \cdot m)\}$$

The gradient of the risk becomes

$$-\nabla_m R_m = \mu \, E[\phi\,(\sigma(x \cdot m), \Theta_m)\,\sigma'x]$$

where σ' represents the derivative of σ at the point $(x \cdot m)$. Note that the multiplication by σ' reduces sensitivity to outliers of the differential equation since for outliers σ' is close to zero. The gradient descent is valid, provided that the risk is bounded from below.

Based on this formulation, a network of Q identical nodes may be constructed. All the neurons in this network receive the same input and inhibit each other, so as to extract several features in parallel. The relation between this network and the network studied by Cooper and Scofield (1988) is discussed in Intrator and Cooper (1991). The activity of neuron k in the network is defined as $c_k = \sigma(x \cdot m_k - \alpha_k)$, where m_k is the synaptic weight vector of neuron k, and α_k is its threshold. The *inhibited* activity and threshold of the kth neuron are given by $\tilde{c}_k = c_k - \eta \sum_{j \neq k} c_j$, $\tilde{\Theta}_m^k = E[\tilde{c}_k^2]$. A more general inhibitory pattern such as a Mexican hat is possible with minor changes in the mathematical details.

We omit the derivation of the synaptic modification equations, and present only the resulting stochastic modification equations for a synaptic vector m_k in a lateral inhibition network of nonlinear neurons:

$$\dot{m}_k = \mu \, [\phi(\tilde{c}_k, \tilde{\Theta}_m^k)\sigma'(\tilde{c}_k) - \eta \sum_{j \neq k} \phi(\tilde{c}_j, \tilde{\Theta}_m^j)\sigma'(\tilde{c}_j)]x$$

The lateral inhibition network performs a direct search of Q-dimensional projections in parallel, and therefore may find a richer structure that a step wise approach may miss (see example 14.1 in Huber 1985).

3 Comparison with Other Feature Extraction Methods

The above feature extraction method has been applied so far to various high-dimensional classification problems: extracting rotation invariant features from 3D wire-like objects (Intrator and Gold 1991) based on a set of sophisticated psychophysical experiments (Edelman and Bülthoff 1991); feature extraction from the TIMIT speech data base using Lyon's Cochlea model (Intrator and Tajchman 1991). The dimensionality of the feature extraction problem for these experiments was 3969 and 5500 dimensions, respectively. It is surprising that a very moderate amount of training data was needed for extracting robust features as will be shown below. In this section we briefly describe a linguistically motivated feature extraction experiment from stop consonants. We compare classification performance of the proposed method to a network that performs

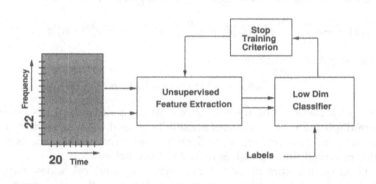

Figure 2: Low-dimensional classifier is trained on features extracted from the high-dimensional data. Training of the feature extraction network stops when the misclassification rate drops below a predetermined threshold on either the same training data (cross-validatory test) or on different testing data.

dimensionality reduction based on minimization of misclassification error (using backpropagation with MSE criterion). In the latter we regard the hidden unit representation as a new reduced feature representation of the input space. Classification on the new feature space was done using backpropagation.[2]

The unsupervised feature extraction/classification method is presented in Figure 2. The pixel images corresponding to speech data, are shown in Figure 3. Similar approaches using the RCE and backpropagation network have been carried out by Reilly et al. (1988).

The following describes the linguistic motivation of the experiment. Consider the six stop consonants [p,k,t,b,g,d], which have been a subject of recent research in evaluating neural networks for phoneme recognition (see review in Lippmann 1989). According to phonetic feature theory, these stops possess several common features, but only two distinguishing phonetic features, place of articulation and voicing (see Lieberman and Blumstein 1988, for a review and related references on phonetic feature theory). This theory suggests an experiment in which features extracted from unvoiced stops can be used to distinguish place of articulation in voiced stops as well. It is of interest if these features can be found from a single speaker, how sensitive they are to voicing and whether they are speaker invariant.

The speech data consists of 20 consecutive time windows of 32 msec with 30 msec overlap, aligned to the beginning of the burst. In each time window, a set of 22 energy levels is computed. These energy levels cor-

[2]See Intrator (1990) for comparison with principal components feature extraction and with k-NN as a classifier.

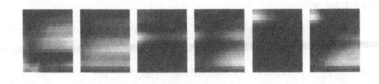

Figure 3: An average of the six stop consonants followed by the vowel [a]. Their order from left to right [pa] [ba] [ka] [ga] [ta] [da]. Time increases from the burst release on the X axis, and frequency increases on the Y axis. Brighter areas correspond to stronger energy.

respond to Zwicker critical band filters (Zwicker 1961). The consonant–vowel (CV) pairs were pronounced in isolation by native American speakers (two male BSS and LTN, and one female JES.) Additional details on biological motivation for the preprocessing, and linguistic motivation related to child language acquisition can be found in Seebach (1990). An average (over 25 tokens) of the six stop consonants followed by the vowel [a] is presented in Figure 3. All the images are smoothed using a moving average. One can see some similarities between the voiced and unvoiced stops especially in the upper left corner of the image (high frequencies beginning of the burst) and the radical difference between them in the low frequencies.

In the experiments reported here, five features were extracted from the 440 dimension original space. Although the dimensionality reduction methods were trained only with the unvoiced tokens of a single speaker, the classifier was trained on (five-dimensional) voiced and unvoiced data from the other speakers as well.

The classification results, which are summarized in Table 1, show that the backpropagation network does well in finding structure useful for classification of the trained data, but this structure is more sensitive to voicing. Classification results using a BCM network suggest that for this specific task structure that is less sensitive to voicing can be extracted, even though voicing has significant effects on the speech signal itself. The results also suggest that these features are more speaker invariant.

The difference in performance between the two feature extractors may be partially explained by looking at the synaptic weight vectors (images) extracted by both methods (Fig. 4): For the backpropagation feature extraction it can be seen that although five units were used, less features were extracted. One of the main distinctions between the unvoiced stops in the training set is the high frequency burst at the beginning of the consonant (the upper left corner). The backpropagation method concentrated mainly on this feature, probably because it is sufficient to base the recognition of the training set on this feature, and the fact that training

Table 1: Percentage of Correct Classification of Place of Articulation in Voiced and Unvoiced Stops.

	Place of articulation classification (B-P)	
	B-P (%)	BCM (%)
BSS /p,k,t/	100	100
BSS /b,g,d/	83.4	94.7
LTN /p,k,t/	95.6	97.7
LTN /b,g,d/	78.3	93.2
JES (both)	88.0	99.4

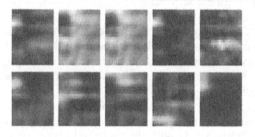

Figure 4: Synaptic weight images of the five hidden units of backpropagation (top), and the five BCM neurons (bottom).

stops when misclassification error falls to zero. On the other hand, the BCM method does not try to reduce the misclassification error and is able to find a richer, linguistically meaningful structure, containing burst locations and format tracking of the three different stops that allowed a better generalization to other speakers and to voiced stops.

The network and its training paradigm present a different approach to speaker independent speech recognition. In this approach the speaker variability problem is addressed by training a network that concentrates mainly on the distinguishing features of a single speaker, as opposed to training a network that concentrates on both the distinguishing and common features, on multispeaker data.

Acknowledgments

I wish to thank Leon N. Cooper for suggesting the problem and for providing many helpful hints and insights. Geoff Hinton made invaluable comments. The application of BCM to speech is discussed in more detail in Seebach (1991) and in a forthcoming article (Seebach and Intrator, in press). Charles Bachmann assisted in running the backpropagation experiments.

Research was supported by the National Science Foundation, the Army Research Office, and the Office of Naval Research.

References

Barron, A. R., and Barron, R. L. 1988. Statistical learning networks: A unifying view. In *Computing Science and Statistics: Proc. 20th Symp. Interface*, E. Wegman, ed., pp. 192–203. American Statistical Association, Washington, DC.

Bear, M. F., and Cooper, L. N 1988. Molecular mechanisms for synaptic modification in the visual cortex: Interaction between theory and experiment. In *Neuroscience and Connectionist Theory*, M. Gluck and D. Rumelhart, eds., pp. 65–94. Lawrence Erlbaum, Hillsdale, NJ.

Bear, M. F., Cooper, L. N, and Ebner, F. F. 1987. A physiological basis for a theory of synapse modification. *Science* **237**, 42–48.

Bellman, R. E. 1961. *Adaptive Control Processes*. Princeton University Press, Princeton, NJ.

Bienenstock, E. L., Cooper, L. N, and Munro, P. W. 1982. Theory for the development of neuron selectivity: Orientation specificity and binocular interaction in visual cortex. *J. Neurosci.* **2**, 32–48.

Clothiaux, E. E., Cooper, L. N, and Bear, M. F. 1991. Synaptic plasticity in visual cortex: Comparison of theory with experiment. *J. Neurophysiol.* To appear.

Cooper, L. N, and Scofield, C. L. 1988. Mean-field theory of a neural network. *Proc. Natl. Acad. Sci. U.S.A.* **85**, 1973–1977.

Diaconis, P., and Freedman, D. 1984. Asymptotics of graphical projection pursuit. *Ann. Statist.* **12**, 793–815.

Duda, R. O., and Hart, P. E. 1973. *Pattern Classification and Scene Analysis*. John Wiley, New York.

Edelman, S., and Bülthoff, H. H. 1991. Canonical views and the representation of novel three-dimensional objects. To appear.

Friedman, J. H. 1987. Exploratory projection pursuit. *J. Amer. Statist. Assoc.* **82**, 249–266.

Friedman, J. H., and Tukey, J. W. 1974. A projection pursuit algorithm for exploratory data analysis. *IEEE Trans. Comput.* **C**(23), 881–889.

Geman, S., Bienenstock, E., and Doursat, R. 1991. Neural networks and the bias-variance dilemma. To appear.

Hinton, G. E., and Nowlan, S. J. 1990. The bootstrap Widrow-Hoff rule as a cluster-formation algorithm. *Neural Comp.* **2**(3), 355–362.

Huber, P. J. 1985. Projection pursuit (with discussion). *Ann. Statist.* **13**, 435–475.

Intrator, N., 1990. Feature extraction using an unsupervised neural network. In *Proceedings of the 1990 Connectionist Models Summer School*, D. S. Touretzky, J. L. Ellman, T. J. Sejnowski, and G. E. Hinton, eds., pp. 310–318. Morgan Kaufmann, San Mateo, CA.

Intrator, N., and Cooper, L. N 1991. Objective function formulation of the BCM theory of visual cortical plasticity: Statistical connections, stability conditions. *Neural Networks*. To appear.

Intrator, N., and Gold, J. I. 1991. Three-dimensional object recognition of gray level images: The usefulness of distinguishing features. To appear.

Intrator, N., and Tajchman, G. 1991. Supervised and unsupervised feature extraction from a cochlear model for speech recognition. In *Neural Networks for Signal Processing — Proceedings of the 1991 IEEE Workshop*, B. H. Juang, S. Y. Kung, and C. A. Kamm, eds., pp. 460–469.

Kruskal, J. B. 1972. Linear transformation of multivariate data to reveal clustering. In *Multidimensional Scaling: Theory and Application in the Behavioral Sciences, I, Theory*, R. N. Shepard, A. K. Romney, and S. B. Nerlove, eds., pp. 179–191. Seminar Press, New York and London.

Lieberman, P., and Blumstein, S. E. 1988. *Speech Physiology, Speech Perception, and Acoustic Phonetics*. Cambridge University Press, Cambridge.

Linsker, R. 1988. Self-organization in a perceptual network. *IEEE. Comp.* **88**, 105–117.

Lippmann, R. P. 1989. Review of neural networks for speech recognition. *Neural Comp.* **1**, 1–38.

Miller, K. D. 1988. Correlation-based models of neural development. In *Neuroscience and Connectionist Theory*, M. Gluck and D. Rumelhart, eds., pp. 267–353. Lawrence Erlbaum, Hillsdale, NJ.

Oja, E. 1982. A simplified neuron model as a principal component analyzer. *Math. Biol.* **15**, 267–273.

Reilly, D. L., Scofield, C. L., Cooper, L. N, and Elbaum, C. 1988. Gensep: A multiple neural network with modifiable network topology. *INNS Conf. Neural Networks*.

Seebach, B. S. 1991. Evidence for the development of phonetic property detectors in a neural net without innate knowledge of linguistic structure. Ph.D. dissertation, Brown University.

Seebach, B. S., and Intrator, N. A neural net model of perinatal inductive acquisition of phonetic features.

Sejnowski, T. J. 1977. Storing covariance with nonlinearly interacting neurons. *J. Math. Biol.* **4**, 303–321.

von der Malsburg, C. 1973. Self-organization of orientation sensitivity cells in the striate cortex. *Kybernetik* **14**, 85–100.

Zwicker, E. 1961. Subdivision of the audible frequency range into critical bands (frequenzgruppen). *J. Acoust. Soc. Am.* **33**(2): 248.

12

Learning Mixture Models of Spatial Coherence

Suzanna Becker
Geoffrey E. Hinton
Department of Computer Science, University of Toronto,
Toronto, Ontario, Canada M5S 1A4

We have previously described an unsupervised learning procedure that discovers spatially coherent properties of the world by maximizing the information that parameters extracted from different parts of the sensory input convey about some common underlying cause. When given random dot stereograms of curved surfaces, this procedure learns to extract surface depth because that is the property that is coherent across space. It also learns how to interpolate the depth at one location from the depths at nearby locations (Becker and Hinton 1992b). In this paper, we propose two new models that handle surfaces with discontinuities. The first model attempts to detect cases of discontinuities and reject them. The second model develops a mixture of expert interpolators. It learns to detect the locations of discontinuities and to invoke specialized, asymmetric interpolators that do not cross the discontinuities.

1 Introduction

Standard backpropagation is implausible as a model of perceptual learning because it requires an external teacher to specify the desired output of the network. We have shown (Becker and Hinton 1992b) how the external teacher can be replaced by internally derived teaching signals. These signals are generated by using the assumption that different parts of the perceptual input have common causes in the external world. Small modules that look at separate but related parts of the perceptual input discover these common causes by striving to produce outputs that agree with each other (see Fig. 1a). The modules may look at different modalities (e.g., vision and touch), or the same modality at different times (e.g., the consecutive 2-D views of a rotating 3-D object), or even spatially adjacent parts of the same image.

In previous work, we showed that when our learning procedure is applied to adjacent patches of images, it allows a neural network that has no prior knowledge of depth to discover stereo disparity in random dot stereograms of curved surfaces. A more general version of the method allows the network to discover the best way of interpolating the depth at one location from the depths at nearby locations. We first summarize this earlier work, and then introduce two new models that allow coherent predictions to be made in the presence of discontinuities. The first assumes a model of the world in which patterns are drawn from two possible classes: one which can be captured by a simple model of coherence, and one which is unpredictable. This allows the network to reject cases containing discontinuities. The second method allows the network to develop multiple models of coherence, by learning a mixture of depth interpolators for curved surfaces with discontinuities. Rather than rejecting cases containing discontinuities, the network develops a set of location-specific discontinuity detectors, and appropriate interpolators for each class of discontinuities. An alternative way of learning the same representation for this problem, using an unsupervised version of the competing experts algorithm described by Jacobs *et al.* (1991), is described in Becker and Hinton (1992a).

2 Learning Spatially Coherent Features in Images

Using a modular architecture as shown in Figure 1a, a network can learn to model a spatially coherent surface, by extracting mutually predictable features from neighboring image patches. The goal of the learning is to produce good agreement between the outputs of modules that receive input from neighboring patches. The simplest way to get the outputs of two modules to agree is to use the squared difference between the outputs as a cost function, and to adjust the weights in each module so as to minimize this cost. Unfortunately, this usually causes each module to produce the same constant output that is unaffected by the input to the module and therefore conveys no information about it. We would like the outputs of two modules to agree closely (i.e., to have a small expected squared difference) *relative* to how much they both vary as the input is varied. When this happens, the two modules must be responding to something that is common to their two inputs. In the special case when the outputs, d_a, d_b, of the two modules are scalars, a good measure of agreement is

$$I = 0.5 \log \frac{V(d_a + d_b)}{V(d_a - d_b)} \tag{2.1}$$

where V is the variance over the training cases. Under the assumption that d_a and d_b are both versions of the same underlying gaussian signal that have been corrupted by independent gaussian noise, it can be shown that I is the mutual information (Shannon and Weaver 1964) between the underlying signal and the average of d_a and d_b. By maximizing I we force the two modules to extract as pure a version as possible of the underlying common signal.

2.1 The Basic Stereo Net. We have shown how this principle can be applied to a multilayer network that learns to extract depth from ran-

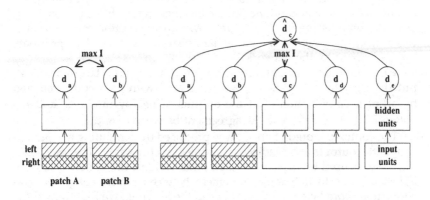

Figure 1: (a) Two modules that receive input from corresponding parts of stereo images. The first module receives input from stereo patch A, consisting of a horizontal strip from the left image (striped) and a corresponding strip from the right image (hatched). The second module receives input from an adjacent stereo patch B. The modules try to make their outputs, d_a and d_b, convey as much information as possible about some underlying signal (i.e., the depth) which is common to both patches. (b) The architecture of the interpolating network, consisting of multiple copies of modules like those in (a) plus a layer of interpolating units. The network tries to maximize the information that the locally extracted parameter d_c and the contextually predicted parameter $\hat{d}_c$ convey about some common underlying signal. We actually used 10 modules and the central 6 modules tried to maximize agreement between their outputs and contextually predicted values. We used weight averaging to constrain the interpolating function to be identical for all modules.

dom dot stereograms (Becker and Hinton 1992b). Each network module received input from a patch of a left image and a corresponding patch of a right image, as shown in Figure 1a. Adjacent modules received input from adjacent stereo image patches, and learned to extract depth by trying to maximize agreement between their outputs. The real-valued depth (relative to the plane of fixation) of each patch of the surface gives rise to a disparity between features in the left and right images; because that disparity is the only property that is coherent across each stereo image, the output units of modules were able to learn to accurately detect relative depth.

2.2 The Interpolating Net. The basic stereo net uses a very simple model of coherence in which an underlying parameter at one location is assumed to be approximately equal to the parameter at a neighboring location. This model is fine for the depth of frontoparallel surfaces but it is far from the best model of slanted or curved surfaces. Fortunately, we can use a far more general model of coherence in which the parameter at one location is assumed to be an unknown linear function of the parameters at nearby locations. The particular linear function that is appropriate can be learned by the network.

We used a network of the type shown in Figure 1b. The depth computed locally by a module, d_c, was compared with the depth predicted by a linear combination $\hat{d}_c$ of the outputs of nearby modules, and the network tried to maximize the agreement between d_c and $\hat{d}_c$.

The contextual prediction, $\hat{d}_c$, was produced by computing a weighted sum of the outputs of *two* adjacent modules on either side. The interpolating weights used in this sum, and all other weights in the network, were adjusted so as to maximize agreement between locally computed and contextually predicted depths. To speed the learning, we first trained the lower layers of the network as before, so that agreement was maximized between neighboring locally computed outputs. This made it easier to learn good interpolating weights. When the network was trained on stereograms of cubic surfaces, it learned interpolating weights of -0.147, 0.675, 0.656, -0.131 (Becker and Hinton 1992b). Given noise free estimates of local depth, the optimal linear interpolator for a cubic surface is -0.167, 0.667, 0.667, -0.167.

3 Mixture Models of Coherence

The models described above were based on the assumption of a single type of coherence in images. We assumed there was some parameter of the image that was either constant for nearby patches, or varied smoothly across space. In natural scenes, these simple models of coherence may not always hold. There may be widely varying amounts of curvature, from smooth surfaces, to highly curved spherical or cylindrical objects. There may be coherent structure at several spatial scales; for example, a rough surface like a brick wall is highly convoluted at a fine spatial scale, while at a coarser scale it is planar. And at boundaries between objects, or between different parts of the same object, there will be discontinuities in coherence. It would be better to have multiple models of coherence, which could account for a wider range of surfaces. One way to handle multiple models is to have a mixture of distributions (McLachlan and Basford 1988). In this section, we introduce a new way of employing mixture models to account for a greater variety of situations. We extend the learning procedure described in the previous section based on these models.

3.1 Throwing out Discontinuities. If the surface is continuous, the depth at one patch can be accurately predicted from the depths of two patches on either side. If, however, the training data contains cases in

which there are depth discontinuities (see Fig. 2) the interpolator will also try to model these cases and this will contribute considerable noise to the interpolating weights and to the depth estimates. One way of reducing this noise is to treat the discontinuity cases as outliers and to throw them out. Rather than making a hard decision about whether a case is an outlier, we make a soft decision by using a mixture model. For each training case, the network compares the locally extracted depth, d_c, with the depth predicted from the nearby context, $\hat{d}_c$. It assumes that $d_c - \hat{d}_c$ is drawn from a zero-mean gaussian if it is a continuity case and from a uniform distribution if it is a discontinuity case, as shown in Figure 3. It can then estimate the probability of a continuity case:

$$p_{\text{cont}}(d_c - \hat{d}_c) = \frac{N[d_c - \hat{d}_c, 0, \hat{V}_{\text{cont}}(d_c - \hat{d}_c)]}{N[d_c - \hat{d}_c, 0, \hat{V}_{\text{cont}}(d_c - \hat{d}_c)] + k_{\text{discont}}} \tag{3.1}$$

where N is a gaussian, and k_{discont} is a constant representing a uniform density.[1]

We can now optimize the *average* information d_c and $\hat{d}_c$ transmit about their common cause. We assume that no information is transmitted in discontinuity cases, so the average information depends on the probability of continuity and on the variance of $d_c + \hat{d}_c$ and $d_c - \hat{d}_c$ measured only in the continuity cases:

$$I^* = 0.5 \; P_{\text{cont}} \; \log \frac{V_{\text{cont}}(d_c + \hat{d}_c)}{V_{\text{cont}}(d_c - \hat{d}_c)} \tag{3.2}$$

where $P_{\text{cont}} = \langle p_{\text{cont}}(d_c - \hat{d}_c) \rangle$.

We tried several variations of this mixture approach. The network is quite good at rejecting the discontinuity cases, but this leads to only a modest improvement in the performance of the interpolator. In cases where there is a depth discontinuity between d_a and d_b or between d_d and d_e the interpolator works moderately well because the weights on d_a or d_e are small. Because of the term P_{cont} in equation 3.2 there is pressure to include these cases as continuity cases, so they probably contribute noise to the interpolating weights. In the next section we show how to avoid making a forced choice between rejecting these cases or treating them just like all the other continuity cases.

---

[1] We empirically select a good (fixed) value of k_{discont}, and we choose a starting value of $\hat{V}_{\text{cont}}(d_c - \hat{d}_c)$ (some proportion of the initial variance of $d_c - \hat{d}_c$), and gradually shrink it during learning. The learning algorithm's performance is fairly robust with respect to variations in the choice of k_{discont}; the main effect of changing this parameter is to sharpen or flatten the network's probabilistic decision function for labeling cases as continuous or discontinuous (equation 3.1). The choice of $\hat{V}_{\text{cont}}(d_c - \hat{d}_c)$, on the other hand, turns out to affect the learning algorithm more critically; if this variance is too small, many cases will be treated as discontinuous, and the network may converge to very large weights which overfit only a small subset of the training cases. There is no problem, however, if this variance is too large initially; in this case, all patterns are treated as continuous, and as the variance is shrunk during learning, some discontinuous cases are eventually detected.

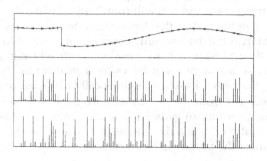

Figure 2: (Top) A curved surface strip with a discontinuity created by fitting 2 cubic splines through randomly chosen control points, 25 pixels apart, separated by a depth discontinuity. Feature points are randomly scattered on each spline with an average of 0.22 features per pixel. (Bottom) A stereo pair of "intensity" images of the surface strip formed by taking two different projections of the feature points, filtering them through a gaussian, and sampling the filtered projections at evenly spaced sample points. The sample values in corresponding patches of the two images are used as the inputs to a module. The depth of the surface for a particular image region is directly related to the disparity between corresponding features in the left and right patch. Disparity ranges continuously from −1 to +1 image pixels. Each stereo image was 120 pixels wide and divided into 10 receptive fields 10 pixels wide and separated by 2 pixel gaps, as input for the networks shown in Figure 1. The receptive field of an interpolating unit spanned 58 image pixels, and discontinuities were randomly located a minimum of 40 pixels apart, so only rarely would more than one discontinuity lie within an interpolator's receptive field.

3.2 Learning a Mixture of Interpolators. The presence of a depth discontinuity somewhere within a strip of five adjacent patches does not necessarily destroy the predictability of depth across these patches. It may just restrict the range over which a prediction can be made. So instead of throwing out cases that contain a discontinuity, the network could try to develop a number of different, specialized models of spatial coherence across several image patches. If, for example, there is a depth discontinuity between d_c and d_e in Figure 1b, an extrapolator with weights of $-1.0, +2.0, 0, 0$ would be an appropriate predictor of d_c. The network could also try to detect the locations of discontinuities, and use this information as the basis for deciding which model to apply on a given case. This information is useful not only in making clean decisions about which coherence model to apply, but it also provides valuable cues for interpreting the scene by indicating the locations of object boundaries in the image. Thus, we can use both the interpolated depth map, as well

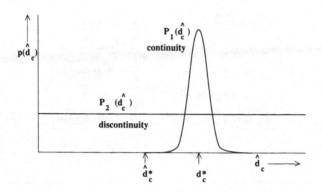

Figure 3: The probability distribution of $\hat{d}_c$, $P_1(\hat{d}_c)$, is modeled as a mixture of two distributions: a gaussian with mean $= d_c^*$ and small variance, and $P_2(\hat{d}_c)$, a uniform distribution. Sample points for $\hat{d}_c$ and d_c, $\hat{d}_c^*$ and d_c^* are shown. In this case, $\hat{d}_c^*$ and d_c^* are far apart so $\hat{d}_c^*$ is more likely to have been drawn from P_2.

as the locations of depth discontinuities, in subsequent stages of scene interpretation.

A network can learn to discover multiple coherence models using a set of competing interpolators. Each interpolator tries, as before, to achieve high agreement between its output and the depth extracted locally by a module. Additionally, each interpolator tries to account for as many cases as possible by maximizing the probability that its model holds. The objective function maximized by the network is the sum over models, i, of the agreement between the output of the ith model, $\hat{d}_{ic}$, and the predicted depth, d_c, weighted by the probability of the ith model:

$$I^{**} = \sum_i \langle p_i \rangle \, \log \frac{V^i(\hat{d}_{ic} + d_c)}{V^i(\hat{d}_{ic} - d_c)} \tag{3.3}$$

where the V^is represent variances given that the ith model holds. The probability that the ith model is applicable on each case α, p_i^α, can be computed independently of how well the interpolators are doing;[2] this can be done by adding extra "controller" units to the network, as shown in Figure 4, whose sole purpose is to compute the probability, p_i, that each interpolator's model holds. The weights of both the controllers and the interpolating experts can be learned simultaneously, so as to maximize

---

[2]More precisely, this computed probability is *conditionally independent* of the interpolators' performance on a particular case, with independence being conditioned on a fixed set of weights. As the reviewer has pointed out, when the weights change over the course of learning, there is an interdependence between the probabilities and interpolated quantities via the shared objective function.

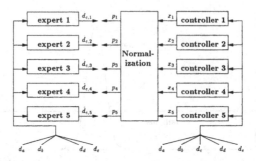

Figure 4: An architecture for learning a mixture model of curved surfaces with discontinuities, consisting of a set of interpolators and discontinuity detectors. We actually used a larger modular network and equality constraints between the weights of corresponding units in different modules, with 6 copies of the architecture shown here. Each copy received input from different but overlapping parts of the input.

I^{**}. By assigning a controller to each expert interpolator, each controller should learn to detect a discontinuity at a particular location (or the absence of a discontinuity in the case of the interpolator for pure continuity cases). And each interpolating unit should learn to capture the particular type of coherence that remains in the presence of a discontinuity at a particular location.

The outputs of the controllers are normalized, so that they represent a probability distribution over the interpolating experts' models. We can think of these normalized outputs as the probability with which the system selects a particular expert. Each controller's output is a normalized exponential function of its *squared* total input, x_i:

$$p_i = \frac{e^{x_i^2/T \, \hat{\sigma}(x_i)^2}}{\sum_j e^{x_j^2/T \, \hat{\sigma}(x_j)^2}} \tag{3.4}$$

Squaring the total input makes it possible for each unit to detect a depth edge at a particular location, independently of the direction of contrast change. We normalize the squared total input in the exponential by an estimate of its variance, $\hat{\sigma}(x_j)^2 = k \sum_{ji} w_{ji}^2$. (This estimate of the variance of the total weighted input is exact if the unweighted individual inputs are independent, gaussian, and have equal variances of size k.) This discourages any one unit from trying to model all of the cases simply by having huge weights. The controllers get to see all five local depth estimates, $d_a \dots d_e$. As before, each interpolating expert computes a linear function of four contextually extracted depths, $\hat{d}_{ic} = w_{ia}d_a + w_{ib}d_b + w_{id}d_d + w_{ie}d_e$, in order to try to predict the centrally extracted depth d_c.

We first trained the network using the original continuous model, as described in Section 2, on a training set of 1000 images with discontinuities, until the lower layers of the network became well tuned to depth. So the interpolators were initially pretrained using the continuity model, and all the interpolators learned similar weights. We then froze the weights in the lower layers, added a small amount of noise to the interpolators' weights (uniform in $[-0.1, 0.1]$), and applied the mixture model to improve the interpolators and train the controller units. We ran the learning procedure for 10 runs, each run starting from different random initial weights and proceeding for 10 conjugate gradient learning iterations. The network learned similar solutions in each case.

A typical set of weights on one run is shown in Figure 5. The graph on the right in this figure shows that four of the controller units are tuned to discontinuities at different locations. The weights for the first interpolator (shown in the top left) are nearly symmetrical, and the corresponding controller's weights (shown immediately to the right) are very small; the graph on the right shows that this controller (shown as a solid line plot) mainly responds in cases when there is no discontinuity. The second interpolator (shown in the left column, second from the top) predominantly uses the leftmost three depths; the corresponding controller for this interpolator (immediately right of the top left interpolator's weights) detects discontinuities between the rightmost two depths, d_c and d_d. Similarly, the remaining controllers detect discontinuities to the right or left of d_c; each controller's corresponding interpolator uses the depths on the opposite side of the discontinuity to predict d_c.

4 Discussion

We have described two ways of modeling spatially coherent features in images of scenes with discontinuities. The first approach was to simply try to discriminate between patterns with and without discontinuities, and throw away the former. In theory, this approach is promising, as it provides a way of making the algorithm more robust against outlying data points. We then applied the idea of multiple models of coherence to a set of interpolating units, again using images of curved surfaces with discontinuities. The competing controllers in Figure 4 learned to explicitly represent which regularity applies in a particular region. The output of the controllers was used to compute a probability distribution over the various competing models of coherence.

The representation learned by this network has a number of advantages. We now have a measure of the probability that there is a discontinuity that is independent of the prediction error of the interpolator. So we can tell how much to trust each interpolator's estimate on each case. It should be possible to distinguish clear cases of discontinuities from cases that are simply noisy, by the entropy of the controllers' outputs.

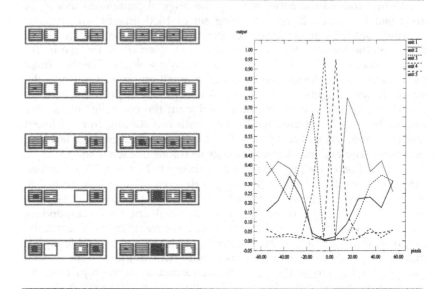

Figure 5: (a) Typical weights learned by the five competing interpolators and corresponding five discontinuity detectors. Positive weights are shown in white, and negative weights in black. (b) The mean probabilities computed by each discontinuity detector are plotted against the distance from the center of the units' receptive field to the nearest discontinuity. The probabilistic outputs are averaged over an ensemble of 1000 test cases. If the nearest discontinuity is beyond ±30 pixels, it is outside the units' receptive field and the case is therefore a continuity example.

Furthermore, the controller outputs tell us not only that a discontinuity is present, but exactly where it lies. This information is important for segmenting scenes, and should be a useful representation for later stages of unsupervised learning. Like the raw depth estimates, the location of depth edges should exhibit coherence across space, at larger spatial scales. It should therefore be possible to apply the same algorithm recursively to the outputs of the controllers, to find object boundaries in two-dimensional stereo images.

The approach presented here should be applicable to other domains that contain a mixture of alternative local regularities across space or time. For example, a rigid shape causes a linear constraint between the locations of its parts in an image, so if there are many possible shapes, there are many alternative local regularities (Zemel and Hinton 1991).

Acknowledgments

This research was funded by grants from NSERC and the Ontario Information Technology Research Centre. Hinton is Noranda fellow of the Canadian Institute for Advanced Research. Thanks to John Bridle and Steve Nowlan for helpful discussions.

References

Becker, S., and Hinton, G. E. 1992a. Learning to make coherent predictions in domains with discontinuities. In *Advances in Neural Information Processing Systems 4*. Morgan Kaufmann, San Mateo, CA.

Becker, S., and Hinton, G. E. 1992b. A self-organizing neural network that discovers surfaces in random-dot stereograms. *Nature (London)* **355**, 161–163.

Jacobs, R. A., Jordan, M. I., Nowlan, S. J., and Hinton, G. E. 1991. Adaptive mixtures of local experts. *Neural Comp.* **3**(1), 79–87.

McLachlan, G. J., and Basford, K. E. 1988. *Mixture Models: Inference and Applications to Clustering*. Marcel Dekker, New York.

Shannon, C. E., and Weaver, W. 1964. *The Mathematical Theory of Communication*. The University of Illinois Press, Urbana, IL.

Zemel, R. S., and Hinton, G. E. 1991. Discovering viewpoint-invariant relationships that characterize objects. In *Advances in Neural Information Processing Systems 3*, pp. 299–305. Morgan Kaufmann, San Mateo, CA.

13

Bayesian Self-Organization Driven by Prior Probability Distributions

Alan L. Yuille
Stelios M. Smirnakis
Lei Xu
Division of Applied Sciences, Harvard University, Cambridge, MA 02138, USA

Recent work by Becker and Hinton (1992) shows a promising mechanism, based on maximizing mutual information assuming spatial coherence, by which a system can self-organize to learn visual abilities such as binocular stereo. We introduce a more general criterion, based on Bayesian probability theory, and thereby demonstrate a connection to Bayesian theories of visual perception and to other organization principles for early vision (Atick and Redlich 1990). Methods for implementation using variants of stochastic learning are described.

1 Introduction

The input intensity patterns received by the human visual system are typically complicated functions of the object surfaces and light sources in the world. It seems probable, however, that humans perceive the world in terms of surfaces and objects (Nakayama and Shimojo 1987). Thus the visual system must be able to extract information from the input intensities that is relatively independent of the actual intensity values. Such abilities may not be present at birth and hence must be learned. It seems, for example, that binocular stereo develops at about the age of 2 to 3 months (Held 1987).

Becker and Hinton (1992) describe an interesting mechanism for self-organizing a system to achieve this. The basic idea is to assume spatial coherence of the structure to be extracted and to train a neural network by maximizing the mutual information between neurons with spatially disjoint receptive fields (see Fig. 1). For binocular stereo, for example, the surface being viewed is assumed flat (see Becker and Hinton 1992, for generalizations of this assumption) and hence has spatially constant disparity. The intensity patterns, however, do not have any simple spatial behavior. Adjusting the synaptic strengths of the network to maximize the mutual information between neurons with nonoverlapping receptive fields, for an ensemble of images, causes the neurons to extract features that are spatially coherent, thereby obtaining the disparity.

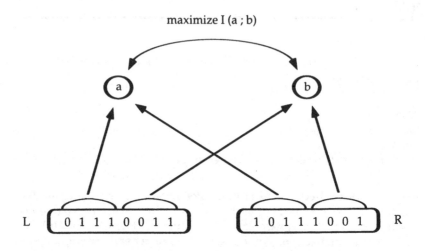

maximize I (a ; b)

Figure 1: In Hinton and Becker's initial scheme, maximization of mutual information between neurons with spatially disjoint receptive fields leads to disparity tuning, provided they train on spatially coherent patterns (i.e., those for which disparity changes slowly with spatial position).

We argue that this approach has three key ingredients:

1. It uses strong prior knowledge about the output variables, i.e., it assumes that the disparities are spatially constant. If this assumption is not valid then the performance of the system will degrade.

2. It represents the desired outputs as functions of the inputs by a multilayer perceptron with adjustable weights.

3. It proposes a criterion, mutual information maximization, motivated by the prior knowledge (see point 1) to determine the weights.

The approach relies heavily on prior assumptions about the form of the outputs. This is similar to Bayesian theories of visual perception that also rely (Clark and Yuille 1990) on prior assumptions about properties of the world, such as binocular disparities. Such priors are needed because of the ill-posed nature of vision (Poggio *et al.* 1985) and can be thought of as *natural constraints* (Marr 1982).

This similarity motivates the following questions. Can we reformulate Becker and Hinton's theory so that it can be applied directly to learning Bayesian theories of vision? More precisely, assuming a prior of the type commonly used in vision, can we find an optimization criterion and learning algorithm such that we can learn the corresponding Bayesian theory?

This note shows that it is indeed possible to reformulate Becker and Hinton to make it compatible with Bayesian theories. In particular, their algorithm for stereo corresponds to one of the standard priors used for Bayesian stereo theories (see Section 3). The key idea is to force the activity distribution of the outputs, S, to be close to a prespecified prior distribution $P_p(S)$. Our approach is general and is related to the work performed by Atick and Redlich (1990) for modeling the early visual system. In previous work (Yuille *et al.* 1993) we proved that applying our approach to linear filtering problems leads to a solution that is the square root of the Wiener filter in Fourier space. A similar result has been derived (Redlich, private communication) from the principles described in Atick and Redlich (1990).

We should clarify what we mean by "learning a Bayesian theory." A Bayesian theory for estimating a scene property S from input D consists of three elements: (1) a prior for the property $P_p(S)$, (2) a likelihood function $P_l(D \mid S)$, and (3) an algorithm for estimating $S^*(D) = \arg\max_S P_l(D \mid S)P_p(S)$.[1] Because we assume that the prior is known we are essentially learning the likelihood function and the algorithm. Our approach, after training, will yield a neural net, or some other function approximation scheme, that computes $S^*(D)$. In related work (Smirnakis and Yuille 1994) we assume that both prior and likelihood are known and train a network to learn the algorithm.

This can be contrasted to alternative ways for learning Bayesian theories. Hidden Markov models (Paul 1990) (see Section 5) learn both the priors and the likelihood functions. A general purpose optimization algorithm, dynamic programming, is then used to compute the MAP, or some alternative, estimator. This approach can be highly effective, though dynamic programming is efficient only for one-dimensional problems and functional forms for the prior and likelihood are required. Kersten *et al.* (1987) describe Bayesian learning with a teacher that yields the algorithm $S^*(D) = \arg\max_S P_l(D \mid S)P_p(S)$. But as Becker and Hinton have shown, a teacher is not always necessary.

We will take the viewpoint that the prior $P_p(S)$ is assumed known in advance by the visual system (perhaps by being specified genetically) and will act as a self-organizing principle. Later we will discuss ways that this might be relaxed.

2 Theory

We assume that the input D is a function $F(n, \alpha)$ of a *signal* α that the system wants to determine and a *distractor* n. These quantities are vectors indexed by spatial location (see Fig. 2). For example, α might correspond to the disparities of a pair of binocular stereo images and n to the intensity

---

[1]This corresponds to the commonly used maximum a posteriori (MAP) estimator. Other estimators may be preferable, but we will consider only MAP in this paper.

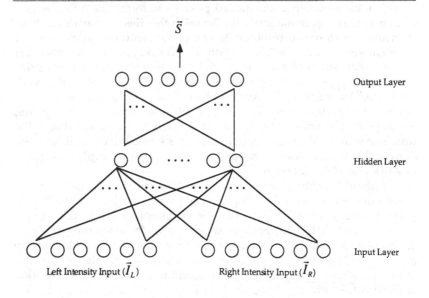

Figure 2: Note that the vectors $\mathbf{I}_L$ and $\mathbf{I}_R$ represent the intensities falling on the left and right retinas respectively, and are indexed by spatial location. $\mathbf{S}$ represents the vector of the disparities to be extracted. That is, the output S_i of output unit i represents the disparity at spatial location i. By setting some of the synapses to zero we obtain the disjoint receptive fields of the Becker and Hinton paradigm (Fig. 1).

patterns. The variables have distributions $P_n(\mathbf{n})$ and $P_p(\alpha)$, respectively. Note that $\mathbf{D}$ and $P_p(\alpha)$ are assumed to be known but $P_n(\mathbf{n})$ and the functional form of $F(\mathbf{n}, \alpha)$ are unknown.

The input distribution is given by

$$P_D(\mathbf{D}) = \int \int \delta[\mathbf{D} - F(\mathbf{n}, \alpha)] P_n(\mathbf{n}) P_p(\alpha)[d\alpha][d\mathbf{n}]$$

and can be observed by the system.

Let the output of the system be $\mathbf{S} = \mathbf{G}(\mathbf{D}, \gamma)$ where $\mathbf{G}$ is a function of a set of parameters γ to be determined. For example, the function $\mathbf{G}(\mathbf{D}, \gamma)$ could be represented by a multilayer perceptron with γ being the synaptic weights. By approximation theory, it can be shown that a large variety of neural networks can approximate any input–output function arbitrarily well given enough hidden nodes (Hornik $et\ al.$ 1991). We can combine these formulas to give

$$\mathbf{S} = \mathbf{G}[F(\mathbf{n}, \alpha), \gamma] \qquad\qquad (2.1)$$

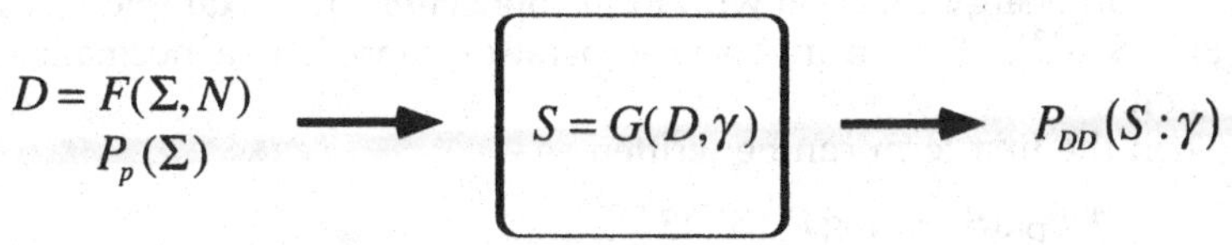

$$D = F(\Sigma, N) \quad\longrightarrow\quad \boxed{S = G(D, \gamma)} \quad\longrightarrow\quad P_{DD}(S : \gamma)$$
$$P_p(\Sigma)$$

$$KL(\gamma) = \int P_{DD}(S : \gamma) \log(\frac{P_{DD}(S : \gamma)}{P_p(S)}) dS$$

Figure 3: The parameters γ are adjusted to minimize the Kullback–Leibler distance between the prior (P_p) distribution of the true signal (Σ) and the derived distribution (P_{DD}) of the network output (S).

The aim of self-organizing the network is to ensure that the parameters γ are chosen so that the outputs S are as close to the α (or some simple transformation of the αs) as possible. We claim that this can be achieved by adjusting the parameters γ so as to make the derived distribution of the outputs $P_{DD}(S : \gamma) = \int \delta[S - G(D, \gamma)]P_D(D)[dD]$ as close as possible to $P_p(S)$.

This can be seen to be a consistency condition for a Bayesian theory. From Bayes's formula we obtain the condition:

$$\int P(S \mid D)P_D(D)[dD] = \int P(D \mid S)P_p(S)[dD] = P_p(S) \qquad (2.2)$$

This is equivalent to our condition provided we identify $P(S \mid D)$ with $\delta[S - G(D, \gamma)]$.

To make this more precise we must define a measure of similarity between the two distributions $P_p(S)$ and $P_{DD}(S : \gamma)$. An attractive measure is the Kullback–Leibler distance (the entropy of P_{DD} relative to P_p):

$$KL(\gamma) = \int P_{DD}(S : \gamma) \log \frac{P_{DD}(S : \gamma)}{P_p(S)}[dS] \qquad (2.3)$$

Thus our theory (see Fig. 3) corresponds to adjusting the parameters γ to minimize the Kullback–Leibler distance between $P_p(S)$ and $P_{DD}(S : \gamma)$. This measure can be divided into two parts: (1) $- \int P_{DD}(S : \gamma) \log P_p(S)[dS]$ and (2) $\int P_{DD}(S : \gamma) \log P_{DD}(S : \gamma)[dS]$. As we now show both terms have very intuitive interpretations.

Suppose that $P_p(S)$ can be expressed as a Markov random field [i.e., the spatial distribution of $P_p(S)$ has a local neighborhood structure, as is commonly assumed in Bayesian models of vision]. Then, by the

Hammersely–Clifford theorem, we can write $P_p(\mathbf{S}) = e^{-\beta E_p(\mathbf{S})}/Z$ where $E_p(\mathbf{S})$ is an energy function with local connections [for example, $E_p(\mathbf{S}) = \sum_i (S_i - S_{i+1})^2$], β is an inverse temperature, and Z is a normalization constant.

Then the first term can be written as

$$-\int P_{DD}(\mathbf{S} : \gamma) \log P_p(\mathbf{S})[d\mathbf{S}]$$

$$= \int\int \delta[\mathbf{S} - \mathbf{G}(\mathbf{D}, \gamma)]P_D(\mathbf{D})\beta E_p(\mathbf{S})[d\mathbf{D}][d\mathbf{S}] + \log Z$$

$$= \int \beta E_p[\mathbf{G}(\mathbf{D}, \gamma)]P_D(\mathbf{D})[d\mathbf{D}] + \log Z$$

$$= \beta\langle E_p[\mathbf{G}(\mathbf{D}, \gamma)]\rangle_D + \log Z \tag{2.4}$$

We can ignore the $\log Z$ term since it is a constant (independent of γ). Minimizing the first term with respect to γ will therefore try to minimize the energy of the outputs averaged over the inputs—$\langle E_p[\mathbf{G}(\mathbf{D}, \gamma)]\rangle_D$— which is highly desirable [since it has a close connection to the minimal energy principles in Poggio et al. (1985), and Clark and Yuille (1990)]. It is important, however, to avoid the trivial solution $\mathbf{G}(\mathbf{D}, \gamma) = constant$ or solutions where $\mathbf{G}(\mathbf{D}, \gamma)$ is very small for most inputs. Fortunately these solutions will be discouraged by the second term.

The second term $\int P_{DD}(\mathbf{D}, \gamma) \log P_{DD}(\mathbf{D}, \gamma)[d\mathbf{D}]$ can be interpreted as the negative of the entropy of the derived distribution of the output. Minimizing it with respect to γ is a maximum entropy principle that will encourage variability in the outputs $G(\mathbf{D}, \gamma)$ and hence prevent the trivial solutions.

The two terms combine to determine the γ so that the energy of the output variables is minimized while maximizing their variability. This is closely related to Becker and Hinton's method of maximizing the mutual information between pairs of output variables—essentially assuming a spatially constant prior distribution for $\mathbf{S}$. At the same time it is reminiscent of other organizational principles for early vision based on information theory (Atick and Redlich 1990).

How can one guarantee that the optimal solution to our criteria will indeed extract the signal? This will depend on a number of factors: (1) the forms of the functions $\mathbf{F}$ and $\mathbf{G}$, (2) the forms of the probability distributions $P_n(\mathbf{n})$ and $P_p(\alpha)$, and (3) whether the prior P_p is indeed correct or not.

It is straightforward to write down the conditions for the derived distribution to be equal to the prior distribution (assuming that the prior is correct). This is a stronger condition than requiring the Kullback–Leibler distance to be minimal (though, if equality is possible, minimizing Kullback–Leibler would lead to it). It is

$$P_p(\mathbf{S}) = \int\int \delta\{\mathbf{S} - \mathbf{G}[\mathbf{F}(\mathbf{n}, \alpha), \gamma]\} P_n(\mathbf{n})P_p(\alpha)[d\alpha][d\mathbf{n}] \tag{2.5}$$

If one could find γ^* so that $\mathbf{G}[\mathbf{F}(\mathbf{n}, \alpha), \gamma^*] = \alpha$, $\forall \mathbf{n}, \alpha$ then the equation could be solved exactly. The condition $\mathbf{G}[\mathbf{F}(\mathbf{n}, \alpha), \gamma^*] = \alpha$, however, is too strong. It requires that the function **G**, which can be thought of as a nonlinear filter, is able to completely eliminate the dependence on **n**.

We have assumed that the correct prior is known by the system, perhaps by being specified genetically. An alternative possibility is that the prior itself is learned by a method reminiscent of Occam's razor: the goodness of the prior is evaluated based on the Kullback–Leibler distance after self-organization, and a more complex prior is chosen if this distance is large (see also Mumford 1992).

3 Connection to Becker and Hinton

In this section, we show that the case of disparity extraction implemented by Becker and Hinton based on their principle of mutual information maximization arises as a special case of our formalism, by choosing a particular prior. The Becker and Hinton method (Becker and Hinton 1992) for extracting the disparity involves maximizing the mutual information between two network output units S_1, S_2 with spatially disjoint receptive fields, under the assumption that disparity is spatially coherent. S_1 and S_2 denote the scalar values of two units in the output layer of a neural network, indexed by spatial location. The mutual information between S_1, S_2 is given by

$$\begin{aligned}
I(S_1, S_2; \gamma) &= -\langle \log P_{DD}(S_1; \gamma) \rangle - \langle \log P_{DD}(S_2; \gamma) \rangle \\
&\quad + \langle \log P_{DD}(S_1, S_2; \gamma) \rangle \\
&= H(S_1; \gamma) - H(S_1 \mid S_2; \gamma)
\end{aligned} \tag{3.1}$$

From this equation we see that we want to maximize the entropy, $H(S_1; \gamma)$, of S_1 while minimizing the conditional entropy, $H(S_1 \mid S_2; \gamma)$, of S_1 given S_2, which forces S_1 to be a deterministic function of S_2 (alternatively, by symmetry, we can interchange the roles of S_1 and S_2). For the discussion below we will use our criterion to reproduce the case in which this last term forces $S_1 \approx S_2$.

By contrast, in our version (see Fig. 4) we propose to minimize the expression $\langle \log P_{DD}(S_1, S_2; \gamma) \rangle - \int \log P_p(S_1, S_2) P_{DD}(S_1, S_2; \gamma) [d\mathbf{S}]$. If we ensure that the prior $P_p(S_1, S_2) \propto e^{-\tau(S_1 - S_2)^2}$, then, for large τ, our second term will force $S_1 \approx S_2$ and our first term will maximize the entropy of the joint distribution of S_1, S_2. We argue that this is effectively the same as Becker and Hinton (1992), since maximizing the joint entropy of S_1, S_2 with S_1 constrained to equal S_2 is equivalent to maximizing the individual entropies of S_1 and S_2 with the same constraint.

To be more concrete, we consider Becker and Hinton's implementation of the mutual information maximization principle in the case of units with continuous outputs. They assume that the outputs of units $1, 2$ are gaussian[2] and perform steepest descent to maximize the symmetrized

---

[2]We assume for simplicity that these gaussians have zero mean.

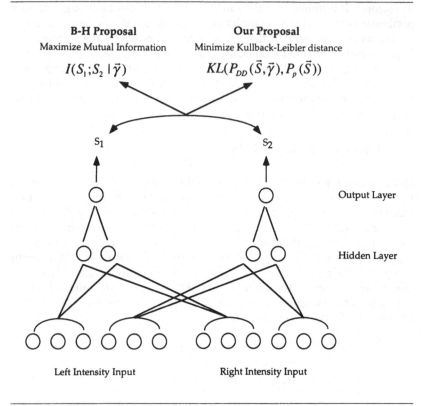

Figure 4: Comparing our theory with Becker and Hinton's. Observe that setting $P_p(S_1, S_2) \propto e^{-\tau(S_1 - S_2)^2}$ forces $S_1 \approx S_2$ for large τ, implementing their assumption that the disparity is spatially coherent.

form of the mutual information between S_1 and S_2:

$$
\begin{aligned}
I(S_1, S_2) &= \log \frac{V(S_1)}{V(S_1 - S_2)} + \log \frac{V(S_2)}{V(S_1 - S_2)} \\
&= \log V(S_1) + \log V(S_2) - 2 \log V(S_1 - S_2)
\end{aligned}
\tag{3.2}
$$

where $V(\cdot)$ stands for variance over the set of inputs. They assume that the difference between the two outputs can be expressed as uncorrelated additive noise, $S_1 = S_2 + N$. Therefore, their criterion amounts to maximizing

$$
E_{BH}[V(S_2), V(N)] = \log\{V(S_2) + V(N)\} + \log V(S_2) - 2 \log V(N)
\tag{3.3}
$$

For our scheme we make similar assumptions about the distributions of S_1 and S_2. We then see that, up to additive constants independent of γ,

$\langle \log P_{DD}(S_1, S_2) \rangle = -1/2 \log\{\langle S_1^2 \rangle \langle S_2^2 \rangle - \langle S_1 S_2 \rangle^2\} = -1/2 \log\{V(S_2)V(N)\}$
[since $\langle S_1 S_2 \rangle = \langle (S_2 + N)S_2 \rangle = V(S_2)$ and $\langle S_1^2 \rangle = V(S_2) + V(N)$]. We now
observe that if we choose the prior distribution $P_p(S_1, S_2) \propto e^{-\tau(S_1 - S_2)^2}$ our
criterion corresponds to minimizing $E_{YSX}[V(S_2), V(N)]$ where

$$E_{YSX}[V(S_2), V(N)] = -\log V(S_2) - \log V(N) + \tau V(N) \qquad (3.4)$$

It is easy to see that maximizing $E_{BH}[V(S_2), V(N)]$ will try to make
$V(S_2)$ as large as possible and force $V(N)$ to zero [recall that, by definition,
$V(N) \geq 0$]. On the other hand, minimizing our energy will try to make
$V(S_2)$ as large as possible and will force $V(N)$ to $1/\tau$. Since τ appears as
the inverse of the variance of the gaussian prior for $\mathbf{S} = (S_1, S_2)$, making
τ large will force the prior distribution to approach $\delta(S_1 - S_2)$. Thus, in
the case of large τ, our method has the same effect as the Becker and
Hinton algorithm.

For this to be true, it is important to choose a network architecture
satisfying the requirement that the output units representing disparity
have spatially disjoint receptive fields (see Fig. 4). If this were not the
case, the output units would run the risk of getting entrained on the receptive field overlap, provided it has the right probability structure. Even
though we did not pursue this issue in the above analysis, it is, in principle, possible to implement such architectural constraints by defining a
prior distribution on the weights of the network.

Note that, in principle, maximizing the mutual information between
S_1, S_2 can only determine the network output up to transformations that
leave the mutual information invariant. Which solution the network will
settle at depends on the specifics of the implementation and on initial
conditions. For instance, in the Becker and Hinton example the network
sometimes settles so that $S_1 \approx S_2$, and sometimes so that $S_1 \approx -S_2$. This
may not be always desirable. In this context, the ability to choose a prior
affords a natural way to restrict the possible space of solutions.

4 Reformulating for Implementation in a General Setting

Our proposal requires us to minimize the Kullback–Leibler distance (equation 2.3) with respect to γ. In the previous section, we showed that Becker
and Hinton's implementation of the mutual information maximization
principle for disparity extraction arose as a special case of our formalism, for a particular prior. Therefore, their simulation already represents
a concrete example of how our scheme can be implemented. In the
present section, we endeavor to expand further by outlining two general
implementation strategies based on variants of stochastic learning:

First observe that by substituting the form of the derived distribution,
$P_{DD}(\mathbf{S} : \gamma) = \int \delta[\mathbf{S} - \mathbf{G}(\mathbf{D}, \gamma)] P_D(\mathbf{D})[d\mathbf{D}]$, into equation 2.3 and integrating
out the $\mathbf{S}$ variable we obtain

$$KL(\gamma) = \int P_D(\mathbf{D}) \log \frac{P_{DD}[\mathbf{G}(\mathbf{D}, \gamma) : \gamma]}{P_p[\mathbf{G}(\mathbf{D}, \gamma)]}[d\mathbf{D}] \qquad (4.1)$$

This is the form of the Kullback–Liebler distance that we assume in the implementation strategies we describe below:

1. Assuming a representative sample $\{\mathbf{D}^\mu : \mu \in \Lambda\}$ of inputs we can approximate $KL(\gamma)$ by $\sum_{\mu \in \Lambda} \log\{P_{DD}[\mathbf{G}(\mathbf{D}^\mu, \gamma) : \gamma]/P_p[\mathbf{G}(\mathbf{D}^\mu, \gamma)]\}$. We can now, in principle, perform stochastic learning using backpropagation: pick inputs $\mathbf{D}^\mu$ at random and update the weights γ using $\log\{P_{DD}[\mathbf{G}(\mathbf{D}^\mu, \gamma) : \gamma]/P_p[\mathbf{G}(\mathbf{D}^\mu, \gamma)]\}$ as the error function.

To do this, however, we need expressions for $P_{DD}[\mathbf{G}(\mathbf{D}^\mu, \gamma) : \gamma]$ and its derivative with respect to γ. If the function $\mathbf{G}(\mathbf{D}, \gamma)$ can be restricted to being 1-1 (artificially increasing the dimensionality of the output space if necessary) then we can obtain analytic expressions $P_{DD}[\mathbf{G}(\mathbf{D}, \gamma) : \gamma] = P_D(\mathbf{D})/|\det(\partial \mathbf{G}/\partial \mathbf{D})|$ and $\{\partial \log P_{DD}[\mathbf{G}(\mathbf{D}, \gamma) : \gamma]/\partial\gamma\} = -(\partial \mathbf{G}/\partial \mathbf{D})^{-1} (\partial^2 \mathbf{G}/\partial \mathbf{D} \partial\gamma)$, where -1 denotes the matrix inverse.

To see this we observe that

$$P_{DD}(\mathbf{S} : \gamma) = \int \delta[\mathbf{S} - \mathbf{G}(\mathbf{D}, \gamma)]P_D(\mathbf{D})[d\mathbf{D}]$$

$$= \frac{P_D(\mathbf{D}^*)}{|\det(\partial \mathbf{G}/\partial \mathbf{D})(\mathbf{D}^*, \gamma)|} \quad (4.2)$$

where $\mathbf{D}^* = G^{-1}(\mathbf{S}, \gamma)$ and we assume that the function G is 1-1. It follows directly that

$$P_{DD}[\mathbf{G}(\mathbf{D}, \gamma) : \gamma] = \frac{P_D(\mathbf{D})}{|\det(\partial \mathbf{G}/\partial \mathbf{D})(\mathbf{D}, \gamma)|} \quad (4.3)$$

Substituting back into the K–L measure (equation 4.1) means that we must minimize with respect to γ the cost function $E[\gamma, \mathbf{D}]$ averaged over a sample of $\mathbf{D}$ (where we have dropped terms that are independent of γ):

$$E[\gamma, \mathbf{D}] = -\log\left|\det \frac{\partial \mathbf{G}}{\partial \mathbf{D}}(\mathbf{D}, \gamma)\right| + \beta E_p[\mathbf{G}(\mathbf{D}, \gamma)] \quad (4.4)$$

We implement this by stochastic learning. Pick an input $\mathbf{D}$ at random, set $\gamma_{new} = \gamma_{old} - \zeta(\partial E/\partial \gamma)$ (where ζ is the learning rate), and repeat.

This involves calculating $\partial E/\partial \gamma$. After some algebra we find that

$$\frac{\partial}{\partial \gamma_a} \log\left|\det\left\{\frac{\partial \mathbf{G}}{\partial \mathbf{D}}(\mathbf{D}, \gamma)\right\}\right| = \sum_{j,k} \left(\frac{\partial G_j}{\partial D_k}\right)^{-1} \frac{\partial^2 G_k}{\partial D_j \partial \gamma_a} \quad (4.5)$$

where -1 denotes the matrix inverse.

The contribution from the second term will simply be $\beta(\partial E/\partial \mathbf{G})$ $(\partial \mathbf{G}/\partial \gamma_a)$.

This analysis has assumed that $\mathbf{G}$ is a 1-1 function and requires, as a necessary condition, that the input and output spaces have the same dimension. This could often be ensured by adding additional output units or input units with fixed synaptic strengths.

2. Alternatively we can perform additional sampling to estimate $P_{DD}[G(D, \gamma) : \gamma]$ and $\{\partial \log P_{DD}[G(D, \gamma) : \gamma]/\partial \gamma\}$ directly from their integral representations. [This second approach is similar to Becker and Hinton (1992), though they are concerned with estimating only the first and second moments of these distributions.] The Kullback–Leibler measure corresponds to minimizing $KL(\gamma) = \sum_\mu E(\gamma, D^\mu)$, where $E(\gamma, D^\mu) = \log P_{DD}[G(D^\mu, \gamma) : \gamma] + \beta E_p[G(D^\mu, \gamma)]$.

Thus calculating the gradient of $E(\gamma, D^\mu)$ requires evaluating the expression $\{\partial P_{DD}[G(D^\mu, \gamma) : \gamma]/\partial \gamma\}/P_{DD}[G(D^\mu, \gamma) : \gamma]$. To estimate these quantities we make the approximation:

$$P_{DD}[G(D^\mu, \gamma) : \gamma] \approx \sum_\nu \frac{1}{\left[\sqrt{(2\pi)}\sigma\right]^N} e^{-(1/2\sigma^2)|G(D^\mu, \gamma) - G(D^\nu, \gamma)|^2} \qquad (4.6)$$

where $\{D^\nu\}$ are a representative set of samples from $P_D(D)$ and σ is a constant. This reduces to the previous expression, the first part of equation 4.2, in the limit as $\sigma \mapsto 0$ and as the size of the sample set tends to infinity.

A formula for $\{\partial P_{DD}[G(D^\mu, \gamma) : \gamma]/\partial \gamma\}$ can be obtained by differentiating (4.6) with respect to γ. This gives

$$\frac{\partial P_{DD}[G(D^\mu, \gamma) : \gamma]}{\partial \gamma_a}$$

$$\approx \sum_\nu \frac{1}{\left[\sqrt{(2\pi)}\sigma\right]^N} \times \left\{-\frac{1}{\sigma^2}\right\}$$

$$\times \sum_i \left\{\frac{\partial G_i(D^\mu, \gamma)}{\partial \gamma_a} - \frac{\partial G_i(D^\nu, \gamma)}{\partial \gamma_a}\right\} \{G_i(D^\mu, \gamma) - G_i(D^\nu, \gamma)\}$$

$$\times e^{-(1/2\sigma^2)|G(D^\mu, \gamma) - G(D^\nu, \gamma)|^2} \qquad (4.7)$$

The learning proceeds by picking a sample D^μ from $P_D(D)$ and then an additional set of samples $\{D^\nu\}$ to approximate the integrals 4.6 and 4.7 and hence enable us to calculate the gradient of $E(\gamma, D^\mu)$ and update the weights. Then the process repeats.

Note that this approach has the advantage of circumventing the demand that the dimensions of the input and output spaces be equal, i.e., that G be 1-1, and is more generally applicable.

5 Relationship to Hidden Markov Models and Maximum Likelihood Estimation

It is instructive to contrast our work to alternative learning approaches and, in particular, to hidden Markov models (HMMs)[3] (Paul 1990).

---

[3] Approaches closely related to HMMs are being used for learning stereo (Geiger, personal communication).

HMMs have been very successful in speech processing where models
are trained for each recognizable speech segment. Here, however, we are
considering training only a single HMM.

In an HMM there are hidden states and observables that, in our nota-
tion, correspond to $\mathbf{S}$ and $\mathbf{D}$, respectively. An HMM assumes (1) a prior
model $P(\mathbf{S} \mid \beta)$, where the β are parameters to be learned, and (2) an
imaging model $P(\mathbf{D} \mid \mathbf{S}, \alpha)$, where the α are parameters to be learned.
Together these generate probabilities $P(\mathbf{D} \mid \alpha, \beta) = \sum_S P(\mathbf{D} \mid \mathbf{S}, \alpha)P(\mathbf{S} \mid \beta)$
for the observables as functions of the parameters.[4] Similar expressions
arise in MLE parameter estimation (Ripley 1992).

To learn the priors and likelihood functions we must estimate the
parameters α and β. This requires a set of data $\{\mathbf{D}^\mu\}$, indexed by μ,
that we assume is a representative sample from the distribution $P(\mathbf{D})$ of
the observables. We then train the system by maximum likelihood estimation (MLE). More precisely, we select the parameters α and β that
maximize $\prod_\mu P(\mathbf{D}^\mu \mid \alpha, \beta)$ or, equivalently, that maximize $\sum_\mu \log P(\mathbf{D}^\mu \mid$
$\alpha, \beta)$. As the sample size tends to infinity this becomes equivalent
to maximizing $\sum_\mathbf{D} P(\mathbf{D}) \log[P(\mathbf{D} \mid \alpha, \beta)$ or, equivalently, to maximizing
$\sum_\mathbf{D} P(\mathbf{D}) \log P(\mathbf{D} \mid \alpha, \beta)/P(\mathbf{D})]$ [since $P(\mathbf{D})$ is independent of α and β].
Thus, in the infinite sample size limit, we are simply *minimizing* the
Kullback–Leibler measure $(\sum_\mathbf{D} P(\mathbf{D}) \log[P(\mathbf{D})/P(\mathbf{D} \mid \alpha, \beta)])$ between the
observed distribution $P(\mathbf{D})$ and the distribution $P(\mathbf{D} \mid \alpha, \beta)$ derived by
the model.

By contrast, we propose a Kullback–Leibler measure of similarity on
the outputs, or hidden states, $\mathbf{S}$, rather than on the input states. The
MLE justification for this leads to minimizing the Kullback–Leibler dis-
tance $\sum_S P(\mathbf{S}) \log[P(\mathbf{S})/P(\mathbf{S} \mid \gamma)]$, where γ represents the parameters of
the network.

HMMs assume a class of prior probabilities, parameterized by β,
rather than the single model that we have assumed. However, we can
readily generalize our model to deal with this case by replacing $P_p(\mathbf{S})$
by a parameterized family of distributions $P_p(\mathbf{S} \mid \tau)$. We must now minimize the Kullback–Leibler distance between $P_p(\mathbf{S} \mid \tau)$ and the derived
distribution $P_{DD}(\mathbf{S} : \gamma)$ with respect to γ and τ simultaneously.

6 Conclusion

The goal of this note was to introduce a Bayesian approach to self-
organization using prior assumptions about the signal as an organizing principle. We argued that it was a natural generalization of the
criterion of maximizing mutual information assuming spatial coherence
(Becker and Hinton 1992). Using our principle it should be possible to

---

[4]HMMs have other important properties that are not directly relevant here. For
example, the functional forms of $P(\mathbf{S} \mid \beta)$ and $P(\mathbf{D} \mid \mathbf{S}, \alpha)$ are chosen to ensure that
highly efficient algorithms are available to perform these computations (Paul 1990).

self-organize Bayesian theories of vision, assuming that the priors are known, the network is capable of representing the appropriate functions, and the learning algorithm converges. There will also be problems if the probability distributions of the true signal and the distractor are too similar.

If the prior is not correct then it may be possible to detect this by evaluating the goodness of the Kullback–Leibler fit after learning.[5] This suggests a strategy whereby the system increases the complexity of the priors until the Kullback–Leibler fit is sufficiently good [this is somewhat similar to an idea proposed by Mumford (1992)]. This is related to the idea of competitive priors in vision (Clark and Yuille 1990). One way to implement this would be for the prior probability itself to have a set of adjustable parameters that would enable it to adapt to different classes of scenes.

Our approach differs from standard MLE by acting on the distributions of the output variables rather than the inputs. Unlike MLE our approach will directly yield an algorithm for computing the outputs. It is still unclear, however, for what class of problems our approach is applicable. For example, it seems unlikely to work if the dimensions of the outputs is a lot lower than that of the inputs.

We proposed two variants of stochastic learning that are suitable for implementing our theory. They relate, in particular, to Becker and Hinton's approach. As a further illustration of our approach we derived elsewhere (Yuille *et al.* 1993) the filter that our criterion would give for filtering out additive gaussian noise (possibly the only analytically tractable case). This turned out to be the square root of the Wiener filter in Fourier space.

Acknowledgments

We would like to thank ARPA for an Air Force contract F49620-92-J-0466. Conversations with Dan Kersten and David Mumford were highly appreciated. We would also like to thank the reviewers for their insightful comments.

References

Atick, J. J., and Redlich, A. N. 1990. Towards a theory of early visual processing. *Neural Comp.* **2**, 308–320.
Barlow, H. B. 1993. What is the computational goal of the neocortex? In *Large Scale Neuronal Theories of the Brain*, C. Koch, ed. MIT Press, Cambridge, MA.

---

[5]This is reminiscent of Barlow's suspicious coincidence detectors (Barlow 1993), where we might hope to determine if two variables x and y are independent or not by calculating the Kullback–Leibler distance between the joint distribution $P(x, y)$ and the product of the individual distributions $P(x)P(y)$.

Becker, S., and Hinton, G. E. 1992. Self-organizing neural network that discovers surfaces in random-dot stereograms. *Nature (London)* **355**, 161–163.

Clark, J. J., and Yuille, A. L. 1990. *Data Fusion for Sensory Information Processing Systems*. Kluwer, Boston.

Held, R. 1987. Visual development in infants. In *The Encyclopedia of Neuroscience*, Vol. 2. Birkhauser, Boston.

Hornik, K., Stinchcombe, S., and White, H. 1991. Multilayer feed-forward networks are universal approximators. *Neural Networks* **4**, 251–257.

Kersten, D., O'Toole, A. J., Sereno, M. E., Knill, D. C., and Anderson, J. A. 1987. Associative learning of scene parameters from images. *Opt. Soc. Am.* **26**, 4999–5006.

Marr, D. 1982. *Vision*. W. H. Freeman, San Francisco.

Mumford, D. 1992. *Pattern Theory: A Unifying Perspective*. Mathematics Preprint. Harvard University.

Nakayama, K., and Shimojo, S. 1987. Experiencing and perceiving visual surfaces. *Science* **257**, 1357–1363.

Paul, D. B. 1990. Speech recognition using hidden Markov models. *Lincoln Lab. J.* **3**, 41–62.

Poggio, T., Torre, V., and Koch, C. 1985. Computational vision and regularization theory. *Nature (London)* **317**, 314–319.

Ripley, B. D. 1992. Classification and clustering in spatial and image data. In *Analyzing and Modeling Data and Knowledge*, M. Schader, ed. Springer-Verlag, Berlin.

Smirnakis, S. M., and Yuille, A. L. 1994. Neural implementation of Bayesian vision theories by unsupervised learning. *CNS Conf. Proc.*, in press.

Yuille, A. L., Smirnakis, S. M., and Xu, L. 1993. Bayesian self-organization. *NIPS Conf. Proc.*

14

Finding Minimum Entropy Codes

H.B. Barlow
T.P. Kaushal
G.J. Mitchison
Physiological Laboratory, Downing Street, Cambridge CB2 3EG, England

To determine whether a particular sensory event is a reliable predictor of reward or punishment it is necessary to know the prior probability of that event. If the variables of a sensory representation normally occur independently of each other, then it is possible to derive the prior probability of any logical function of the variables from the prior probabilities of the individual variables, without any additional knowledge; hence such a representation enormously enlarges the scope of definable events that can be searched for reliable predictors. Finding a Minimum Entropy Code is a possible method of forming such a representation, and methods for doing this are explored in this paper. The main results are (1) to show how to find such a code when the probabilities of the input states form a geometric progression, as is shown to be nearly true for keyboard characters in normal text; (2) to show how a Minimum Entropy Code can be approximated by repeatedly recoding pairs, triples, etc. of an original 7-bit code for keyboard characters; (3) to prove that in some cases enlarging the capacity of the output channel can lower the entropy.

1 Reasons for Minimum Entropy Coding

When any combination of sensory stimuli — a sensory event — occurs the brain needs to know whether it is an expected, common, usual event, or an unexpected, rare, unusual event. It is evident that the brain works this out for itself because animals make startle or alerting reponses to unusual stimuli, and the following explanation of the need to attend to the unusual is also fairly obvious. One of the brains's most important jobs is to find predictive or causal relationships between the sensory events that impinge on it, the motor actions it takes, and the rewards and punishments these lead to. Now unexpected rewards and punishments are somewhat unusual, and for an animal with good knowledge of its environment they are presumably very unusual, so it follows that the sensory events it is seeking as new but reliable predictors are themselves somewhat or very unusual. For the purpose of learning something new the vast majority of sensory events can be ignored, but it is necessary to know the prior probability of what is happening in order to select the small minority of events that might form reliable new predictors.

Another way of seeing the importance of prior probabilities is to consider what is needed to detect "suspicious coincidences," which are the clues for detecting causal relations not only in detective stories but also in real life. Obviously the co-occurrence of two events is not in the least suspicious if they both occur frequently, so it is essential to know that the constituent events are rare before one can reach any conclusion at all about the significance of a coincidence that might point to a previously unsuspected causal factor.

A sensory event is signaled by the joint activity of a good many nerve cells, and it is therefore necessary to know the prior probability, not just of the signals from individual cells, but of combinations and perhaps other logical functions of such signals. There is only one condition under which this can be done, short of having available a past record of the occurrence of every combination that occurs, and that is for the activities of each of the nerve cells to be independent of all others in the sensory environment to which the animal is accustomed. Minimum Entropy Coding aims to achieve this by measuring the entropies of individual representative variables and choosing the reversible code for which the sum is a minimum. The summed entropy seems an easily computed measure for assessing putative codes, and the aim of this article is to explore methods of putting the idea into practice.

The general idea of Minimum Entropy Coding has been discussed by Watanabe (1981, 1985) and the principle is described in a previous article (Barlow 1989); the aim is to find a set of symbols to represent the messages such that, in the normal environment, the occurrence of each symbol is independent of the occurrence of any of the others. If such a set can be found it is called a factorial code, since the probabilities of the 1s and 0s in the code word are factors of the probability of the input state the word represents. In such a coded representation any nonindependence between two symbols signals the occurrence of a new, hitherto undiscovered, association, whereas with nonindependent codes one must always take into account the associative structure of the normal messages from the environment. The idea of minimum entropy coding comes from thoughts about redundancy reducing codes (Attneave 1954; Barlow 1960; Watanabe 1981; 1985) and is related to decorrelation (Barlow and Földiák 1989); such a code separates knowledge of the environment derived from the redundancy of past messages from the information in the current inputs, and its specification stores the knowledge that is required for the detection of new associations.

In the previous article the principle was explained using for an example the coding of keyboard characters in 7 binary digits, as in the familiar 7-bit ASCII code. The advantages of this choice are its familiarity and simplicity, the fact that the characters occur nonrandomly with known frequencies (Kučera and Francis 1967; Zettersten 1978), and the ready availability of samples of English text with normal statistical structure. An appendix shows some of the more general mathematical properties of minimum entropy codes, while below we discuss how the 7-bit coding can actually be done, and what its results are.

2 Finding the Codes

The requirement is to code keyboard characters that occur with probabilities A_j on to 7 binary outputs that occur as nearly as possible independently of each other when transmitting normal messages. The entropy calculated from the probabilities of the input states is $E(A) = -\sum A_j \log A_j$, and for a code $\mathbf{b}$ this is normally less than the sum of the bit entropies $e(A, \mathbf{b})$ given by

$$e(A, \mathbf{b}) = -\sum p_i \log p_i - \sum q_i \log q_i$$

where $p_i = 1 - q_i$ is the probability of the ith bit taking the value 1 in the encoded form of ordinary text. The aim is to find a reversible code that minimizes $e(A, \mathbf{b})$. We assume that $p_i < q_i$, which is a trivial restriction since substituting its logical complement for an output simply interchanges p_i and q_i.

2.1 The Number of Possible Codes. Consider a list of the input states in any order, and number them with a seven digit binary number 0000000, 0000001, 0000010, 0000011, ... , 1111111. Changing the order of input states in the list changes the code, and any reversible code can be produced by a list in appropriate order; hence the number of reversible codes is the number of permutations of a list of 2^7, that is $(2^7)!$. But many of the above codes are equivalent from the point of view of redundancy. One can substitute the complement for each output, interchanging the values of p and q and obviously leaving the entropy unchanged. Since this can be done independently for each of the outputs one must divide by 2^7. In addition, one can permute all the outputs without changing the entropy sum so one must also divide by 7!. Thus the total number of nonequivalent codes is $(2^7)!/(2^7 \cdot 7!)$, still a very large number.

2.2 Finding the Code with the Minimum Sum of Bit Entropies. We have failed to find a general method, other than searching through all codes and calculating the summed entropy for each, which the number of codes makes impractical. We have so far tried three methods that are described briefly below. Minimizing the sum of 7 quantities that obey the constraints of the bit probabilities of a reversible code has the flavor of a problem suitable for a network solution, but this has not yet been tried.

One approach is to minimize the average probability of a bit being active, since given that $p_i < 1/2$, the lower it is the less its individual

Code	Sum of bit entropies $e(A, \mathbf{b})$	Redundancy R (%)
Minimum bit probability	4.50	3.7
Binary sequence	4.37	0.7
ASCII	5.42	24.9
Random-1	6.89	58.8
Random-2	6.77	56.0
Random-3	6.74	55.3

Table 1: Entropies and Redundancies of Different Codes. Character entropy $E(A) = 4.34$ bits. Redundancy $R = [e(A, b) - E(A)]/E(A)$.

contribution is to the summed entropy. This can be done as follows. First measure the probabilities of each of the input states and rank them in order of decreasing probability. The most probable is assigned the output with all 0s, the next 7 are assigned to the outputs with just one bit active, the next 21 to those with 2 active, the next 35 to those with 3 active, and so on. We call these *Minimum Bit Probability codes*. Although this gives the lowest average number of active outputs, it does not necessarily minimize the sum of bit entropies (see Appendix).

Table 1 shows the values of the average entropy $E(A)$ obtained from the character frequencies in a portion of a scientific text, and the sum of bit entropies for the same text coded in this way. For a factorial code they would be equal, and it will be seen that the sum of the bit entropies comes quite close to the character entropy.

Another code can be obtained by listing input state probabilities as before and then numbering them in an ordinary binary sequence. This *Binary Sequence Coding* gives a factorial code provided that the probabilities of the input states form a geometric progression (see Appendix).

It will be seen from table 1 that this code reduces the summed bit entropies to very nearly the same as the character entropy, the residual redundancy being only 0.7%. Thus, it is very nearly a factorial code. The reasons for this success are that the character probabilities form a geometric progression, as shown in Figure 1, for which binary sequence coding yields a factorial code.

We can compare these codes with the regular 7-bit ASCII code, the entropies for which are also shown in Table 1. Though this was not defined with any idea of minimizing entropy in mind, the summed bit entropy is in fact a great deal less than 7, because the more frequently used letters have fewer active bits.

2.3 Subsection Coding. In order to test how successfully the next set of recoding procedures minimized the entropy we needed to start with a 7-bit binary code with maximum entropy, so we have generated

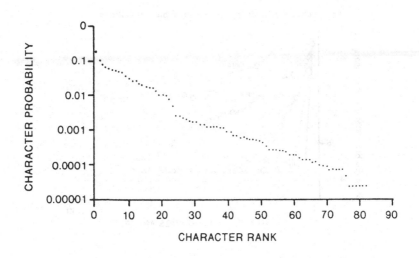

Figure 1: The ranked character probabilities plot close to a straight line on these log-linear axes, showing that the ranked probabilities form a geometric progression. The text sample analyzed was a portion of a scientific text similar to this paper, and was composed of approximately 42,000 printable ASCII characters. Similar distributions are commonly found (Kuçera and Francis 1967; Zettersten 1978).

random codes in which the binary numbers up to 1111111 were assigned at random to the input states; three examples of such codes are included in Table 1.

Minimum bit probability and binary sequence codes are based on measurements of the frequencies of the 128 different input states of a 7-bit code. This is not difficult to do, but it would become impossible if one were dealing with the very large input channels that feed the brain, so we have been very interested in how well one can achieve a minimum entropy code by repeated recoding of small subsections. The codes listed in Table 2 as *pairs* were formed by taking 2 bits at a time, recoding on the principle of mimimum bit probability or binary sequence coding, and doing this repeatedly until no further improvement occurred. Similar codes were formed taking 3, 4, or 5 at a time for those marked, *triples, quadruples,* and *quintuples.* For the minimum bit probability code, Figure 2a graphs the summed bit entropies as a function of the number of recoding attempts, taking different numbers of bits at a time; Figure 2b does likewise for the binary sequence code. It will be seen that recoding small subsets of elements is surprisingly ineffective in producing low entropy codes, and many repetitions are needed to approach low values.

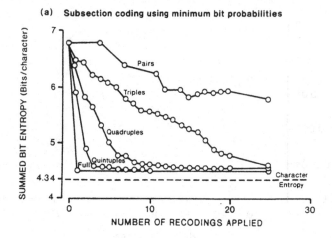

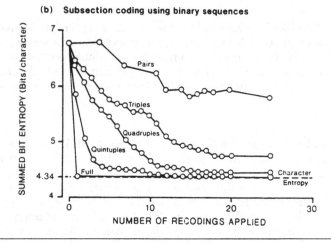

Figure 2: Coding subsections of the input. These graphs show the gradual reduction in entropy that is typically achieved by repeatedly recoding subsections of the 7-bit input. In (a) a Minimum Bit Probability code was applied to pairs, triples, etc. of bits; the group of bits $(b_i, b_j, b_k, \ldots)$ chosen for recoding was the one that maximized $P(b_i \ \& \ b_j \ \& \ b_k \ldots) - P(b_i) \cdot P(b_j) \cdot P(b_k) \ldots$. A χ^2 criterion was also tried, without improvement. Coding was repeatedly applied to pairs, triples, etc. until there was no further reduction of the summed bit entropy. The procedure in (b) was the same, except that a binary sequence code was applied to the pair, triple, etc. selected for recoding. The character entropy, marked on the graphs at 4.34 bits/character, is the theoretical minimum that can be achieved by any recoding, and the better the coding, the closer and faster the curves will fall to this baseline. As can be seen in (b), the full width (7-bit) binary sequence code achieves this goal in a single step.

	Code			
	Minimum bit probability		Binary sequence	
Subsection	$e(A, \mathbf{b})$	R (%)	$e(A, \mathbf{b})$	R (%)
Pairs	5.76	32.7	5.76	32.7
Triples	4.61	6.2	4.75	9.4
Quadruples	4.55	4.8	4.44	2.3
Quintuples	4.51	3.9	4.37	0.7
All 7 bits	4.50	3.7	4.37	0.7

Table 2: Entropies and Redundancies of Subsection Codes: Recoding of Random-2 by Subsection Method. Entropy of Random-2 code = 6.77 bits; character entropy $E(A) = 4.34$ bits; redundancy $R = [e(A, \mathbf{b}) - E(A)]/E(A)$.

2.4 Expansive Coding. It is shown in the appendix that coding on to an expanded channel can in some cases decrease the entropy. This is unexpected, because in such cases some of the output states do not occur and this represents additional redundancy. Furthermore, the recoding tends to introduce negative dependencies between some of the output variables, and when this happens the code cannot be a true minimum entropy code. Nonetheless, when we compare the efficiency of association formation with various coded representations we plan to include such expanded codes since they have some plausibility as the type of coding that the cerebral cortex does.

3 Conclusions

The 7-bit coding of keyboard characters has served to illustrate the problem of finding minimum entropy codes. In this example there happens to be a good approximation to a factorial code because the probabilities of the input states form an approximate geometric progression, but it does not lead to a code in which the individual bits have any readily interpretable significance: for instance the bits in the code do not correspond to significant features of the characters, such as being vowels or numbers (see Table 3). A minimum entropy code would come into its own when the states being coded have a natural combinatorial character, but it is unknown how far this is true of the world of sensory data.

Although in this case the code does not impose a particularly informative classification or categorization on the characters, it nevertheless has the advantages promised in the introduction, namely that the probability of the characters can be predicted from the probabilities of the bits that represent them. Translating this to the field of sensory events,

Rank	Character	Code 6543210	Probability	Rank	Character	Code 6543210	Probability
0	'space'	0000000	0.17595	41	, ,	0101001	0.00070
1	e	0000001	0.09843	42	O	0101010	0.00066
2	t	0000010	0.07817	43	C	0101011	0.00063
3	i	0000011	0.06272	44	O	0101100	0.00061
4	o	0000100	0.06214	45	R	0101101	0.00056
5	a	0000101	0.05791	46	j	0101110	0.00054
6	n	0000110	0.05773	47	|	0101111	0.00052
7	s	0000111	0.05620	48	/	0110000	0.00047
8	r	0001000	0.04375	49	E	0110001	0.00045
9	h	0001001	0.03604	50	F	0110010	0.00042
10	l	0001010	0.03050	51	:	0110011	0.00033
11	c	0001011	0.02610	52	'	0110100	0.00028
12	u	0001100	0.02610	53	D	0110101	0.00028
13	d	0001101	0.02345	54	M	0110110	0.00028
14	f	0001110	0.01953	55	H	0110111	0.00026
15	m	0001111	0.01796	56	L	0111000	0.00026
16	b	0010000	0.01768	57	z	0111001	0.00021
17	p	0010001	0.01768	58	6	0111010	0.00019
18	g	0010010	0.01231	59	Q	0111011	0.00019
19	y	0010011	0.01032	60	w	0111100	0.00019
20	w	0010100	0.01025	61	=	0111101	0.00016
21	v	0010101	0.00943	62	!	0111110	0.00014
22	'	0010110	0.00753	63	3	0111111	0.00014
23	.	0010111	0.00490	64	G	1000000	0.00014
24	N	0011000	0.00253	65	+	1000001	0.00012
25	k	0011001	0.00251	66	U	1000010	0.00012
26	I	0011010	0.00195	67	4	1000011	0.00009
27	T	0011011	0.00195	68	?	1000100	0.00009
28	x	0011100	0.00181	69	X	1000101	0.00009
29	q	0011101	0.00176	70	5	1000110	0.00007
30	)	0011110	0.00171	71	8	1000111	0.00007
31	(	0011111	0.00150	72	9	1001000	0.00007
32	V	0100000	0.00148	73	>	1001001	0.00007
33	P	0100001	0.00129	74	K	1001010	0.00007
34	-	0100010	0.00122	75	#	1001011	0.00005
35	1	0100011	0.00117	76	%	1001100	0.00002
36	S	0100100	0.00117	77	7	1001101	0.00002
37	B	0100101	0.00117	78	<	1001110	0.00002
38	A	0100110	0.00108	79	J	1001111	0.00002
39	;	0100111	0.00098	80	[	1010000	0.00002
40	2	0101000	0.00096	81	]	1010001	0.00002

Probability of each bit

Bit	Probability
6	0.001196
5	0.018945
4	0.110085
3	0.247532
2	0.368637
1	0.401721
0	0.439799

Table 3: Actual Binary Sequence Code

if these were represented by variables that occurred independently under normal circumstances, one's ability to detect unusual or suspicious coincidences would be enormously enhanced.

4 Mathematical Appendix (G.J. Mitchison) _____

Suppose we are given a set of states whose probabilities are A_j (with $\sum A_j = 1$), and a code $\mathbf{b}$ that assigns to each character a binary string. In the coding problem considered in the main text the states are keyboard characters. Let the ith bit of the code for the jth state be denoted by b_{ij}. The probability of the ith bit taking the value 1, summed over all the states, is denoted by p_i. Formally

$$p_i = \sum_{b_{ij}=1} A_j \tag{4.1}$$

and we define $q_i = 1-p_i$. We say that $\mathbf{b}$ is a factorial code if the probability of each state A_j is the product of the probabilities that the bits have the values in the code for A_j. Formally,

$$A_j = \pi_j \tag{4.2}$$

where

$$\pi_j = \prod_{b_{ij}=1} p_i \cdot \prod_{b_{ij}=0} q_i$$

It is assumed here that there is a state for each possible polynomial π_j, i.e., that there are 2^N states, where N is the number of bits.

The state entropy $E(A)$ is defined by $E(A) = -\sum A_j \log A_j$. The sum of the bit entropies, $e(A, \mathbf{b})$, is defined by $e(A, \mathbf{b}) = -\sum p_i \log p_i - \sum q_i \log q_i$.

Proposition 1. $e(A, \mathbf{b}) \geq E(A)$, with $e(A, \mathbf{b}) = E(A)$ if and only if $\mathbf{b}$ is factorial.

This proposition is proved in Watanabe (1985). Intuitively, it means that the capacity of the bits of the code is greater than that of the states they represent, except in the case of a factorial code where the states are represented by a product of independent bits. The following short proof uses an adaptation, suggested by Dr. C.J. St C. Webber (private communication), of an argument in Jones (1979):

Proof. Using (4.1) and the definition of p_i following (4.2) we can write:

$$
\begin{aligned}
e(A, \mathbf{b}) - E(A) &= -\sum p_i \log p_i - \sum q_i \log q_i + \sum A_j \log A_j \\
&= -\sum_{b_{ij}=1} \left(\sum A_j\right) \log p_i - \sum_{b_{ij}=0} \left(\sum A_j\right) \log q_i \\
&\quad + \sum A_j \log A_j \\
&= -\sum A_j \log(\pi_j/A_j)
\end{aligned}
$$

It is easy to check that $\log x \leq x - 1$ for $x > 0$, with equality only for $x = 1$. Thus:

$$- \sum A_j \log(\pi_j/A_j) \geq - \sum A_j(\pi_j/A_j - 1) = \sum A_j - \sum \pi_j = 1 - 1 = 0$$

using the fact that $\sum \pi_j = \prod(p_i + q_i) = 1$. Equality occurs if and only if $\pi_j = A_j$ for all j, which means that $\mathbf{b}$ is factorial.

This result implies that, for any set $\{A_j\}$ that has a factorial code, any code $\mathbf{b}$ which minimizes the entropy $e(A, \mathbf{b})$ will also be factorial. Minimizing $e(A, \mathbf{b})$ can therefore be regarded as a strategy for finding a code that is "as factorial as possible." Of course, not every set of 2^N state probabilities has a factorial code. In fact, the factorial codes have dimension N (one for each choice of the N p_is) and the sets of A_j with $\sum A_j = 1$ have dimension $2^N - 1$, so it is highly unlikely that an arbitrary set $\{A_j\}$ will have a factorial code. However, one case of interest is the following:

Proposition 2. *If $A_j = Kx^j$, for $i = 1 \ldots 2^N$, for some x, with K chosen so that $\sum A_j = 1$, then A has a factorial code.*

Proof. Define p_i by $p_i/q_i = x^{2^{i-1}}$, for $i = 1$ to N. Then, for the binary sequence code, $\pi_j = Q \cdot x^j$, where $\sum Q x^j = 1$. It follows that $Q = K$ and $A_j = \pi_j$, so A has a factorial code.

This result illustrates the difference between minimizing the sum of bit entropies $e(A, \mathbf{b})$ and minimizing $\sum p_i$, the total probability of the bits. To achieve the latter one should assign the binary string consisting entirely of zeros to the largest A_j, the strings with just one "1" to the next smallest A_js, and so on. The factorial code for input states with probabilities in a geometric progression does not follow this sequence.

Until now we have assumed that there are N bits and 2^N states. More generally, one could try to code M states on N bits, where $N \geq \log_2 M$, with the convention that one assigns a probability of zero to the codewords that are not used. A simple example shows that a lower entropy can sometimes be obtained by coding on to more than the minimum possible number of bits. Let the state probabilities be $a, a, Ka^2, 1 - 2a - Ka^2$, where $0 < a < 1$ and $1 - 2a - Ka^2 > 0$. One can consider two codings:

0 0	with probability	$1 - 2a - Ka^2$
0 1		a
1 0		a
1 1		Ka^2

and

0 0 0	with probability	$1 - 2a - Ka^2$
0 0 1		a
0 1 0		a
1 0 0		Ka^2

It is straightforward to check that when a is small enough for terms in a^3 and higher powers to be neglected, then the second (expansive) coding gives a lower entropy when $\log_e K > 3$.

One can prove other results of this kind. For instance, if there are M states, $M - 1$ of which have the same probability a, then the expansive coding on $M - 1$ bits that assigns a codeword with a single 1 to each state of probability a and the all-zero codeword to the state with probability $1 - (M - 1)a$, gives minimum entropy provided a is small enough. For suppose there were a coding on L bits with $L < M - 1$, and let the bit probabilities p_i be ak_i, where the k_i are integers. Since there must be at least one bit which is set to 1 in two or more codewords it follows that $\sum k_i \geq M$. For small bit probabilities we can approximate the bit entropy by $- \sum p_i \log p_i$. Then the difference Δe between the bit entropies for the coding on L bits and that on $M - 1$ bits is approximately $\Delta e = - \sum ak_i \log(ak_i) + (M-1)a \log a \geq -a \log a - a \sum k_i \log k_i$. Since each $k_i < M$ the maximum value of $\sum k_i \log k_i$ is $M^2 \log M$, so $\Delta e > 0$ provided that $- \log a > M^2 \log M$ or $a < (1/M)^{M^2}$.

References

Attneave, F. 1954. Informational aspects of visual perception. *Psychol. Rev.* **61**, 183–193.

Barlow, H.B. 1960. The coding of sensory messages. pp. 331–360. In *Current Problems in Animal Behaviour*, W.H. Thorpe and O.L. Zangwill, eds., Cambridge University Press, Cambridge.

Barlow, H.B. 1989. Unsupervised learning. *Neural Comp.* **1**, 295–311.

Barlow, H.B., and Földiák, P.F. 1989. Adaptation and decorrelation in the cortex. In *The Computing Neuron*, R. Durbin, C. Miall, and G.J. Mitchison, eds. Addison-Wesley, New York.

Jones, D.S. 1979. *Elementary Information Theory*. Oxford University Press, London.

Kučera, H., and Francis, W.N. 1967. *Computational Analysis of Present day American English*. Brown University Press, Providence, RI.

Watanabe, S. 1981. Pattern recognition as a quest for minimum entropy. *Pattern Recognit.* **13**, 381–387.

Watanabe, S. 1985. *Pattern Recognition: Human and Mechanical*. Wiley, New York.

Zettersten, A. 1978. *A Word Frequency List Based on American English Press Re-portage*. Universitetsforlaget, 1 Kopenhavn, Akademisk Forlag, Copenhagen.

15

Learning Population Codes by Minimizing Description Length

Richard S. Zemel*
Computational Neurobiology Laboratory, The Salk Institute,
10010 North Torrey Pines Rd., La Jolla, CA 92037 USA

Geoffrey E. Hinton
Department of Computer Science, University of Toronto,
6 King's College Road, Toronto, Ontario M5S 1A4, Canada

The minimum description length (MDL) principle can be used to train the hidden units of a neural network to extract a representation that is cheap to describe but nonetheless allows the input to be reconstructed accurately. We show how MDL can be used to develop highly redundant population codes. Each hidden unit has a location in a low-dimensional *implicit* space. If the hidden unit activities form a bump of a standard shape in this space, they can be cheaply encoded by the center of this bump. So the weights from the input units to the hidden units in an autoencoder are trained to make the activities form a standard bump. The coordinates of the hidden units in the implicit space are also learned, thus allowing flexibility, as the network develops a discontinuous topography when presented with different input classes.

1 Introduction

Most existing unsupervised learning algorithms can be understood using the minimum description length (MDL) principle (Rissanen 1989). Given an ensemble of input vectors, the aim of the learning algorithm is to find a method of coding each input vector that minimizes the total cost, in bits, of communicating the input vectors to a receiver. There are three terms in the total description length:

- The **code-cost** is the number of bits required to communicate the code that the algorithm assigns to each input vector.

- The **model-cost** is the number of bits required to specify how to reconstruct input vectors from codes (e.g., the hidden-to-output weights).

---

*Present address: Carnegie Mellon University, Department of Psychology, Pittsburgh, PA 15213 USA.

- The **reconstruction-error** is the number of bits required to fix up any errors that occur when the input vector is reconstructed from its code.

Formulating the problem in terms of a communication model allows us to derive an objective function for a network (note that we are not actually sending the bits). For example, in competitive learning (vector quantization), the code is the identity of the winning hidden unit, so by limiting the system to $\mathcal{H}$ units we limit the average code-cost to at most $\log_2 \mathcal{H}$ bits. The reconstruction-error is proportional to the squared difference between the input vector and the weight-vector of the winner, and this is what competitive learning algorithms minimize. The model-cost is usually ignored.

The representations produced by vector quantization contain very little information about the input (at most $\log_2 \mathcal{H}$ bits on average). To get richer representations we must allow many hidden units to be active at once and to have varying activity levels. Principal components analysis (PCA) achieves this for linear mappings from inputs to codes. It can be viewed as a version of MDL in which we limit the code-cost by having only a few hidden units, and ignore the model-cost and the accuracy with which the hidden activities must be coded. An autoencoder that tries to reconstruct the input vector on its output units will perform a version of PCA if the output units are linear. We can obtain novel and interesting unsupervised learning algorithms using this MDL approach by considering various alternative methods of communicating the hidden activities. The algorithms can all be implemented by backpropagating the derivative of the code-cost for the hidden units in addition to the derivative of the reconstruction-error backpropagated from the output units.

Any method that communicates each hidden activity separately and independently will tend to lead to *factorial* codes because any mutual information between hidden units will cause redundancy in the communicated message, so the pressure to keep the message short will squeeze out the redundancy. In Zemel (1993) and Hinton and Zemel (1994), we present algorithms derived from this MDL approach aimed at developing factorial codes. Although factorial codes are interesting, they are not robust against hardware failure nor do they resemble the population codes found in some parts of the brain. Our aim in this paper is to show how the MDL approach can be used to develop population codes in which the activities of hidden units are highly correlated.

2 Population Codes

2.1 Constraint Surfaces. Unsupervised algorithms contain an implicit assumption about the nature of the structure or constraints underlying the input set. For example, competitive learning algorithms are suited to datasets in which each input can be attributed to one of a set

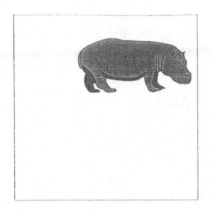 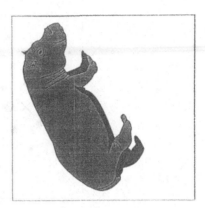

Figure 1: Two example images where only a few dimensions of variability underlie seemingly unrelated vectors of pixel intensity values.

of possible causes. In the algorithm we present here, we assume that each input can be described as a point in a low-dimensional continuous *constraint space*.

An example is shown in Figure 1. If we imagine a high-dimensional input representation produced by digitizing these images, many bits would be required to describe each instance of the hippopotamus. But a particular image among a set of images of the hippo from multiple viewpoints can be concisely represented by first describing a canonical hippo, and then encoding the instance as a point in the constraint space spanned by the four 2D viewing parameters: (x, y)-position, orientation, and scale. Other examples exist in biology, e.g., recent studies have found that in monkey motor cortex, the direction of movement in 3D space of a monkey's arm is encoded by the activities of populations of cells, each of which responds based on its preferred direction of motion (Georgopoulos *et al.* 1986). Averaging each cell's preferred motion directions weighted by its activity accurately predicts the direction of movement that the animal makes. In these examples, knowledge of an underlying lower-dimensional constraint surface allows for compact descriptions of stimuli or responses. Our goal is to find and represent the constraint space underlying high-dimensional data samples.

2.2 Representing Underlying Dimensions Using Population Codes.
In order to represent inputs as points drawn from a constraint space, we choose a *population code* style of representation. In a population code, each code unit is associated with a position in what we call the *implicit*

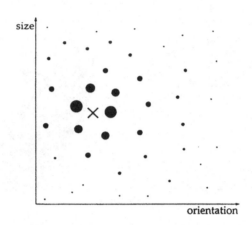

Figure 2: The population code for an instance in a two-dimensional implicit space. The position of each blob corresponds to the position of a unit within the population, and the blob size corresponds to the unit's activity. Here one dimension describes the size and the other the orientation of a shape. We can determine the instantiation parameters of this particular shape by computing the center of gravity of the blob activities, marked here by an "X."

space, and the code units' pattern of activity conveys a single point in this space. This implicit space should correspond to the constraint space. For example, suppose that each code unit is assigned a position in a 2D implicit space, where one dimension corresponds to the size of the shape and the second to its orientation (see Fig. 2). A population of code units broadly tuned to different positions can represent any particular instance of the shape by their relative activity levels.

This example illustrates that population codes involve *three* quite different spaces:

1. the input-vector space (the pixel intensities in the example);

2. the hidden-vector space (where each hidden, or code unit entails an additional dimension);

3. the implicit space, which is of lower dimension than the other two spaces.

In a learning algorithm for population codes, the implicit space is intended to come to smoothly represent the underlying dimensions of variability in the inputs, i.e., the constraint space.

For instance, in a Kohonen network (Kohonen 1982), the hidden unit with the greatest total input has an activity of one, while the others are zero. Yet these hidden units are also assigned positions in implicit space based on a neighborhood function that determines the degree of interaction between a pair of units according to their distance. The active unit then maps the input to a particular point in this implicit space. Here the implicit space topology is defined a priori through fixed neighborhood relations, and the algorithm then adjusts weights so that neighbors in implicit space respond to similar inputs. Similarly, in a one-dimensional version of the elastic-net algorithm (Durbin and Willshaw 1987), the code units are assigned positions along a ring; these units are then pulled toward the inputs, but are also pulled toward their ring neighbors. In the Traveling Salesman Problem, for example, the inputs are cities, and code units adjacent in implicit space represent consecutive cities in the tour, so that the active unit for a given input city describes its order in the tour.

Population codes have several computational advantages, in addition to their obvious biological relevance. The codes contain some redundancy and hence have some degree of fault-tolerance. A population code as described above reflects structure in the input, in that similar inputs are mapped to nearby implicit positions, if the implicit dimensionality matches the intrinsic dimensionality of the input. They also possess a hyperacuity property, as the number of implicit positions that can be represented far exceeds the number of code units; this makes population codes well-suited to describing values along a continuous dimension.

3 Learning Population Codes with MDL

Autoencoders are a general way of addressing issues of coding. The hidden unit activities for an input are the codes for that input that are produced by the input-hidden weights, and reconstruction from the code is done by the hidden-output mapping. To allow an autoencoder to develop population codes for an input set, we need some additional structure in the hidden layer that will allow a code vector to be interpreted as a point in implicit space. While most topographic-map formation algorithms (e.g., the Kohonen and elastic-net algorithms) define the topology of this implicit space by fixed neighborhood relations, in our algorithm we use a more explicit representation. Each hidden unit has weights coming from the input units that determine its activity level. But in addition to these weights, it has another set of adjustable parameters that represents its coordinates in the implicit space. To determine what implicit position is represented by a vector of hidden activities, we can average together the implicit coordinates of the hidden units, weighting each coordinate vector by the activity level of the unit.

Suppose, for example, that each hidden unit is connected to an 8 × 8 retina and has two implicit coordinates that represent the size and orientation of a particular kind of shape on the retina, as in our earlier example. If we plot the hidden activity levels in the implicit space (not the

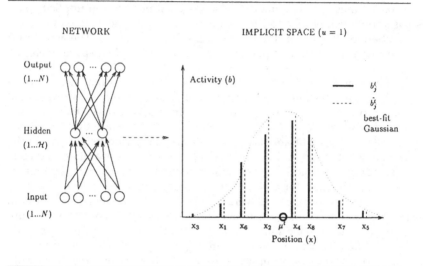

Figure 3: Each of the $\mathcal{H}$ hidden units in the autoencoder has an associated position in implicit space. Here we show a 1D implicit space. The activity b_j^t of each hidden unit j on case t is shown by a solid line. The network fits the best gaussian to this pattern of activity in implicit space. The predicted activity, $\hat{b}_j^t$, of unit j under this gaussian is based on the distance from x_j to the mean μ^t; it serves as a target for b_j^t.

input space), we would like to see a bump of activity of a standard shape (e.g., a gaussian) whose center represents the instantiation parameters of the shape (Fig. 3 depicts this for a 1D implicit space).

If the activities form a perfect gaussian bump of fixed variance we can communicate them by simply communicating the coordinates of the mean of the gaussian; this is very economical if there are many less implicit coordinates than hidden units.

It is important to realize that the activity of a hidden unit is actually caused by the input-to-hidden weights, but by setting these weights appropriately we can make the activity match the height under the gaussian in implicit space. If the activity bump is not quite perfect, we must also encode the *bump-error*—the misfit between the actual activity levels and the levels predicted by the gaussian bump. The cost of encoding this misfit is what forces the activity bump in implicit space to approximate a gaussian.

The reconstruction-error is then the deviation of the output from the input. This reconstruction ignores implicit space; the output activities depend only on the vector of hidden activities and weights.

3.1 Activations and Objective Function. Let a_i^t be the activity of input unit i on case t. The actual activity of a hidden unit j is then

$$b_j^t = \exp\left(\sum_i w_{ji} a_i^t\right) \Big/ \sum_{h=1}^{H} \exp\left(\sum_i w_{hi} a_i^t\right) \tag{3.1}$$

Note that the unit's actual activity is independent of its position x_j in implicit space. Its expected activity is its normalized value under the predicted gaussian bump:

$$\hat{b}_j^t = \exp\left[-(x_j - \mu^t)^2/2\sigma^2\right] \Big/ \sum_{i=1}^{\mathcal{H}} \exp\left[-(x_i - \mu^t)^2/2\sigma^2\right] \tag{3.2}$$

where μ^t is the mean of the bump and σ its width, which we assume is fixed throughout training. The activity c_k^t of output unit k is just the weighted sum of its inputs. The network has full interlayer connectivity.

Currently, we ignore the model-cost, and assume a fixed cost for specifying the bump mean on each case, so the description length to be minimized is

$$\begin{aligned} E^t &= B^t + R^t \\ &= \sum_{j=1}^{\mathcal{H}} (b_j^t - \hat{b}_j^t)^2/2V_B + \sum_{k=1}^{N} (a_k^t - c_k^t)^2/2V_R \end{aligned} \tag{3.3}$$

where V_B and V_R are the fixed variances of the gaussians used for coding the bump-errors[2] and the reconstruction-errors.

We have explored several methods for computing μ^t, the mean of the bump. Simply computing the center of gravity of the hidden units' positions, weighted by their activity, produces a bias toward points in the center of implicit space. Instead, on each case, a separate minimization determines μ^t; it is the position in implicit space that minimizes B^t given $\{x_j, b_j^t\}$.

Both the network weights and the implicit coordinates of the hidden units are adapted simultaneously. We minimize E with respect to the weights by backpropagating the derivatives of the reconstruction-error from the output units, and then add in the derivatives of the bump-error at the hidden layer. The implicit coordinates affect the bump-error through the computation of the predicted hidden activities (see equation 3.2).

4 Experimental Results

4.1 Parameters. The algorithm includes three adjustable parameters. The width of the gaussian bump in implicit space, σ, is set in each experiment to be approximately 1/4 of the width of the space. In many

---

[2]Note that this gaussian assumption for encoding the bump-error is an approximation to the true distribution. Both b_j^c and $\hat{b}_j^c$ are bounded between 0.0 and 1.0, so the error is bounded between -1.0 and 1.0, and the true distribution has a mean of 0.0 and falls off exponentially in both directions to these bounds.

learning algorithms that include a gaussian fitting step, such as the Kohonen algorithm, the elastic-net, and the mixture-of-gaussians, this width is initially large and is then annealed down to a minimum width during training; this approach did not significantly improve this algorithm's performance. The second and third parameters are V_B and V_R, the variances of the gaussians for coding the reconstruction and activity costs. The relative values of these two terms act as regularization parameters, trading off the weighting of the two costs.

Two architectural parameters also play important roles in this algorithm. The first is the number of hidden units. To accurately and robustly represent a wide range of values in implicit space, the network must contain a sufficient number of hidden units to make a true population code. The second parameter is related to the first—the number of dimensions in implicit space. Clearly many more units are required to form population codes as we increase the dimensionality of implicit space. In the experiments below, we predetermine the appropriate number of dimensions for the input set; in the Discussion section we describe an extension that will allow the network to automatically determine the appropriate dimensionality.

We train the networks in these experiments using a batch conjugate gradient optimization technique, with a line-search. The results described below represent best-case performance, as the algorithm occasionally gets stuck in local minima. In these experiments, if the network contains a sufficient number of hidden units, and the input is devoid of noise, then the algorithm should be able to force the cost function to zero (since we are ignoring the cost of communicating the bump means). This makes it relatively easy to determine when a solution is a local minimum.

4.2 Experiment 1: Learning to Represent Position. Each 8×8 real-valued input image contains a rigid object, which is composed of two gaussian blobs of intensity at its ends (see Fig. 4). The image is generated by randomly choosing a point between 0.0 and 1.0 to be the center of the object. The two ends of the object are then a fixed distance from this center (each is approximately 0.2 units displaced from the center, where the entire image is 1.0 units wide). Each end is then composed of the difference of two gaussian blobs of intensity: one of standard deviation 0.1 units, and a second with a standard deviation of 0.25 units, which acts to sharpen up the edges of the object. This simple object has four degrees of freedom, as each instantiation has a unique (x, y)-position, orientation (within a 180° range), and size (based on the spacing between the ends). These four parameters describe the variability due to seeing the same rigid 2D object from different viewpoints in the fronto-parallel plane. To avoid edge effects, the input space was represented using wraparound. We also use wraparound in the implicit space, which creates a toroidal shape, i.e., the points at 2π radians are neighbors of the points at 0 radians.

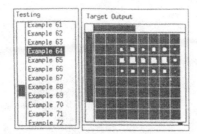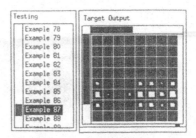

Figure 4: Each 8×8 real-valued input image for the first experiment contains an instance of a dipole. The dipole has four continuous degrees-of-freedom: (x, y)-position, orientation, and size. This figure shows two sample images from the test set. The image on the right shows that the input space is represented using wraparound.

In the first experiment, only the (x, y)-position of the object is varied from image to image. The training set consists of 400 examples of this shape in random positions; we test generalization with a test set of 100 examples, located at the gridpoints of the 10×10 grid covering the space of possible positions. The network begins with random weights, and each of 100 hidden units has random 2D implicit coordinates. The system converges to a minimum of the objective function after 25 epochs. The *generalization length* (the mean description length of the test set) on this experiment is 0.52 bits, indicating that the algorithm was able virtually to eliminate the bump and reconstruction errors.

Each hidden unit develops a *receptive field* so that it responds to objects in a limited neighborhood of the underlying constraint space that corresponds to its learned position in implicit space (see Fig. 5). This arises due to the constraint that the implicit pattern of activity should be bump-like. The algorithm successfully learns the underlying constraint surface in this dataset; the implicit space forms a relatively smooth, stable map of the generating surface (Fig. 6), i.e., a small change in the (x, y)-coordinates of the object produces a corresponding small change in the mean's coordinates in implicit space.

4.3 Experiment 2: Learning a Three-Dimensional Constraint Surface. In the second experiment, we also vary the orientation of the shape. The training set contains 1000 images of the same object with three random instantiation parameters, i.e., its position and orientation are drawn randomly from the range of (x, y)-coordinates and $180°$ of orientation. The test set contains 512 examples, made up of all gridpoints in an evenly

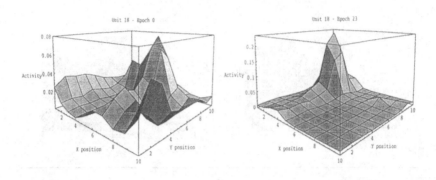

Figure 5: This figure shows the receptive field in implicit space for two hidden units. Here the two dimensions in implicit space correspond to x and y positions. The left panel shows that before learning, the units respond randomly to 100 different test patterns, generated by positioning a shape in the image at each point in a 10×10 grid. The right panel shows that after learning, the units respond to objects in a particular position, and their activity level falls off smoothly as the object position moves away from the center of the learned receptive field.

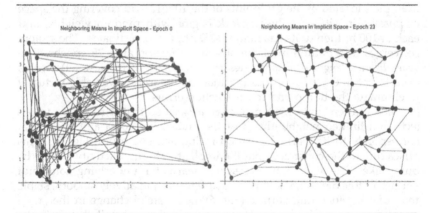

Figure 6: This figure shows the implicit positions of the bump means for the test set before and after training. In the 100 testing examples, the object is located at the gridpoints of a 10×10 grid covering the space of possible positions. In this figure, lines connect the means between a given test image and its four neighbors on this grid. Note that implicit space has a toroidal shape, i.e., the points at 2π radians are neighbors of the points at 0 radians. The lines connecting these wraparound neighbors have been left off of this figure to improve its clarity.

spaced grid that divides each of the three underlying dimensions into eight intervals.

We give each hidden unit three implicit coordinates, and also increase the number of hidden units to 225. Since this network has a larger ratio of hidden to input units, we increase the bump variance ($V_B = 2.5$) to maintain a balance between the two costs. The network converges after 60 epochs of training on the 1000 images. The generalization length is 1.16 bits per image. The hidden unit activities again form a population code that allows the input to be accurately reconstructed. The three dimensions of the implicit space correspond to a recoding of the object instantiation parameters, such that smooth changes in the object's parameters produce similar changes in the implicit space codes. While the algorithm often gets stuck in local minima when we decrease the number of hidden units below 200, this problem virtually disappears with sufficient hidden units. The algorithms defined using this MDL approach can effectively remove the excess units once good representations for the input set have been discovered with the initial large pool of units.

4.4 Experiment 3: Learning a Discontinuous Constraint Surface. A third experiment employs a training set where each image contains either a horizontal or vertical bar, in some random position. The training set contains 200 examples of each bar, and the test set contains 100 examples of each, evenly spaced at 10 locations along both dimensions of the underlying constraint surface, the (x, y)-position of the shape.

This task is a what/where problem: the underlying constraint surface has the two continuous dimensions of position, but it also has a binary value that describes which object (horizontal or vertical) is in the image. Even though we only give each of the 100 hidden units two implicit coordinates in this experiment, they are able to discover a representation of all three of these underlying dimensions. The algorithm requires 112 epochs to reduce the generalization length to 1.4 bits. This generalization length is nearly three times that of Experiment 1, where the network had the same number of hidden units trained on a single shape in various positions. The decrease in representational quality can be attributed to this additional "what" dimension of the training set.

After training, we find that one set of hidden units has moved to one corner of implicit space, and represents the position of instances of one shape, while the other group has moved to an opposite corner and represents the position of the other shape (see Fig. 7). The network sometimes finds solutions where rather than identity being the primary dimension in implicit space, the units instead cluster according to the shape location, and the representation of identity is patchy within this ordering. A wide variety of this solution type can be found, based on parameters such as the within-shape versus between-shape correlations. For the training set used in this experiment, this second solution typically has a higher generalization length (≈ 1.8 bits).

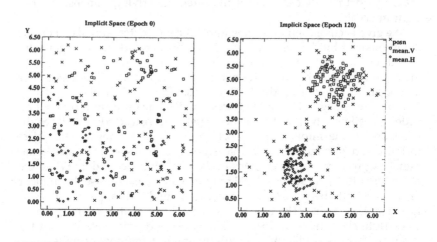

Figure 7: This figure shows the positions of the hidden units and the means in the 2D implicit space before and after training on the horizontal/vertical task. In each plot, an "x" marks the implicit position of a hidden unit; a box marks the implicit mean of the bump formed for an input image containing a vertical bar; and a diamond marks the mean of a horizontal bar image. The network has learned a topology where the means in the top right of the second plot all correspond to images containing vertical bars, while the other set corresponds to horizontal bar images. The different shapes are thus separated in implicit space. Note that some hidden units are far from all the means; these units do not play a role in the coding of the input, and are free to be recruited for other types of input cases.

A Kohonen network typically finds this second type of representation in which position is the primary implicit dimension. We have run a Kohonen network with 100 output units on this horizontal/vertical task. The network always forms a patchy topographic map, where the underlying constraint surface is captured in a local fashion by the map. While initializing the Kohonen algorithm with a large neighborhood size and using a long annealing schedule may enable it to learn the other representation, the key point is that learning this sort of mapping is difficult, which is probably due to the fact that the implicit space topology remains fixed while the network learns to associate points in implicit space with points in input space. The fact that the hidden units *learn* their implicit coordinates in our algorithm allows more flexibility than any system in which these coordinates are fixed in advance.

A related problem to this what/where task is the development of ocular dominance and retinotopic maps in striate visual cortex. Inputs from the two eyes' retinae are mapped in V1 such that neighboring retinal positions innervate nearby neurons in V1, and these nearby neurons also tend to respond to input from one eye or the other. In this mapping, location is the primary dimension, and the binary dimension, ocularity, is secondary; the resulting map resembles the patchy structure found by the Kohonen network. Obermayer *et al.* (1991) showed how a Kohonen algorithm trained on this task could develop a similar map. Goodhill and Willshaw (1990) discussed the solutions that may be found using an elastic net algorithm, while Dayan (1993) analyzed how the neighborhood relations in the elastic net could determine the learned topology. Each of these papers analyzes the dependence of the map structure on certain key underlying input parameters; these analyses apply to the task described here as well.

5 Related Work

This new algorithm bears some similarities to several earlier algorithms, particularly topographic map formation algorithms such as the Kohonen and elastic-net algorithms. Like these algorithms, our method aims to create a map where the constructed, or implicit, space corresponds to the underlying constraint space of the inputs; this structure is created primarily by indirect local learning.

Several important differences exist between our method and these earlier algorithms. The key difference is that our algorithm explicitly encourages the hidden unit activity to form a population code in implicit space rather than developing these codes implicitly through neighborhood interaction during learning.

In addition, the population code in these methods is in effect formed in input space. Each unit's weights are moved toward the input patterns, whereas our method moves the weights based on the implicit space coding as well as the reconstruction error.[3]

In Saund (1989), hidden unit patterns of activity in an autoencoder are trained to form gaussian bumps, where the center of the bump is intended to correspond to the position in an underlying dimension of the inputs. Ossen (1992) proposed a similar objective, and our activation function for the hidden layer also resembles the one he used. Yet the objective function in our algorithm is quite different due to the implicit space construction. An additional crucial difference exists: in these

---

[3]In Luttrell's (1990) interpretation of Kohonen's algorithm in terms of a communication model, the algorithm minimizes the expected distortion between the decoding of an encoded input with added noise, and the input itself. This minimization produces the Kohonen learning rule, moving neighbors of the winner toward the input patterns, when the encoding is calculated by ignoring the added noise and finding the point that the decoding maps closest to the input.

earlier algorithms,[4] the implicit space topology is statically determined a priori by the ordering of the hidden units, while units in our model learn their implicit coordinates. Learning this topology lends additional flexibility to our algorithm.

6 Discussion and Current Directions

We have shown how MDL can be used to develop nonfactorial, redundant representations. The objective function is derived from a communication model where rather than communicating each hidden unit activity independently, we instead communicate the location of a gaussian bump in a low-dimensional implicit space. If the hidden units are appropriately tuned in this space, their activities can then be inferred from the bump location.

When the underlying dimensions of variability in a set of input images are the instantiation parameters of an object, this implicit space comes to correspond to these parameters. Since the implicit coordinates of the hidden units are also learned, the network develops separate population codes when presented with different objects.

While we have tested the algorithm on noisier versions of the datasets described above, and have found that the solution quality gracefully degrades with added noise, we have not described any results of applying it to more realistic data. Instead we have chosen to emphasize this hand-crafted data in order to determine the quality of network solution. The primary contributions of this paper are theoretical: we introduce a method of encouraging a particular functional form of activity for the hidden units, and also demonstrate an objective based on compact coding that nevertheless encourages redundancy in the codes. It would be interesting to consider generalizations of this algorithm that derive from positing other functional forms for the hidden unit activity patterns.

Our method can easily be applied to networks with multiple hidden layers, where the implicit space is constructed at the last hidden layer before the output and derivatives are then backpropagated; this allows the implicit space to correspond to arbitrarily high-order input properties. Alternatively, instead of using multiple hidden layers to extract a single code for the input, one could use a hierarchical system in which the code-cost is computed at every layer.

A limitation of this approach (as well as the aforementioned approaches) is the need to predefine the dimensionality of implicit space. We are currently working on an extension that will allow the learning algorithm to determine for itself the appropriate number of dimensions

---

[4]A recent variation of Kohonen's algorithm (Martinetz and Schulten 1991) learns the implicit coordinates (still in input space), and also allows different parts of implicit space to have different dimensionalities. Bregler and Omohundro (1994) present a method of learning the dimensionality using local linear patches.

in implicit space. We start with many dimensions but include the cost of specifying μ^t in the description length. This depends on how many implicit coordinates are used. If all of the hidden units have the same value for one of the implicit coordinates, it costs nothing to communicate that value for each bump. In general, the cost of an implicit coordinate depends on the ratio between its variance (over all the different bumps) and the accuracy with which it must be communicated. So the network can save bits by reducing the variance for unneeded coordinates. This creates a smooth search space for determining how many implicit coordinates are needed.

Acknowledgments

We thank Peter Dayan, Klaus Obermayer, and Terry Sejnowski for their help. This research was supported by grants from NSERC, the Ontario Information Technology Research Center, and the Institute for Robotics and Intelligent Systems. Geoffrey Hinton is the Noranda Fellow of the Canadian Institute for Advanced Research.

References

Bregler, C., and Omohundro, S. M. 1994. Surface learning with applications to lipreading. In *Advances in Neural Information Processing Systems 6*, pp. 43–50. Morgan Kaufmann, San Mateo, CA.

Dayan, P. 1993. Arbitrary elastic topologies and ocular dominance. *Neural Comp.* 5(3), 392–401.

Durbin, R., and Willshaw, D. 1987. An analogue approach to the travelling salesman problem. *Nature (London)* 326, 689–691.

Georgopoulos, A. P., Schwartz, A. B., and Kettner, R. E. 1986. Neuronal population coding of movement direction. *Science* 243, 1416–1419.

Goodhill, G. J., and Willshaw, D. J. 1990. Application of the elastic net algorithm to the formation of ocular dominance stripes. *Network* 1, 41–61.

Hinton, G. E., and Zemel, R. S. 1994. Autoencoders, minimum description length, and Helmholtz free energy. In *Advances in Neural Information Processing Systems 6*, J. D. Cowan, G. Tesauro, J. Alspector, eds., pp. 3–10. Morgan Kaufmann, San Mateo, CA.

Kohonen, T. 1982. Self-organized formation of topologically correct feature maps. *Biol. Cybern.* 43, 59–69.

Luttrell, S. P. 1990. Derivation of a class of training algorithms. *IEEE Transact. Neural Networks* 1, 1229–1232.

Martinetz, T., and Schulten, K. 1991. A 'neural gas' network learns topologies. *Proc. ICANN-91*, 397–402.

Obermayer, S. J., Ritter, H., and Schulten, K. 1991. A neural network model for the formation of the spatial structure of retinotopic maps, orientation and ocular dominance columns. In *Artificial Neural Networks I*, T. Kohonen, O. Simula, and J. Kangas, eds., pp. 505–511. North Holland, Amsterdam.

Ossen, A. 1992. *Learning topology-preserving maps using self-supervised backpropagation on a parallel machine.* Tech. Rep. TR-92-059, International Computer Science Institute.

Rissanen, J. 1989. *Stochastic Complexity in Statistical Inquiry.* World Scientific Publishing Co., Singapore.

Saund, E. 1989. Dimensionality-reduction using connectionist networks. *IEEE Transact. Pattern Anal. Machine Intelligence* **11**(3), 304–314.

Zemel, R. S. 1993. A minimum description length framework for unsupervised learning. Ph.D. thesis, University of Toronto.

16

The Helmholtz Machine

Peter Dayan
Geoffrey E. Hinton
Radford M. Neal
Department of Computer Science, University of Toronto,
6 King's College Road, Toronto, Ontario M5S 1A4, Canada

Richard S. Zemel
CNL, The Salk Institute, PO Box 85800, San Diego, CA 92186-5800 USA

Discovering the structure inherent in a set of patterns is a fundamental aim of statistical inference or learning. One fruitful approach is to build a parameterized stochastic generative model, independent draws from which are likely to produce the patterns. For all but the simplest generative models, each pattern can be generated in exponentially many ways. It is thus intractable to adjust the parameters to maximize the probability of the observed patterns. We describe a way of finessing this combinatorial explosion by maximizing an easily computed lower bound on the probability of the observations. Our method can be viewed as a form of hierarchical self-supervised learning that may relate to the function of bottom-up and top-down cortical processing pathways.

1 Introduction

Following Helmholtz, we view the human perceptual system as a statistical inference engine whose function is to infer the probable causes of sensory input. We show that a device of this kind can learn how to perform these inferences without requiring a teacher to label each sensory input vector with its underlying causes. A *recognition* model is used to infer a probability distribution over the underlying causes from the sensory input, and a separate *generative* model, which is also learned, is used to train the recognition model (Zemel 1994; Hinton and Zemel 1994; Zemel and Hinton 1995).

As an example of the generative models in which we are interested, consider the shift patterns in Figure 1, which are on four 1×8 rows of binary pixels. These were produced by the two-level stochastic hierarchical generative process described in the figure caption. The task of learning is to take a set of examples generated by such a process and induce the model. Note that underlying any pattern there are multiple

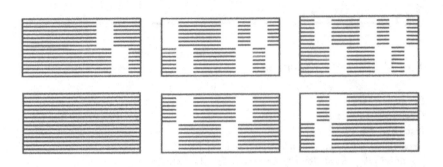

Figure 1: Shift patterns. In each of these six patterns the bottom row of square pixels is a random binary vector, the top row is a copy shifted left or right by one pixel with wraparound, and the middle two rows are copies of the outer rows. The patterns were generated by a two-stage process. First the direction of the shift was chosen, with left and right being equiprobable. Then each pixel in the bottom row was turned on (white) with a probability of 0.2, and the corresponding shifted pixel in the top row and the copies of these in the middle rows were made to follow suit. If we treat the top two rows as a left retina and the bottom two rows as a right retina, detecting the direction of the shift resembles the task of extracting depth from simple stereo images of short vertical line segments. Copying the top and bottom rows introduces extra redundancy into the images that facilitates the search for the correct generative model.

simultaneous causes. We call each possible set of causes an *explanation* of the pattern. For this particular example, it is possible to infer a unique set of causes for most patterns, but this need not always be the case.

For general generative models, the causes need not be immediately evident from the surface form of patterns. Worse still, there can be an exponential number of possible explanations underlying each pattern. The computational cost of considering all of these explanations makes standard maximum likelihood approaches such as the Expectation–Maximization algorithm (Dempster *et al.* 1977) intractable. In this paper we describe a tractable approximation to maximum likelihood learning implemented in a layered hierarchical connectionist network.

2 The Recognition Distribution

The log probability of generating a particular example, d, from a model with parameters θ is

$$\log p(d \mid \theta) = \log \left[\sum_\alpha p(\alpha \mid \theta) p(d \mid \alpha, \theta) \right] \qquad (2.1)$$

where the α are explanations. If we view the alternative explanations of an example as alternative configurations of a physical system there is a precise analogy with statistical physics. We define the energy of explanation α to be

$$E_\alpha(\theta, d) = -\log p(\alpha \mid \theta) p(d \mid \alpha, \theta) \qquad (2.2)$$

The posterior probability of an explanation given d and θ is related to its energy by the equilibrium or Boltzmann distribution, which at a temperature of 1 gives

$$P_\alpha(\theta, d) = \frac{p(\alpha \mid \theta) p(d \mid \alpha, \theta)}{\sum_{\alpha'} p(\alpha' \mid \theta) p(d \mid \alpha', \theta)} = \frac{e^{-E_\alpha}}{\sum_{\alpha'} e^{-E_{\alpha'}}} \qquad (2.3)$$

where indices θ and d in the last expression have been omitted for clarity. Using E_α and P_α equation 2.1 can be rewritten in terms of the Helmholtz free energy, which is the difference between the expected energy of an explanation and the entropy of the probability distribution across explanations.

$$\log p(d \mid \theta) = -\left[\sum_\alpha P_\alpha E_\alpha - \left(-\sum_\alpha P_\alpha \log P_\alpha \right) \right] \qquad (2.4)$$

So far, we have not gained anything in terms of computational tractability because we still need to compute expectations under the posterior distribution P, which, in general, has exponentially many terms and cannot be factored into a product of simpler distributions. However, we know (Thompson 1988) that any probability distribution over the explanations will have at least as high a free energy as the Boltzmann distribution (equation 2.3). Therefore we can restrict ourselves to some class of tractable distributions and still have a lower bound on the log probability of the data. Instead of using the true posterior probability distribution, P, for averaging over explanations, we use a more convenient probability distribution, Q. The log probability of the data can then be written as

$$\log p(d \mid \theta) = -\sum_\alpha Q_\alpha E_\alpha - \sum_\alpha Q_\alpha \log Q_\alpha + \sum_\alpha Q_\alpha \log[Q_\alpha / P_\alpha] \quad (2.5)$$

$$= -F(d; \theta, Q) + \sum_\alpha Q_\alpha \log[Q_\alpha / P_\alpha] \qquad (2.6)$$

where F is the free energy based on the incorrect or nonequilibrium posterior Q.

Making the dependencies explicit, the last term in equation 2.5 is the Kullback–Leibler divergence between $Q(d)$ and the posterior distribution, $P(\theta, d)$ (Kullback 1959). This term cannot be negative, so by ignoring it we get a lower bound on the log probability of the data given the model.

In our work, distribution Q is produced by a separate *recognition* model that has its own parameters, ϕ. These parameters are optimized at the same time as the parameters of the generative model, θ, to maximize the overall fit function $-\mathcal{F}(d; \theta, \phi) = -F[d; \theta, Q(\phi)]$. Figure 2 shows

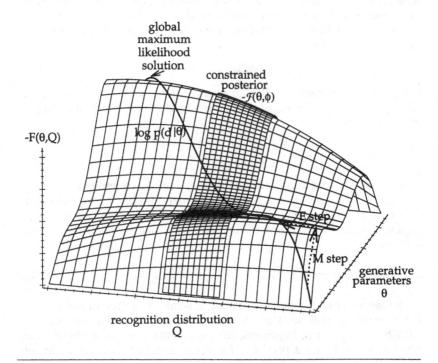

Figure 2: Graphic view of our approximation. The surface shows a simplified example of $-F(\theta, Q)$ as a function of the generative parameters θ and the recognition distribution Q. As discussed by Neal and Hinton (1994), the Expectation-Maximization algorithm ascends this surface by optimizing alternately with respect to θ (the M-step) and Q (the E-step). After each E-step, the point on the surface lies on the line defined by $Q_\alpha = P_\alpha$, and on this line, $-F = \log p(d \mid \theta)$. Using a factorial recognition distribution parameterized by ϕ restricts the surface over which the system optimizes (labeled "constrained posterior"). We ascend the restricted surface using a conjugate gradient optimization method. For a given θ, the difference between $\log p(d \mid \theta) = \max_Q \{-F(\theta, Q)\}$ and $-F(\theta, Q)$ is the Kullback–Leibler penalty in equation 2.5. That EM gets stuck in a local maximum here is largely for graphic convenience, although neither it, nor our conjugate gradient procedure, is guaranteed to find its respective global optima. Showing the factorial recognition as a connected region is an arbitrary convention; the actual structure of the recognition distributions cannot be preserved in one dimension.

graphically the nature of the approximation we are making and the relationship between our procedure and the EM algorithm. From equation 2.5, maximizing $-F$ is equivalent to maximizing the log probability

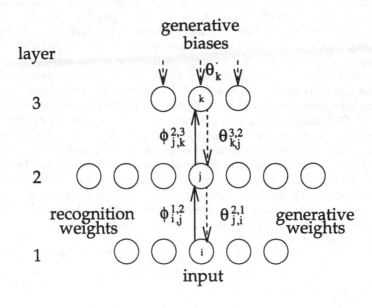

Figure 3: A simple three layer Helmholtz machine modeling the activity of 5 binary inputs (layer 1) using a two-stage hierarchical model. Generative weights (θ) are shown as dashed lines, including the generative biases, the only such input to the units in the top layer. Recognition weights (ϕ) are shown with solid lines. Recognition and generative activation functions are described in the text.

of the data minus the Kullback–Leibler divergence, showing that this divergence acts like a penalty on the traditional log probability. The recognition model is thus encouraged to be a good approximation to the true posterior distribution P. However, the same penalty also encourages the generative model to change so that the true posterior distributions will be close to distributions that can be represented by the recognition model.

3 The Deterministic Helmholtz Machine

A *Helmholtz machine* (Fig. 3) is a simple implementation of these principles. It is a connectionist system with multiple layers of neuron-like binary stochastic processing units connected hierarchically by two sets of weights. Top-down connections θ implement the generative model. Bottom-up connections ϕ implement the recognition model.

The key simplifying assumption is that the recognition distribution for a particular example d, $Q(\phi, d)$, is *factorial* (separable) in each layer. If there are h stochastic binary units in a layer ℓ, the portion of the distribution $P(\theta, d)$ due to that layer is determined by $2^h - 1$ probabilities. However, $Q(\phi, d)$ makes the assumption that the actual activity of any one unit in layer ℓ is independent of the activities of all the other units in that layer, given the activities of all the units in the lower layer, $\ell - 1$, so the recognition model needs only specify h probabilities rather than $2^h - 1$. The independence assumption allows $\mathcal{F}(d; \theta, \phi)$ to be evaluated efficiently, but this computational tractability is bought at a price, since the true posterior is unlikely to be factorial: the log probability of the data will be underestimated by an amount equal to the Kullback–Leibler divergence between the true posterior and the recognition distribution.

The generative model is taken to be factorial in the same way, although one should note that factorial generative models rarely have recognition distributions that are themselves exactly factorial.

Recognition for input example d entails using the bottom-up connections ϕ to determine the probability $q_j^\ell(\phi, d)$ that the jth unit in layer ℓ has activity $s_j^\ell = 1$. The recognition model is inherently stochastic—these probabilities are functions of the $0, 1$ activities $s_i^{\ell-1}$ of the units in layer $\ell - 1$. We use

$$q_j^\ell(\phi, \mathbf{s}^{\ell-1}) = \sigma \left(\sum_i s_i^{\ell-1} \phi_i^{\ell-1,\ell} {}_{,j} \right) \tag{3.1}$$

where $\sigma(x) = 1/[1 + \exp(-x)]$ is the conventional sigmoid function, and $\mathbf{s}^{\ell-1}$ is the vector of activities of the units in layer $\ell - 1$. All units have recognition biases as one element of the sums, all the activities at layer ℓ are calculated after all the activities at layer $\ell - 1$, and s_i^1 are the activities of the input units. It is essential that there are no feedback connections in the recognition model.

In the terms of the previous section, α is a complete assignment of s_j^ℓ for all the units in all the layers other than the input layer (for which $\ell = 1$). The multiplicative contributions to the probability of choosing that assignment using the recognition weights are q_j^ℓ for units that are on and $1 - q_j^\ell$ for units that are off:

$$Q_\alpha(\phi, d) = \prod_{\ell > 1} \prod_j \left[q_j^\ell(\phi, \mathbf{s}^{\ell-1}) \right]^{s_j^\ell} \left[1 - q_j^\ell(\phi, \mathbf{s}^{\ell-1}) \right]^{1 - s_j^\ell} \tag{3.2}$$

The Helmholtz free energy $\mathcal{F}$ depends on the generative model through $E_\alpha(\theta, d)$ in equation 2.2. The top-down connections θ use the activities $\mathbf{s}^{\ell+1}$ of the units in layer $\ell + 1$ to determine the factorial generative probabilities $p_j^\ell(\theta, \mathbf{s}^{\ell+1})$ over the activities of the units in layer ℓ. The obvious rule to use is the sigmoid:

$$p_j^\ell(\theta, \mathbf{s}^{\ell+1}) = \sigma \left(\sum_i s_k^{\ell+1} \theta_k^{\ell+1,\ell} {}_{,j} \right) \tag{3.3}$$

including a generative bias (which is the only contribution to units in the topmost layer). Unfortunately this rule did not work well in practice for the sorts of inputs we tried. Appendix A discusses the more complicated method that we actually used to determine $p_j^\ell(\theta, \mathbf{s}^{\ell+1})$. Given this, the overall generative probability of α is

$$p(\alpha \mid \theta) = \prod_{\ell > 1} \prod_j \left[p_j^\ell(\theta, \mathbf{s}^{\ell+1}) \right]^{s_j^\ell} \left[1 - p_j^\ell(\theta, \mathbf{s}^{\ell+1}) \right]^{1-s_j^\ell} \tag{3.4}$$

We extend the factorial assumption to the input layer $\ell = 1$. The activities $\mathbf{s}^2$ in layer 2 determine the probabilities $p_j^1(\theta, \mathbf{s}^2)$ of the activities in the input layer. Thus

$$p(d \mid \alpha, \theta) = \prod_j \left[p_j^1(\theta, \mathbf{s}^2) \right]^{s_j^1} \left[1 - p_j^1(\theta, \mathbf{s}^2) \right]^{1-s_j^1} \tag{3.5}$$

Combining equations 2.2, 3.4, and 3.5, and omitting dependencies for clarity,

$$
\begin{aligned}
E_\alpha(\theta, d) &= -\log p(\alpha \mid \theta) p(d \mid \alpha, \theta) && (3.6) \\
&= -\sum_{\ell \geq 1} \sum_j s_j^\ell \log p_j^\ell + \left(1 - s_j^\ell \right) \log \left(1 - p_j^\ell \right) && (3.7)
\end{aligned}
$$

Putting together the two components of $\mathcal{F}$, an unbiased estimate of the value of $\mathcal{F}(d; \theta, \phi)$ based on an explanation α drawn from Q_α is

$$
\begin{aligned}
\mathcal{F}_\alpha(d; \theta, \phi) &= E_\alpha + \log Q_\alpha && (3.8) \\
&= \sum_\ell \sum_j s_j^\ell \log \frac{q_j^\ell}{p_j^\ell} + \left(1 - s_j^\ell \right) \log \frac{1 - q_j^\ell}{1 - p_j^\ell} && (3.9)
\end{aligned}
$$

One could perform stochastic gradient ascent in the negative free energy across all the data $-\mathcal{F}(\theta, \phi) = -\sum_d \mathcal{F}(d; \theta, \phi)$ using equation 3.9 and a form of REINFORCE algorithm (Barto and Anandan 1985; Williams 1992). However, for the simulations in this paper, we made a number of mean-field inspired approximations, in that we replaced the stochastic binary activities s_j^ℓ by their mean values under the recognition model q_j^ℓ. We took

$$q_j^\ell(\phi, \mathbf{q}^{\ell-1}) = \sigma \left(\sum_i q_i^{\ell-1} \phi_{i\,j}^{\ell-1,\ell} \right) \tag{3.10}$$

we made a similar approximation for p_j^ℓ, which we discuss in Appendix A, and we then averaged the expression in equation 3.9 over α to give the overall free energy:

$$-\mathcal{F}(\theta, \phi) = \sum_d \sum_\ell \sum_j \mathrm{KL} \left[q_j^\ell(\phi, \mathbf{q}^{\ell-1}), p_j^\ell(\theta, \mathbf{q}^{\ell+1}) \right] \tag{3.11}$$

where the innermost term in the sum is the Kullback–Leibler divergence between generative and recognition distributions for unit j in layer ℓ for example d:

$$\mathrm{KL}[q, p] = q \log \frac{q}{p} + (1 - q) \log \frac{1 - q}{1 - p}$$

Weights θ and ϕ are trained by following the derivatives of $\mathcal{F}(\theta, \phi)$ in equation 3.11. Since the generative weights θ do not affect the actual activities of the units, there are no cycles, and so the derivatives can be calculated in closed form using the chain rule. Appendix B gives the appropriate recursive formulas.

Note that this deterministic version introduces a further approximation by ignoring correlations arising from the fact that under the real recognition model, the actual activities at layer $\ell + 1$ are a function of the actual activities at layer ℓ rather than their mean values.

Figure 4 demonstrates the performance of the Helmholtz machine in a hierarchical learning task (Becker and Hinton 1992), showing that it is capable of extracting the structure underlying a complicated generative model. The example shows clearly the difference between the generative (θ) and the recognition (ϕ) weights, since the latter often include negative side-lobes around their favored shifts, which are needed to prevent incorrect recognition.

4 The Wake-Sleep Algorithm

The derivatives required for learning in the deterministic Helmholtz machine are quite complicated because they have to take into account the effects that changes in an activity at one layer will have on activities in higher layers. However, by borrowing an idea from the Boltzmann machine (Hinton and Sejnowski 1986; Ackley et al. 1985), we get the wake-sleep algorithm, which is a very simple learning scheme for layered networks of stochastic binary units that approximates the correct derivatives (Hinton et al. 1995).

Learning in the wake-sleep algorithm is separated into two phases. During the wake phase, data d from the world are presented at the lowest layer and binary activations of units at successively *higher* layers are picked according to the recognition probabilities, $q_j^\ell(\phi, \mathbf{s}^{\ell-1})$, determined by the bottom-up weights. The top-down generative weights from layer $\ell + 1$ to layer ℓ are then altered to reduce the Kullback–Leibler divergence between the actual activations and the generative probabilities $p_j^\ell(\theta, \mathbf{s}^{\ell+1})$. In the sleep phase, the recognition weights are turned off and the top-down weights are used to activate the units. Starting at the top layer, activities are generated at successively *lower* layers based on the current top-down weights θ. The network thus generates a random instance from its generative model. Since it has generated the instance, it knows the true underlying causes, and therefore has available the target values for the hidden units that are required to train the bottom-up weights. If the bottom-up and the top-down activation functions are both sigmoid (equations 3.1 and 3.3), then both phases use exactly the same learning rule, the purely local delta rule (Widrow and Stearns 1985).

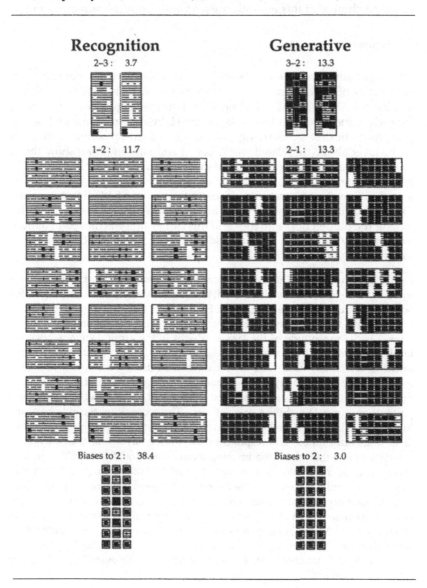

Recognition

2-3 :   3.7

1-2 :   11.7

Biases to 2 :   38.4

Generative

3-2 :   13.3

2-1 :   13.3

Biases to 2 :   3.0

Unfortunately, there is no single cost function that is reduced by these two procedures. This is partly because the sleep phase trains the recognition model to invert the generative model for input vectors that are distributed according to the generative model rather than according to the real data and partly because the sleep phase learning does not follow the correct gradient. Nevertheless, $Q_\alpha = P_\alpha$ at the optimal end point, if it can be reached. Preliminary results by Brendan Frey (personal communication) show that this algorithm works well on some nontrivial tasks.

5 Discussion

The Helmholtz machine can be viewed as a hierarchical generalization of the type of learning procedure described by Zemel (1994) and Hinton and Zemel (1994). Instead of using a fixed independent prior distribution for each of the hidden units in a layer, the Helmholtz machine makes this prior more flexible by deriving it from the bottom-up activities of units in the layer above. In related work, Zemel and Hinton (1995) show that a system can learn a redundant population code in a layer of hidden units, provided the activities of the hidden units are represented by a point in a multidimensional constraint space with pre-specified dimensionality. The role of their constraint space is to capture statistical dependencies among the hidden unit activities and this can again be achieved in a more uniform way by using a second hidden layer in a hierarchical generative model of the type described here.

Figure 4: *Facing page.* The shifter. Recognition and generative weights for a three layer Helmholtz machine's model for the shifter problem (see Fig. 1 for how the input patterns are generated). Each weight diagram shows recognition or generative weights between the given layers (1–2, 2–3, etc.) and the number quoted is the magnitude of the largest weight in the array. White is positive, black negative, but the generative weights shown are the natural logarithms of the ones actually used. The lowest weights in the 2–3 block are the biases to layer 3; the biases to layer 2 are shown separately because of their different magnitude. All the units in layer 2 are either silent, or respond to one or two pairs of appropriately shifted pairs of bits. The recognition weights have inhibitory side lobes to stop their units from responding incorrectly. The units in layer 3 are shift tuned, and respond to the units in layer 2 of their own shift direction. Note that under the imaging model (equation A.2 or A.3), a unit in layer 3 cannot specify that one in layer 2 should be off, forcing a solution that requires two units in layer 3. One aspect of the generative model is therefore not correctly captured. Finding weights equivalent to those shown is hard, requiring many iterations of a conjugate gradient algorithm. To prevent the units in layers 2 and 3 from being permanently turned off early in the learning they were given fixed, but tiny generative biases ($\theta = 0.05$). Additional generative biases to layer 3 are shown in the figure; they learn the overall probability of left and right shifts.

The old idea of analysis-by-synthesis assumes that the cortex contains a generative model of the world and that recognition involves inverting the generative model in real time. This has been attempted for non-probabilistic generative models (MacKay 1956; Pece 1992). However, for stochastic ones it typically involves Markov chain Monte Carlo methods (Neal 1992). These can be computationally unattractive, and their requirement for repeated sampling renders them unlikely to be employed by the cortex. In addition to making learning tractable, its separate recognition model allows a Helmholtz machine to recognize without iterative sampling, and makes it much easier to see how generative models could be implemented in the cortex without running into serious time constraints. During recognition, the generative model is superfluous, since the recognition model contains all the information that is required. Nevertheless, the generative model plays an essential role in defining the objective function $\mathcal{F}$ that allows the parameters ϕ of the recognition model to be learned.

The Helmholtz machine is closely related to other schemes for self-supervised learning that use feedback as well as feedforward weights (Carpenter and Grossberg 1987; Luttrell 1992, 1994; Ullman 1994; Kawato *et al.* 1993; Mumford 1994). By contrast with adaptive resonance theory (Carpenter and Grossberg 1987) and the counter-streams model (Ullman 1994), the Helmholtz machine treats self-supervised learning as a statistical problem—one of ascertaining a generative model that accurately captures the structure in the input examples. Luttrell (1992, 1994) discusses multilayer self-supervised learning aimed at faithful vector quantization in the face of noise, rather than our aim of maximizing the likelihood. The outputs of his separate low level coding networks are combined at higher levels, and thus their optimal coding choices become mutually dependent. These networks can be given a coding interpretation that is very similar to that of the Helmholtz machine. However, we are interested in distributed rather than local representations at each level (multiple cause rather than single cause models), forcing the approximations that we use. Kawato *et al.* (1993) consider forward (generative) and inverse (recognition) models (Jordan and Rumelhart 1992) in a similar fashion to the Helmholtz machine, but without this probabilistic perspective. The recognition weights between two layers do not just invert the generation weights between those layers, but also take into account the prior activities in the upper layer. The Helmholtz machine fits comfortably within the framework of Grenander's pattern theory (Grenander 1976) in the form of Mumford's (1994) proposals for the mapping onto the brain.

As described, the recognition process in the Helmholtz machine is purely bottom-up—the top-down generative model plays no direct role and there is no interaction between units in a single layer. However, such effects are important in real perception and can be implemented using iterative recognition, in which the generative and recognition activations interact to produce the final activity of a unit. This can introduce substantial theoretical complications in ensuring that the activation process is stable and converges adequately quickly, and in determining how the weights should change so as to capture input examples more accurately. An interesting first step toward interaction within layers would be to organize their units into small clusters with local excitation and longer-range inhibition, as is seen in the columnar structure of the brain. Iteration would be confined within layers, easing the complications.

Appendix A: The Imaging Model

The sigmoid activation function given in equation 3.3 turned out not to work well for the generative model for the input examples we tried, such as the shifter problem (Fig. 1). Learning almost invariably got caught in one of a variety of local minima. In the context of a one layer generative model and without a recognition model, Saund (1994; 1995) discussed why this might happen in terms of the underlying imaging model—which is responsible for turning binary activities in what we call layer 2 into probabilities of activation of the units in the input layer. He suggested using a noisy-or imaging model (Pearl 1988), for which the weights $0 \leq \theta_{k\,,j}^{\ell+1,\ell} \leq 1$ are interpreted as probabilities that $s_j^\ell = 1$ if unit $s_k^{\ell+1} = 1$, and are combined as

$$p_j^\ell(\theta, \mathbf{s}^{\ell+1}) = 1 - \prod_k \left(1 - s_k^{\ell+1}\theta_{k\,,j}^{\ell+1,\ell}\right) \tag{A.1}$$

The noisy-or imaging model worked somewhat better than the sigmoid model of equation 3.3, but it was still prone to fall into local minima. Dayan and Zemel (1995) suggested a yet more competitive rule based on the integrated segmentation and recognition architecture of Keeler et $al.$ (1991). In this, the weights $0 \leq \theta_{k\,,j}^{\ell+1,\ell}$ are interpreted as the odds that $s_j^\ell = 1$ if unit $s_k^{\ell+1} = 1$, and are combined as

$$p_j^\ell(\theta, \mathbf{s}^{\ell+1}) = 1 - \frac{1}{1 + \sum_k s_k^{\ell+1}\theta_{k\,,j}^{\ell+1,\ell}} \tag{A.2}$$

For the deterministic Helmholtz machine, we need a version of this activation rule that uses the probabilities $\mathbf{q}^{\ell+1}$ rather than the binary samples $\mathbf{s}^{\ell+1}$. This is somewhat complicated, since the obvious expression $1 - 1/(1 + \sum_k q_k^{\ell+1}\theta_{k\,,j}^{\ell+1,\ell})$ turns out not to work. In the end (Dayan and Zemel 1995) we used a product of this term and the deterministic version of the noisy-or:

$$p_j^\ell(\theta, \mathbf{q}^{\ell+1}) = \left(1 - \frac{1}{1 + \sum_k q_k^{\ell+1}\theta_{k\,,j}^{\ell+1,\ell}}\right)\left[1 - \prod_k \left(1 - q_k^{\ell+1}\frac{\theta_{k\,,j}^{\ell+1,\ell}}{1 + \theta_{k\,,j}^{\ell+1,\ell}}\right)\right] \tag{A.3}$$

Appendix B gives the derivatives of this. We used the exact expected value of equation A.2 if there were only three units in layer $\ell + 1$ because it is computationally inexpensive to work it out.

For convenience, we used the same imaging model (equations A.2 and A.3) for all the generative connections. In general one could use different types of connections between different levels.

Appendix B: The Derivatives

Write $\mathcal{F}(d; \theta, \phi)$ for the contribution to the overall error in equation 3.11 for input example d, including the input layer:

$$
\mathcal{F}(d; \theta, \phi) = \sum_\ell \sum_j -q_j^\ell \log p_j^\ell - \left(1 - q_j^\ell\right) \log \left(1 - p_j^\ell\right) + q_j^\ell \log q_j^\ell
$$
$$
+ \left(1 - q_j^\ell\right) \log \left(1 - q_j^\ell\right)
$$

Then the total derivative for input example d with respect to the activation of a unit in layer ℓ is

$$
\frac{\partial \mathcal{F}(d; \theta, \phi)}{\partial q_j^\ell} = \log \frac{1 - p_j^\ell}{p_j^\ell} \sum \frac{q_j^\ell}{1 - q_j^\ell} + \sum_i \frac{p_i^{\ell-1} - q_i^{\ell-1}}{p_i^{\ell-1}\left(1 - p_i^{\ell-1}\right)} \frac{\partial p_i^{\ell-1}}{\partial q_j^\ell}
$$
$$
+ \sum_{p > \ell} \sum_k \frac{\partial \mathcal{F}(d; \theta, \phi)}{\partial q_k^p} \frac{\partial q_k^p}{\partial q_j^\ell} \tag{B.1}
$$

since changing q_j^ℓ affects the generative priors at layer $\ell - 1$, and the recognition activities at all layers higher than ℓ. These derivatives can be calculated in a single backward propagation pass through the network, accumulating $\partial \mathcal{F}(d; \theta, \phi)/\partial q_k^p$ as it goes. The use of standard sigmoid units in the recognition direction makes $\partial q_k^p / \partial q_j^\ell$ completely conventional. Using equation A.3 makes

$$
\frac{\partial p_i^{\ell-1}}{\partial q_j^\ell} = \frac{\theta_{j,i}^{\ell,\ell-1}}{\left(1 + \sum_a q_a^\ell \theta_{a,i}^{\ell,\ell-1}\right)^2} \left[1 - \prod_a \left(1 - q_a^\ell \frac{\theta_{a,i}^{\ell,\ell-1}}{1 + \theta_{a,i}^{\ell,\ell-1}}\right)\right]
$$
$$
+ \left(1 - \frac{1}{1 + \sum_a q_a^\ell \theta_{a,i}^{\ell,\ell-1}}\right) \frac{\theta_{j,i}^{\ell,\ell-1}}{1 + \theta_{j,i}^{\ell,\ell-1}} \times
$$
$$
\prod_{a \neq j} \left(1 - q_a^\ell \frac{\theta_{a,i}^{\ell,\ell-1}}{1 + \theta_{a,i}^{\ell,\ell-1}}\right) \tag{B.2}
$$

One also needs the derivative

$$
\frac{\partial p_i^{\ell-1}}{\partial \theta_{j,i}^{\ell,\ell-1}} = \frac{q_j^\ell}{\left(1 + \sum_a q_a^\ell \theta_{a,i}^{\ell,\ell-1}\right)^2} \left[1 - \prod_a \left(1 - q_a^\ell \frac{\theta_{a,i}^{\ell,\ell-1}}{1 + \theta_{a,i}^{\ell,\ell-1}} \right) \right]
$$

$$
+ \left(1 - \frac{1}{1 + \sum_a q_a^\ell \theta_{a,i}^{\ell,\ell-1}} \right) \frac{q_j^\ell}{\left(1 + \theta_{j,i}^{\ell,\ell-1}\right)^2} \times
$$

$$
\prod_{a \neq j} \left(1 - q_a^\ell \frac{\theta_{a,i}^{\ell,\ell-1}}{1 + \theta_{a,i}^{\ell,\ell-1}} \right) \tag{B.3}
$$

This is exactly what we used for the imaging model in equation A.3. However, it is important to bear in mind that $p_j^\ell(\theta, \mathbf{s}^{\ell+1})$ should really be a function of the stochastic choices of the units in layer $\ell + 1$. The contribution to the expected cost $\mathcal{F}$ is a function of $\langle \log p_j^\ell(\theta, \mathbf{s}^{\ell+1}) \rangle$ and $\langle \log [1 - p_j^\ell(\theta, \mathbf{s}^{\ell+1})] \rangle$, where $\langle \ \rangle$ indicates averaging over the recognition distribution. These are not the same as $\log \langle p_j^\ell(\theta, \mathbf{s}^{\ell+1}) \rangle$ and $\log \left(1 - \langle p_j^\ell(\theta, \mathbf{s}^{\ell+1}) \rangle \right)$, which is what the deterministic machine uses. For other imaging models, it is possible to take this into account.

Acknowledgments

We are very grateful to Drew van Camp, Brendan Frey, Geoff Goodhill, Mike Jordan, David MacKay, Mike Revow, Virginia de Sa, Nici Schraudolph, Terry Sejnowski, and Chris Williams for helpful discussions and comments, and particularly to Mike Jordan for extensive criticism of an earlier version of this paper. This work was supported by NSERC and IRIS. G. E. H. is the Noranda Fellow of the Canadian Institute for Advanced Research. The current address for R. S. Z. is Baker Hall 330, Department of Psychology, Carnegie Mellon University, Pittsburgh, PA 15213.

References

Ackley, D. H., Hinton, G. E., and Sejnowski, T. J. 1985. A learning algorithm for Boltzmann machines. Cog. Sci. 9, 147–169.

Barto, A. G., and Anandan, P. 1985. Pattern recognizing stochastic learning automata. IEEE Trans. Syst. Man Cybernet. 15, 360–374.

Becker, S., and Hinton, G. E. 1992. A self-organizing neural network that discovers surfaces in random-dot stereograms. Nature (London) 355, 161–163.

Carpenter, G., and Grossberg, S. 1987. A massively parallel architecture for a self-organizing neural pattern recognition machine. Comp. Vision, Graphics Image Process. 37, 54–115.

Dayan, P., and Zemel, R. S. 1995. Competition and multiple cause models. *Neural Comp.* **7**, 565–579.

Dempster, A. P., Laird, N. M., and Rubin, D. B. 1977. Maximum likelihood from incomplete data via the EM algorithm. *Proc. Royal Stat. Soc.* B-39 1–38.

Grenander, U. 1976–1981. *Lectures in Pattern Theory I, II and III: Pattern Analysis, Pattern Synthesis and Regular Structures.* Springer-Verlag, Berlin.

Hinton, G. E., Dayan, P., Frey, B. J., Neal, R. M. 1995. The wake-sleep algorithm for unsupervised neural networks. *Science* **268**, 1158–1160.

Hinton, G. E., and Sejnowski, T. J. 1986. Learning and relearning in Boltzmann machines. In *Parallel Distributed Processing: Explorations in the Microstructure of Cognition. Volume 1: Foundations*, D. E. Rumelhart, J. L. McClelland, and the PDP research group, eds., pp. 282–317. MIT Press, Cambridge, MA.

Hinton, G. E., and Zemel, R. S. 1994. Autoencoders, minimum description length and Helmholtz free energy. In *Advances in Neural Information Processing Systems 6*, J. D. Cowan, G. Tesauro, and J. Alspector, eds., pp. 3–10. Morgan Kaufmann, San Mateo, CA.

Jordan, M. I., and Rumelhart, D. E. 1992. Forward models: Supervised learning with a distal teacher. *Cog. Sci.* **16**, 307–354.

Kawato, M., Hayakama, H., and Inui, T. 1993. A forward-inverse optics model of reciprocal connections between visual cortical areas. *Network* **4**, 415–422.

Keeler, J. D., Rumelhart, D. E., and Leow, W. K. 1991. Integrated segmentation and recognition of hand-printed numerals. In *Advances in Neural Information Processing Systems*, R. P. Lippmann, J. Moody, and D. S. Touretzky, eds., Vol. 3, 557–563. Morgan Kaufmann, San Mateo, CA.

Kullback, S. 1959. *Information Theory and Statistics.* Wiley, New York.

Luttrell, S. P. 1992. Self-supervised adaptive networks. *IEE Proc. Part F* **139**, 371–377.

Luttrell, S. P. 1994. A Bayesian analysis of self-organizing maps. *Neural Comp.* **6**, 767–794.

MacKay, D. M. 1956. The epistemological problem for automata. In *Automata Studies*, C. E. Shannon and J. McCarthy, eds., pp. 235–251. Princeton University Press, Princeton, NJ.

Mumford, D. 1994. Neuronal architectures for pattern-theoretic problems. In *Large-Scale Theories of the Cortex*, C. Koch and J. Davis, eds., pp. 125–152. MIT Press, Cambridge, MA.

Neal, R. M. 1992. Connectionist learning of belief networks. *Artificial Intelligence* **56**, 71–113.

Neal, R. M., and Hinton, G. E. 1994. A new view of the EM algorithm that justifies incremental and other variants. *Biometrika* (submitted).

Pearl, J. 1988. *Probabilistic Reasoning in Intelligent Systems: Networks of Plausible Inference.* Morgan Kaufmann, San Mateo, CA.

Pece, A. E. C. 1992. Redundancy reduction of a Gabor representation: A possible computational role for feedback from primary visual cortex to lateral geniculate nucleus. In *Artificial Neural Networks*, I. Aleksander and J. Taylor, eds., Vol. 2, pp. 865–868. Elsevier, Amsterdam.

Saund, E. 1994. Unsupervised learning of mixtures of multiple causes in binary data. In *Advances in Neural Information Processing Systems*, J. D. Cowan,

G. Tesauro and J. Alspector, eds., Vol. 6, pp. 27–34. Morgan Kaufmann, San Mateo, CA.

Saund, E. 1995. A multiple cause mixture model for unsupervised learning. *Neural Comp.* **7**, 51–71.

Thompson, C. J. 1988. *Classical Equilibrium Statistical Mechanics.* Clarendon Press, Oxford.

Ullman, S. 1994. Sequence seeking and counterstreams: A model for bidirectional information flow in the cortex. In *Large-Scale Theories of the Cortex*, C. Koch and J. Davis, eds., pp. 257–270. MIT Press, Cambridge, MA.

Widrow, B., and Stearns, S. D. 1985. *Adaptive Signal Processing.* Prentice-Hall, Englewood Cliffs, NJ.

Williams, R. J. 1992. Simple statistical gradient-following algorithms for connectionist reinforcement learning. *Machine Learn.* **8**, 229–256.

Zemel, R. S. 1994. *A Minimum Description Length Framework for Unsupervised Learning.* Ph.D. Dissertation, Computer Science, University of Toronto, Canada.

Zemel, R. S., and Hinton, G. E. 1995. Learning population codes by minimizing description length. *Neural Comp.* **7**, 549–564.

17

Factor Analysis Using Delta-Rule Wake-Sleep Learning

Radford M. Neal
Department of Statistics and Department of Computer Science, University of Toronto, Toronto M5S 1A1, Canada

Peter Dayan
Department of Brain and Cognitive Sciences, Massachusetts Institute of Technology, Cambridge, MA, 02139 U.S.A.

We describe a linear network that models correlations between real-valued visible variables using one or more real-valued hidden variables—a factor analysis model. This model can be seen as a linear version of the Helmholtz machine, and its parameters can be learned using the wake-sleep method, in which learning of the primary generative model is assisted by a recognition model, whose role is to fill in the values of hidden variables based on the values of visible variables. The generative and recognition models are jointly learned in wake and sleep phases, using just the delta rule. This learning procedure is comparable in simplicity to Hebbian learning, which produces a somewhat different representation of correlations in terms of principal components. We argue that the simplicity of wake-sleep learning makes factor analysis a plausible alternative to Hebbian learning as a model of activity-dependent cortical plasticity.

1 Introduction

Statistical structure in a collection of inputs can be found using purely local Hebbian learning rules (Hebb, 1949), which capture second-order aspects of the data in terms of principal components (Linsker, 1988; Oja, 1989). This form of statistical analysis has therefore been used to provide a computational account of activity-dependent plasticity in the vertebrate brain (e.g., von der Malsburg, 1973; Linsker, 1986; Miller, Keller, & Stryker, 1989).

There are reasons, however, that principal component analysis may not be an adequate model for the generation of cortical receptive fields (e.g., Olshausen & Field, 1996). Furthermore, a Hebbian mechanism for performing principal component analysis would accord no role to the top-down (feedback) connections that always accompany bottom-up connections (Felleman & Van Essen, 1991). Hebbian learning must also be augmented by extra mechanisms in order to extract more than just the first principal component and in order to prevent the synaptic weights from growing without bound.

In this article, we present the statistical technique of factor analysis as an alternative to principal component analysis and show how factor analysis models can be learned using an algorithm whose demands on synaptic plasticity are as local as those of the Hebb rule.

Our approach follows the suggestion of Hinton and Zemel (1994) (see also Grenander, 1976–1981; Mumford, 1994; Dayan, Hinton, Neal, & Zemel, 1995; Olshausen & Field, 1996) that the top-down connections in the cortex might be constructing a hierarchical, probabilistic "generative" model, in which dependencies between the activities of neurons reporting sensory data are seen as being due to the presence in the world of hidden or latent "factors." The role of the bottom-up connections is to implement an inverse "recognition" model, which takes low-level sensory input and instantiates in the activities of neurons in higher layers a set of likely values for the hidden factors, which are capable of explaining this input. These higher-level activities are meant to correspond to significant features of the external world, and thus to form an appropriate basis for behavior.

We refer to such a combination of generative and recognition models as a Helmholtz machine. The simplest form of Helmholtz machine, with just two layers, linear units, and gaussian noise, is equivalent to the factor analysis model, a statistical method that is used widely in psychology and the social sciences as a way of exploring whether observed patterns in data might be explainable in terms of a small number of unobserved factors. Everitt (1984) gives a good introduction to factor analysis and to other latent variable models.

Even though factor analysis involves only linear operations and gaussian noise, learning a factor analysis model is not computationally straightforward; practical algorithms for maximum likelihood factor analysis (Jöreskog, 1967, 1969, 1977) took many years to develop. Existing algorithms change the values of parameters based on complex and nonlocal calculations. A general approach to learning in Helmholtz machines that is attractive for its simplicity is the wake-sleep algorithm of Hinton, Dayan, Frey, and Neal (1995). We show empirically in this article that maximum likelihood factor analysis models can be learned by the wake-sleep method, which uses just the purely local delta rule in both of its two separate learning phases. The wake-sleep algorithm has previously been applied to the more difficult task of learning nonlinear models with binary latent variables, with mixed results. We have found that good results are obtained much more consistently when the wake-sleep algorithm is used to learn factor analysis models, perhaps because settings of the recognition model parameters that invert the generative model always exist.

In the factor analysis models we look at in this article, the factors are a priori independent, and this simplicity prevents them from reproducing interesting aspects of cortical structure. However, these results contribute to the understanding of wake-sleep learning. They also point to possibilities for modeling cortical plasticity, since the wake-sleep approach avoids many of the criticisms that can be leveled at Hebbian learning.

2 Factor Analysis

Factor analysis with a single hidden factor is based on a generative model for the distribution of a vector of real-valued visible inputs, x, given by

$$x = \mu + gy + \epsilon. \tag{2.1}$$

Here, y is the single real-valued factor, and is assumed to have a gaussian distribution with mean zero and variance one. The vector of "factor loadings," g, which we refer to as the generative weights, expresses the way the visible variables are related to the hidden factor. The vector of overall means, μ, will, for simplicity of presentation, be taken to be zero in this article, unless otherwise stated. Finally, the noise, ϵ, is assumed to be gaussian, with a diagonal covariance matrix, Ψ, which we will write as

$$\Psi = \begin{pmatrix} \tau_1^2 & 0 & \dots & 0 \\ 0 & \tau_2^2 & \dots & 0 \\ & & \dots & \\ 0 & 0 & \dots & \tau_n^2 \end{pmatrix} \tag{2.2}$$

The τ_j^2 are sometimes called the "uniquenesses," as they represent the portion of the variance in each visible variable that is unique to it rather than being explained by the common factor. We will refer to them as the generative variance parameters (not to be confused with the variance of the hidden factor in the generative model, which is fixed at one).

The model parameters, μ, g, and Ψ, define a joint gaussian distribution for both the hidden factor, y, and the visible inputs, x. In a Helmholtz machine, this generative model is accompanied by a recognition model, which represents the conditional distribution for the hidden factor, y, given a particular input vector, x. This recognition model also has a simple form, which for $\mu = 0$, is

$$y = r^T x + v, \tag{2.3}$$

where r is the vector of recognition weights and v has a gaussian distribution with mean zero and variance σ^2. It is straightforward to show that the correct recognition model has $r = [gg^T + \Psi]^{-1}g$ and $\sigma^2 = 1 - g^T[gg^T + \Psi]^{-1}g$, but we presume that directly obtaining the recognition model's parameters in this way is not plausible in a neurobiological model.

The factor analysis model can be extended to include several hidden factors, which are usually assumed to have independent gaussian distributions with mean zero and variance one (though we discuss other possibilities in section 5.2). These factors jointly produce a distribution for the visible variables, as follows:

$$x = \mu + Gy + \epsilon. \tag{2.4}$$

Here, y is the vector of hidden factor values, G is a matrix of generative weights (factor loadings), and ϵ is again a noise vector with diagonal covariance. A linear recognition model can again be found to represent the conditional distribution of the hidden factors for given values of the visible variables. Note that there is redundancy in the definition of the multiple-factor model, caused by the symmetry of the distribution of y in the generative model. A model with generative weights $G' = GU^T$, where U is any unitary matrix (for which $U^T U = I$), will produce the same distribution for x, with the hidden factors $y' = Uy$ again being independent, with mean zero and variance one. The presence of multiple solutions is sometimes seen as a problem with factor analysis in statistical applications, since it makes interpretation more difficult, but this is hardly an issue in neurobiological modeling, since easy interpretability of neural activities is not something that we are at liberty to require.

Although there are some special circumstances in which factor analysis is equivalent to principal component analysis, the techniques are in general quite different (Jolliffe, 1986). Loosely speaking, principal component analysis pays attention to both variance and covariance, whereas factor analysis looks only at covariance. In particular, if one of the components of x is corrupted by a large amount of noise, the principal eigenvector of the covariance matrix of the inputs will have a substantial component in the direction of that input. Hebbian learning will therefore result in the output, y, being dominated by this noise. In contrast, factor analysis uses ϵ_j to model any noise that affects only component j. A large amount of noise simply results in the corresponding τ_j^2 being large, with no effect on the output y. Principal component analysis is also unaffected by a rotation of the coordinate system of the input vectors, whereas factor analysis privileges the particular coordinate system in which the data are presented, because it is assumed in equation 2.2 that it is in this coordinate system that the components of the noise are independent.

3 Learning Factor Analysis Models with the Wake-Sleep Algorithm ____

In this section, we describe wake-sleep algorithms for learning factor analysis models, starting with the simplest such model, having a single hidden factor. We also provide an intuitive justification for believing that these algorithms might work, based on their resemblance to the Expectation-Maximization (EM) algorithm. We have not found a complete theoretical proof that wake-sleep learning for factor analysis works, but we present empirical evidence that it usually does in section 4.

3.1 Maximum Likelihood and the EM Algorithm.

In maximum likelihood learning, the parameters of the model are chosen to maximize the probability density assigned by the model to the data that were observed (the "likelihood"). For a factor analysis model with a single factor, the likelihood, L, based on the observed data in n independent cases, $x^{(1)}, \ldots, x^{(n)}$, is obtained by integrating over the possible values that the hidden factors, $y^{(c)}$, might take on for each case:

$$L(g, \Psi) = \prod_{c=1}^{n} p(x^{(c)} \mid g, \Psi) = \prod_{c=1}^{n} \int p(x^{(c)} \mid y^{(c)}, g, \Psi) \, p(y^{(c)}) \, dy^{(c)} \quad (3.1)$$

where g and Ψ are the model parameters, as described previously, and $p(\cdot)$ is used to write probability densities and conditional probability densities. The prior distribution for the hidden factor, $p(y^{(c)})$, is gaussian with mean zero and variance one. The conditional distribution for $x^{(c)}$ given $y^{(c)}$ is gaussian with mean $\mu + g y^{(c)}$ and covariance Ψ, as implied by equation 2.1.

Wake-sleep learning can be viewed as an approximate implementation of the EM algorithm, which Dempster, Laird, and Rubin (1977) present as a general approach to maximum likelihood estimation when some variables (in our case, the values of the hidden factors) are unobserved. Applications of EM to factor analysis are discussed by Dempster et al. (1977) and by Rubin and Thayer (1982), who find that EM produces results almost identical to those of Jöreskog's (1969) method, including getting stuck in essentially the same local maxima given the same starting values for the parameters.[1]

EM is an iterative method, in which each iteration consists of two steps. In the E-step, one finds the conditional distribution for the unobserved variables given the observed data, based on the current estimates for the model parameters. When the cases are independent, this conditional distribution factors into distributions for the unobserved variables in each case. For the single-factor model, the distribution for the hidden factor, $y^{(c)}$, in a case with observed data $x^{(c)}$, is

$$p(y^{(c)} \mid x^{(c)}, g, \Psi) = \frac{p(y^{(c)}, x^{(c)} \mid g, \Psi)}{\int p(x^{(c)} \mid y, g, \Psi) \, p(y) \, dy}. \quad (3.2)$$

---

[1] It may seem surprising that maximum likelihood factor analysis can be troubled by local maxima, in view of the simple linear nature of the model, but this is in fact quite possible. For example, a local maximum can arise if a single-factor model is applied to data consisting of two pairs of correlated variables. The single factor can capture only one of these correlations. If the initial weights are appropriate for modeling the weaker of the two correlations, learning may never find the global maximum in which the single factor is used instead to model the stronger correlation.

In the M-step, one finds new parameter values, $\mathbf{g}'$ and Ψ', that maximize (or at least increase) the expected log likelihood of the complete data, with the unobserved variables filled in according to the conditional distribution found in the E-step:

$$\sum_{c=1}^{n} \int p(y^{(c)} \mid \mathbf{x}^{(c)}, \mathbf{g}, \Psi) \log\left[p(\mathbf{x}^{(c)} \mid y^{(c)}, \mathbf{g}', \Psi') p(y^{(c)})\right] dy^{(c)}. \qquad (3.3)$$

For factor analysis, the conditional distribution for $y^{(c)}$ in equation 3.2 is gaussian, and the quantity whose expectation with respect to this distribution is required above is quadratic in $y^{(c)}$. This expectation is therefore easily found on a computer. However, the matrix calculations involved require nonlocal operations.

3.2 The Wake-Sleep Approach. To obtain a local learning procedure, we first eliminate the explicit maximization in the M-step of the quantity defined in equation 3.3 in terms of an expectation. We replace this by a gradient-following learning procedure in which the expectation is implicitly found by combining many updates based on values for the $y^{(c)}$ that are stochastically generated from the appropriate conditional distributions. We furthermore avoid the direct computation of these conditional distributions in the E-step by learning to produce them using a recognition model, trained in tandem with the generative model.

This approach results in the wake-sleep learning procedure, with the wake phase playing the role of the M-step in EM and the sleep phase playing the role of the E-step. The names for these phases are metaphorical; we are not proposing neurobiological correlates for the wake and sleep phases. Learning consists of interleaved iterations of these two phases, which in the context of factor analysis operate as follows:

Wake phase: From observed values for the visible variables, $\mathbf{x}$, randomly fill in values for the hidden factors, $\mathbf{y}$, using the conditional distribution defined by the current recognition model. Update the parameters of the generative model to make this filled-in case more likely.

Sleep phase: Without reference to any observation, randomly choose values for the hidden factors, $\mathbf{y}$, from their fixed generative distribution, and then randomly choose "fantasy" values for the visible variables, $\mathbf{x}$, from their conditional distribution given $\mathbf{y}$, as defined by the current parameters of the generative model. Update the parameters of the recognition model to make this fantasy case more likely.

The wake phase of learning will correctly implement the M-step of EM (in a stochastic sense), provided that the recognition model produces the correct conditional distribution for the hidden factors. The aim of sleep phase learning is to improve the recognition model's ability to produce this conditional distribution, which would be computed in the E-step of EM. If values for the recognition model parameters exist that reproduce this conditional distribution exactly and if learning of the recognition model proceeds at a much faster rate than changes to the generative model, so that this correct distribution can continually be tracked, then the sleep phase will effectively implement the E-step of EM, and the wake-sleep algorithm as a whole will be guaranteed to find a (local) maximum of the likelihood (in the limit of small learning rates, so that stochastic variation is averaged out).

These conditions for wake-sleep learning to mimic EM are too stringent for actual applications, however. At a minimum, we would like wake-sleep learning to work for a wide range of relative learning rates in the two phases, not just in the limit as the ratio of the generative learning rate to the recognition learning rate goes to zero. We would also like wake-sleep learning to do something sensible even when it is not possible for the recognition model to invert the generative model perfectly (as is typical in applications other than factor analysis), though one would not usually expect the method to produce exact maximum likelihood estimates in such a case.

We could guarantee that wake-sleep learning behaves well if we could find a cost function that is decreased (on average) by both the wake phase and the sleep phase updates. The cost would then be a Lyapunov function for learning, providing a guarantee of stability and allowing something to be said about the stable states. Unfortunately, no such cost function has been discovered, for either wake-sleep learning in general or wake-sleep learning applied to factor analysis. The wake and sleep phases each separately reduces a sensible cost function (for each phase, a Kullback-Leibler divergence), but these two cost functions are not compatible with a single global cost function. An algorithm that correctly performs stochastic gradient descent in the recognition parameters of a Helmholtz machine using an appropriate global cost function does exist (Dayan & Hinton, 1996), but it involves reinforcement learning methods for which convergence is usually extremely slow.

We have obtained some partial theoretical results concerning wake-sleep learning for factor analysis, which show that the maximum likelihood solutions are second-order Lyapunov stable and that updates of the weights (but not variances) for a single-factor model decrease an appropriate cost function. However, the primary reason for thinking that the wake-sleep algorithm generally works well for factor analysis is not these weak theoretical results but rather the empirical results in section 4. Before presenting these, we discuss in more detail how the general wake-sleep scheme is applied to factor analysis, first for a single-factor model and then for models with multiple factors.

3.3 Wake-Sleep Learning for a Single-Factor Model. A Helmholtz machine that implements factor analysis with a single hidden factor is shown

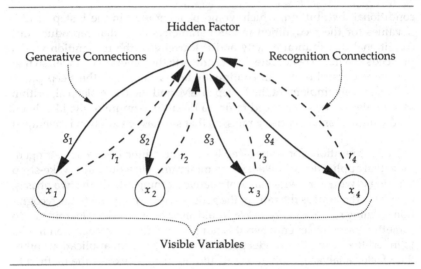

Figure 1: The one-factor linear Helmholtz machine. Connections of the generative model are shown using solid lines, those of the recognition model using
dashed lines. The weights for these connections are given by the g_j and the r_j.

in Figure 1. The connections for the linear network that implements the
generative model of equation 2.1 are shown in the figure using solid lines.
Generation of data using this network starts with the selection of a random
value for the hidden factor, y, from a gaussian distribution with mean zero
and variance one. The value for the jth visible variable, x_j, is then found by
multiplying y by a connection weight, g_j, and adding random noise with
variance τ_j^2. (A bias value, μ_j, could be added as well, to produce nonzero
means for the visible variables.)

The recognition model's connections are shown in Figure 1 using dashed
lines. These connections implement equation 2.3. When presented with values for the visible input variables, x_j, the recognition network produces a
value for the hidden factor, y, by forming a weighted sum of the inputs,
with the weight for the jth input being r_j, and then adding gaussian noise
with mean zero and variance σ^2. (If the inputs have nonzero means, the
recognition model would include a bias for the hidden factor as well.)

The parameters of the generative model are learned in the wake phase, as
follows. Values for the visible variables, $x^{(c)}$, are obtained from the external
world; they are set to a training case drawn from the distribution that we
wish to model. The current version of the recognition network is then used
to stochastically fill in a corresponding value for the hidden factor, $y^{(c)}$, using
equation 2.3. The generative weights are then updated using the delta rule,

as follows:

$$g'_j = g_j + \eta \, (x_j^{(c)} - g_j y^{(c)}) \, y^{(c)}, \tag{3.4}$$

where η is a small positive learning rate parameter. The generative variances, τ_j^2, which make up Ψ, are also updated, using an exponentially weighted moving average:

$$(\tau_j^2)' = \alpha \, \tau_j^2 + (1 - \alpha) \, (x_j^{(c)} - g_j y^{(c)})^2, \tag{3.5}$$

where α is a learning rate parameter that is slightly less than one.

If the recognition model correctly inverted the generative model, these wake-phase updates would correctly implement the M-step of the EM algorithm (in the limit as $\eta \to 0$ and $\alpha \to 1$). The update for g_j in equation 3.4 improves the expected log likelihood because the increment to g_j is proportional to the derivative of the log likelihood for the training case with y filled in, which is as follows:

$$\frac{\partial}{\partial g_j} \left(\log p(\mathbf{x}^{(c)}, y^{(c)} \mid \mathbf{g}, \Psi) \right) = \frac{\partial}{\partial g_j} \left(-\frac{1}{2\tau_j^2} (x_j^{(c)} - g_j y^{(c)})^2 \right) \tag{3.6}$$

$$= \frac{1}{\tau_j^2} (x_j^{(c)} - g_j y^{(c)}) \, y^{(c)}. \tag{3.7}$$

The averaging operation by which the generative variances, τ_j^2, are learned will (for α close to one) also lead toward the maximum likelihood values based on the filled-in values for y.

The parameters of the recognition model are learned in the sleep phase, based not on real data but on "fantasy" cases, produced using the current version of the generative model. Values for the hidden factor, $y^{(f)}$, and the visible variables, $\mathbf{x}^{(f)}$, in a fantasy case are stochastically generated according to equation 2.1, as described at the beginning of this section. The connection weights for the recognition model are then updated using the delta rule, as follows:

$$r'_j = r_j + \eta \, (y^{(f)} - \mathbf{r}^T \mathbf{x}^{(f)}) \, x_j^{(f)}, \tag{3.8}$$

where η is again a small positive learning rate parameter, which might or might not be the same as that used in the wake phase. The recognition variance, σ^2, is updated as follows:

$$(\sigma^2)' = \alpha \, \sigma^2 + (1 - \alpha) \, (y^{(f)} - \mathbf{r}^T \mathbf{x}^{(f)})^2, \tag{3.9}$$

where α is again a learning rate parameter slightly less than one.

These updates are analogous to those made in the wake phase and have the effect of improving the recognition model's ability to produce the correct distribution for the hidden factor. However, as noted in section 3.2, the criterion by which the sleep phase updates "improve" the recognition model does not correspond to a global Lyapunov function for wake-sleep learning as a whole, and we therefore lack a theoretical guarantee that the wake-sleep procedure will be stable and will converge to a maximum of the likelihood, though the experiments in section 4 indicate that it usually does.

3.4 Wake-Sleep Learning for Multiple-Factor Models. A Helmholtz machine with more than one hidden factor can be trained using the wake-sleep algorithm in much the same way as described above for a single-factor model. The generative model is simply extended by including more than one hidden factor. In the most straightforward case, the values of these factors are chosen independently at random when a fantasy case is generated. However, a new issue arises with the recognition model. When there are k hidden factors and p visible variables, the recognition model has the following form (assuming zero means):

$$\mathbf{y} = \mathbf{R}\mathbf{x} + \boldsymbol{\nu} \tag{3.10}$$

where the $k \times p$ matrix $\mathbf{R}$ contains the weights on the recognition connections, and $\boldsymbol{\nu}$ is a k-dimensional gaussian random vector with mean $\mathbf{0}$ and covariance matrix Σ, which in general (i.e., for some arbitrary generative model) will not be diagonal. Generation of a random $\boldsymbol{\nu}$ with such covariance can easily be done on a computer using the Cholesky decomposition of Σ, but in a method intended for consideration as a neurobiological model, we would prefer a local implementation that produces the same effect.

One way of producing arbitrary covariances between the hidden factors is to include a set of connections in the recognition model that link each hidden factor to hidden factors that come earlier (in some arbitrary ordering). A Helmholtz machine with this architecture is shown in Figure 2. During the wake phase, values for the hidden factors are filled in sequentially by random generation from gaussian distributions. The mean of the distribution used in picking a value for factor y_i is the weighted sum of inputs along connections from the visible variables and from the hidden factors whose values were chosen earlier. The variance of the distribution for factor y_i is an additional recognition model parameter, σ_i^2. The $k(k-1)/2$ connections between the hidden factors and the k variances associated with these factors together make up the $k(k+1)/2$ independent degrees of freedom in Σ. Accordingly, a recognition model of this form exists that can perfectly invert any generative model.[2]

---

[2] Another way of seeing this is to note that the joint distribution for the visible vari-

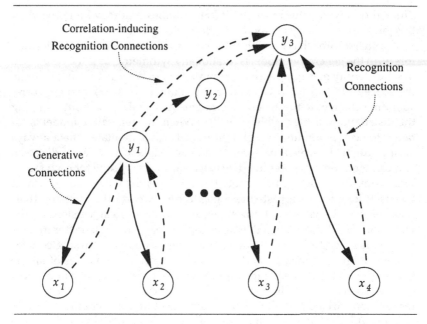

Figure 2: A Helmholtz machine implementing a model with three hidden factors, using a recognition model with a set of correlation-inducing connections. The figure omits some of the generative connections from hidden factors to visible variables and some of the recognition connections from visible variables to hidden factors (indicated by the ellipses). Note, however, that the only connections between hidden factors are those shown, which are part of the recognition model. There are no generative connections between hidden factors.

This method is reminiscent of some of the proposals to allow Hebbian learning to extract more than one principal component (e.g., Sanger, 1989; Plumbley, 1993); various of these also order the "hidden" units. In these proposals, the connections are used to remove correlations between the units so that they can represent different facets of the input. However, for the Helmholtz machine, the factors come to represent different facets of the input because they are jointly rather than separately engaged in capturing the statistical regularities in the input. The connections between the hidden units capture the correlations in the distribution for the hidden factors con-

---

ables and hidden factors is multivariate gaussian. From general properties of multivariate gaussians, the conditional distribution for a hidden factor given values for the visible variables and for the earlier hidden factors must also be gaussian, with some constant variance and with a mean given by some linear function of the other values.

ditional on given values for the visible variables that may be induced by this joint responsibility for modeling the visible variables.

Another approach is possible if the covariance matrix for the hidden factors, $\mathbf{y}$, in the generative model is rotationally symmetric, as is the case when it is the identity matrix, as we have assumed so far. We may then freely rotate the space of factors ($\mathbf{y}' = \mathbf{U}\mathbf{y}$, where $\mathbf{U}$ is a unitary matrix), making corresponding changes to the generative weights ($\mathbf{G}' = \mathbf{G}\mathbf{U}^T$), without changing the distribution of the visible variables. When the generative model is rotated, the corresponding recognition model will also rotate. There always exist rotations in which the recognition covariance matrix, Σ, is diagonal and can therefore be represented by just k variances, σ_i^2, one for each factor. This amounts to forcing the factors to be independent, or factorial, which has itself long been suggested as a goal for early cortical processing (Barlow, 1989) and has generally been assumed in nonlinear versions of the Helmholtz machine. We can therefore hope to learn multiple-factor models using wake-sleep learning in exactly the same way as we learn single-factor models, with equations 2.4 and 3.10 specifying how the values of all the factors $\mathbf{y}$ combine to predict the input $\mathbf{x}$, and vice versa. As seen in the next section, such a Helmholtz machine with only the capacity to represent k recognition variances, with no correlation-inducing connections, is usually able to find a rotation in which such a recognition model is sufficient to invert the generative model.

Note that there is no counterpart in Hebbian learning of this second approach, in which there are no connections between hidden factors. If Hebbian units are not connected in some manner, they will all extract the same single principal component of the inputs.

4 Empirical Results

We have run a number of experiments on synthetic data in order to test whether the wake-sleep algorithm applied to factor analysis finds parameter values that at least locally maximize the likelihood, in the limit of small values for the learning rates. These experiments also provide data on how small the learning rates must be in practice and reveal situations in which learning (particularly of the uniquenesses) can be relatively slow. We also report in section 4.4 the results of applying the wake-sleep algorithm to a real data set used by Everitt (1984). Away from conditions in which the maximum likelihood model is not well specified, the wake-sleep algorithm performs quite competently.

4.1 Experimental Procedure. All the systematic experiments described were done with randomly generated synthetic data. Models for various numbers (p) of visible variables, using various numbers (k) of hidden factors, were tested. For each such model, 10 sets of model parameters were generated, each of which was used to generate 2 sets of training data, the first with 10 cases and the second with 500 cases. Models with the same p and k were then learned from these training sets using the wake-sleep algorithm.

The models used to generate the data were randomly constructed as follows. First, initial values for generative variances (the "uniquenesses") were drawn independently from exponential distributions with mean one, and initial values for the generative weights (the "factor loadings") were drawn independently from gaussian distributions with mean zero and variance one. These parameters were then rescaled so as to produce a variance of one for each visible variable; that is, for a single-factor model, the new generative variances were set to $\tau_j'^2 = f_j^2 \tau_j^2$ and the new generative weights to $g_j' = f_j g_j$, with the f_j chosen such that the new variances for the visible variables, $\tau_j'^2 + g_j'^2$, were equal to one.

In all experiments, the wake-sleep learning procedure was started with the generative and recognition variances set to one and the generative and recognition weights and biases set to zero. Symmetry is broken by the stochastic nature of the learning procedure. Learning was done online, with cases from the training set being presented one at a time, in a fixed sequence. The learning rates for both generative and recognition models were usually set to $\eta = 0.0002$ and $\alpha = 0.999$, but other values of η and α were investigated as well, as described below. In the models used to generate the data, the variables all had mean zero and variance one, but this knowledge was not built into the learning procedure. Bias parameters were therefore present, allowing the network to learn the means of the visible variables in the training data (which were close to zero, but not exactly zero, due to the use of a finite training set).

We compared the estimates produced by the wake-sleep algorithm with the maximum likelihood estimates based on the same training sets produced using the "factanal" function in S-Plus (Version 3.3, Release 1), which uses a modification of Jöreskog's (1977) method. We also implemented the EM factor analysis algorithm to examine in more detail cases in which wake-sleep disagreed with S-Plus. As with most stochastic learning algorithms, using fixed learning rates implies that convergence can at best be to a distribution of parameter values that is highly concentrated near some stable point. One would in general have to reduce the learning rates over time to ensure stronger forms of convergence. The software used in these experiments may be obtained over the Internet.[3]

4.2 Experiments with Single-Factor Models. We first tried using the wake-sleep algorithm to learn single-factor models for three ($p = 3$) and six ($p = 6$) visible variables. Figure 3 shows the progress of learning for a

---

[3] Follow the links from the first author's home page: http://www.cs.utoronto.ca/~radford/

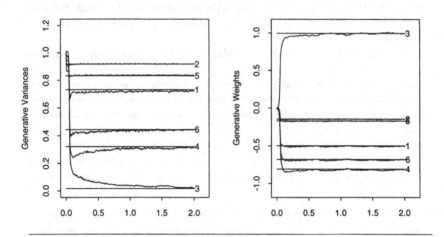

Figure 3: Wake-sleep learning of a single-factor model for six variables. The graphs show the progress of the generative variances and weights over the course of 2 million presentations of input vectors, drawn sequentially from a training set of size 500, with learning parameters of $\eta = 0.0002$ and $\alpha = 0.999$ being used for both the wake and the sleep phases. The training set was randomly generated from a single-factor model whose parameters were picked at random, as described in section 4.1. The maximum likelihood parameter estimates found by S-Plus are shown as horizontal lines.

typical run with $p = 6$, applied to a training set of size 500. The figure shows progress over 2 million presentations of input vectors (4000 presentations of each of the 500 training cases). Both the generative variances and the generative weights are seen to converge to the maximum likelihood estimates found by S-Plus, with a small amount of random variation, as is expected with a stochastic learning procedure. Of the 20 runs with $p = 6$ (based on data generated from 10 random models, with training sets of size 10 and 500), all but one showed similar convergence to the S-Plus estimates within 3 million presentations (and usually much earlier). The remaining run (on a training set of size 10) converged to a different local maximum, which S-Plus found when its maximization routine was started from the values found by wake-sleep.

Convergence to maximum likelihood estimates was sometimes slower when there were only three variables ($p = 3$). This is the minimum number of visible variables for which the single-factor model is identifiable (that is, for which the true values of the parameters can be found given enough data, apart from an ambiguity in the overall signs of the weights). Three of the 10 runs with training sets of size 10 and one of the 10 runs with training sets of size 500 failed to converge clearly within 3 million presentations, but convergence was seen when these runs were extended to 10 million presentations (in one case to a different local maximum than initially found by S-Plus). The slowest convergence was for a training set of size 10 for which the maximum likelihood estimate for one of the generative weights was close to zero (0.038), making the parameters nearly unidentifiable.

All the runs were done with learning rates of $\eta = 0.0002$ and $\alpha = 0.999$, for both the generative and recognition models. Tests on the training sets with $p = 3$ were also done with learning for the recognition model slowed to $\eta = 0.00002$ and $\alpha = 0.9999$—a situation that one might speculate would cause problems, due to the recognition model's not being able to keep up with the generative model. No problems were seen (though the learning was, of course, slower).

4.3 Experiments with Multiple-Factor Models. We have also tried using the wake-sleep algorithm to learn models with two and three hidden factors ($k = 2$ and $k = 3$) from synthetic data generated as described in section 4.1. Systematic experiments were done for $k = 2$, $p = 5$, using models with and without correlation-inducing recognition weights, and for $k = 2$, $p = 8$ and $k = 3$, $p = 9$, in both cases using models with no correlation-inducing recognition weights. For most of the experiments, learning was done with $\eta = 0.0002$ and $\alpha = 0.999$.

The behavior of wake-sleep learning with $k = 2$ and $p = 5$ was very similar for the model with correlation-inducing recognition connections and the model without such connections. The runs on most of the 20 data sets converged within the 6 million presentations that were initially performed; a few required more iterations before convergence was apparent. For two data sets (both of size 10), wake-sleep learning converged to different local maxima than S-Plus. For one training set of size 500, the maximum likelihood estimate for one of the generative variances is very close to one, making the model almost unidentifiable ($p = 5$ being the minimum number of visible variables for identifiability with $k = 2$); this produced an understandable difficulty with convergence, though the wake-sleep estimates still agreed fairly closely with the maximum likelihood values found by S-Plus.

In contrast with these good results, a worrying discrepancy arose with one of the training sets of size 10, for which the two smallest generative variances found using wake-sleep learning differed somewhat from the maximum likelihood estimates found by S-Plus (one of which was very close to zero). When S-Plus was started at the values found using wake-sleep, it did *not* find a similar local maximum; it simply found the same estimates as it had found with its default initial values. However, when the full EM algorithm was started at the estimates found by wake-sleep, it barely changed the parameters for many iterations. One explanation could be that there is a local maximum in this vicinity, but it is for some reason not found by S-Plus. Another possible explanation could be that the likelihood is extremely flat in this region. In neither case would the discrepancy be cause for much worry regarding the general ability of the wake-sleep method to learn these multiple-factor models. However, it is also possible that this is an instance of the problem that arose more clearly in connection with the Everitt crime data, as reported in section 4.4.

Runs using models without correlation-inducing recognition connections were also performed for data sets with $k = 2$ and $p = 8$. All runs converged, most within 6 million presentations, in one case to a different local maximum than S-Plus. We also tried runs with the same model and data sets using higher learning rates ($\eta = 0.002$ and $\alpha = 0.99$). The higher learning rates produced both higher variability and some bias in the parameter estimates, but for most data sets the results were still generally correct.

Finally, runs using models without correlation-inducing recognition connections were performed for data sets with $k = 3$ and $p = 9$. Most of these converged fine. However, for two data sets (both of size 500), a small but apparently real difference was seen between the estimates for the two smallest generative variances found using wake-sleep and the maximum likelihood estimates found using S-Plus. As was the case with the similar situation with $k = 2, p = 5$, S-Plus did not converge to a local maximum in this vicinity when started at the wake-sleep estimates. As before, however, the EM algorithm moved very slowly when started at the wake-sleep estimates, which is one possible explanation for wake-sleep having apparently converged to this point. However, it is also possible that something more fundamental prevented convergence to a local maximum of the likelihood, as discussed in connection with similar results in the next section.

4.4 Experiments with the Everitt Crime Data. We also tried learning a two-factor model for a data set used as an example by Everitt (1984), in which the visible variables are the rates for seven types of crime, with the cases being 16 American cities. The same learning procedure (with $\eta = 0.0002$ and $\alpha = 0.999$) was used as in the experiments above, except that the visible variables were normalized to have mean zero and variance one, and bias parameters were accordingly omitted from both the generative and recognition models.

Fifteen runs with different random number seeds were done, for both models with a correlation-inducing recognition connection between the two factors and without such a connection. All of these runs produced results fairly close to the maximum likelihood estimates found by S-Plus (which match the results of Everitt). In some runs, however, there were small, but clearly real, discrepancies, most notably in the smallest two generative variances, for which the wake-sleep estimates were sometimes nearly zero, whereas the maximum likelihood estimate is zero for only one of them. This behavior is similar to that seen in the three runs where discrepancies were found in the systematic experiments of section 4.3.

These discrepancies arose much more frequently when a correlation-inducing recognition connection was not present (14 out of 15 runs) than when such a connection was included (6 out of 15 runs). Figure 4a shows one of the runs with discrepancies for a model with a correlation-inducing connection present. Figure 4b shows a run differing from that of 4a only in its random seed, but which did find the maximum likelihood estimates. The sole run in which the model without a correlation-inducing recognition connection converged to the maximum likelihood estimates is shown in Figure 4c. Close comparison of Figures 4b and 4c shows that even in this run, convergence was much more labored without the correlation-inducing connection. (In particular, the generative variance for variable 6 approaches zero rather more slowly.)

According to S-Plus, the solution found in the discrepant runs is *not* an alternative local maximum. Furthermore, extending the runs to many more iterations or reducing the learning rates by a large factor does not eliminate the problem. This makes it seem unlikely that the problem is merely slow convergence due to the likelihood of being nearly flat in this vicinity, although, on the other hand, when EM is started at the discrepant wake-sleep estimates, its movement toward the maximum likelihood estimates is rather slow (after 200 iterations, the estimate for the generative variance for variable 4 had moved only about a third of the way from the wake-sleep estimate to the maximum likelihood estimate). It seems most likely therefore that the runs with discrepancies result from a local "basin of attraction" for wake-sleep learning that does not lead to a local maximum of the likelihood.

The discrepancies can be eliminated for the model with a correlation-inducing connection in either of two ways. One way is to reduce the learning rate for the generative parameters (in the wake phase), while leaving the recognition learning rate unchanged. As discussed in section 3.2, there is a theoretical reason to think that this method will lead to the maximum likelihood estimates, since the recognition model will then have time to learn how to invert the generative model perfectly. When the generative learning rates are reduced by setting $\eta = 0.00005$ and $\alpha = 0.99975$, the maximum likelihood estimates are indeed found in eight of eight test runs. The second solution is to impose a constraint that prevents the generative variances from falling below 0.01. This also worked in eight of eight runs. However, these two methods produce little or no improvement when the correlation-inducing connection is omitted from the recognition model (no successes in eight runs with smaller generative learning rates; three successes in eight runs with a constraint on the generative variances). Thus, although models without correlation-inducing connections often work well, it appears that learning is sometimes easier and more reliable when they are present.

Finally, we tried learning a model for this data without first normalizing the visible variables to have mean zero and variance one, but with biases included in the generative and recognition models to handle the nonzero means. This is not a very sensible thing to do; the means of the variables in this data set are far from zero, so learning would at best take a long time, while the biases slowly adjusted. In fact, however, wake-sleep learning fails

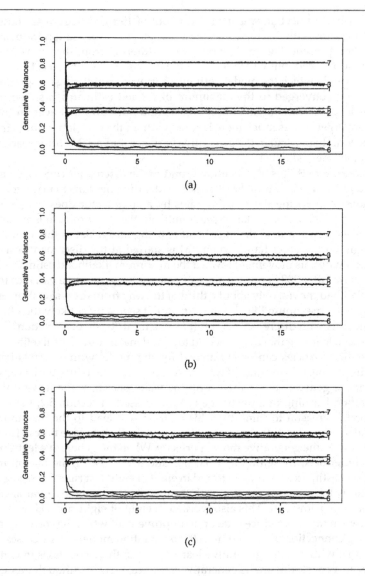

Figure 4: Wake-sleep learning of two-factor models for the Everitt crime data.
The horizontal axis shows the number of presentations in millions. The vertical axis shows the generative variances, with the maximum likelihood values
indicated by horizontal lines. (a) One of the six runs in which a model with a
correlation-inducing recognition connection did not converge to the maximum
likelihood estimates. (b) One of the nine such runs that did find the maximum
likelihood estimates. (c) The only run in which the maximum likelihood estimates were found using a model without a correlation-inducing connection.

rather spectacularly. The generative variances immediately become quite large. As soon as the recognition weights depart significantly from zero, the recognition variances also become quite large, at which point positive feedback ensues, and all the weights and variances diverge.

The instability that can occur once the generative and recognition weights and variances are too large appears to be a fundamental aspect of wake-sleep dynamics. Interestingly, however, it seems that the dynamics may operate to avoid this unstable region of parameter space, since the instability does not occur with the Everitt data if the learning rate is set very low. With a larger learning rate, however, the stochastic aspect of the learning can produce a jump into the unstable region.

5 Discussion

We have shown empirically that wake-sleep learning, which involves nothing more than two simple applications of the local delta rule, can be used to implement the statistical technique of maximum likelihood factor analysis. However, just as it is usually computationally more efficient to implement principal component analysis using a standard matrix technique such as singular-value decomposition rather than by using Hebbian learning, factor analysis is probably better implemented on a computer using either EM (Rubin & Thayer, 1982) or the second-order Newton methods of Jöreskog (1967, 1969, 1977) than by the wake-sleep algorithm. In our view, wake-sleep factor analysis is interesting as a simple and successful example of wake-sleep learning and as a possible model of activity-dependent plasticity in the cortex.

5.1 Implications for Wake-Sleep Learning. The experiments in section 4 show that, in most situations, wake-sleep learning applied to factor analysis leads to estimates that (locally) maximize the likelihood, when the learning rate is set to be small enough. In a few situations, the parameter estimates found using wake-sleep deviated slightly from the maximum likelihood values. More work is needed to determine exactly when and why this occurs, but even in these situations, the estimates found by wake-sleep are reasonably good and the likelihoods are close to their maxima. The sensitivity of learning to settings of parameters such as learning rates appears no greater than is typical for stochastic gradient descent methods. In particular, setting the learning rate for the generative model to be equal to or greater than that for the recognition model did not lead to instability, even though this is the situation in which one might worry that the algorithm would no longer mimic EM (as discussed in section 3.2). However, we have been unable to prove in general that the wake-sleep algorithm for factor analysis is guaranteed to converge to the maximum likelihood solution. Indeed, the empirical results show that any general theoretical proof of correctness would have to contain caveats regarding unstable regions of the parameter space. Such a proof may be impossible if the discrepancies seen in the experiments are indeed due to a false basin of attraction (rather than being an effect of finite learning rates). Despite the lack so far of strong theoretical results, the relatively simple factor analysis model may yet provide a good starting point for a better theoretical understanding of wake-sleep learning for more complex models.

One empirical finding was that it is possible to learn multiple-factor models even when correlation-inducing recognition connections are absent, although the lack of such connections did cause difficulties in some cases. A better understanding of what is going on in this respect would provide insight into wake-sleep learning for more complex models, in which the recognition model will seldom be able to invert the generative model perfectly. Such a complex generative model may allow the data to be modeled in many nearly equivalent ways, for some of which the generative model is harder to invert than for others. Good performance may sometimes be possible only if wake-sleep learning favors the more easily inverted generative models. We have seen that this does usually happen for factor analysis.

5.2 Implications for Activity-Dependent Plasticity. Much progress has been made using Hebbian learning to model the development of structures in early cortical areas, such as topographic maps (Willshaw & von der Malsburg 1976, 1979; von der Malsburg, & Willshaw, 1977), ocular dominance stripes (Miller et al., 1989), and orientation domains (Linkser, 1988; Miller, 1994). However, Hebbian learning suffers from three problems that the equally-local wake-sleep algorithm avoids.

First, because of the positive feedback inherent in Hebbian learning, some form of synaptic normalization is required to make it work (Miller & MacKay, 1994). There is no evidence for synaptic normalization in the cortex. This is not an issue for Helmholtz machines because building a statistical model of the inputs involves negative feedback instead, as in the delta rule.

Second, in order for Hebbian learning to produce several outputs that represent more than just the first principal component of a collection of inputs, there must be connections of some sort between the output units, which force them to be decorrelated. Typically, some form of anti-Hebbian learning is required for these connections (see Sanger, 1989; Földiák, 1989; Plumbley, 1993). The common alternative of using fixed lateral connections between the output units is not informationally efficient. In the Helmholtz machine, the goal of modeling the distribution of the inputs forces output units to differentiate rather than perform the same task. This goal also supplies a clear interpretation in terms of finding the hidden causes of the input.

Third, Hebbian learning does not accord any role to the prominent cortical feature that top-down connections always accompany bottom-up connections. In the Helmholtz machine, these top-down connections play a crucial role in wake-sleep learning. Furthermore, the top-down connections come to embody a hierarchical generative model of the inputs, some form of which appears necessary in any case to combine top-down and bottom-up processing during inference.

Of course, the Helmholtz machine suffers from various problems itself. Although learning rules equivalent to the delta rule are conventional in classical conditioning (Rescorla & Wagner, 1972; Sutton & Barto, 1981) and have also been suggested as underlying cortical plasticity (Montague & Sejnowski, 1994), it is not clear how cortical microcircuitry might construct the required predictions (such as $g_j y^{(c)}$ of equation 3.4) or prediction errors (such as $x_j^{(c)} - g_j y^{(c)}$ of the same equation). The wake-sleep algorithm also requires two phases of activation, with different connections being primarily responsible for driving the cells in each phase. Although there is some suggestive evidence of this (Hasselmo & Bower, 1993), it has not yet been demonstrated. There are also alternative developmental methods that construct top-down statistical models of their inputs using only one, slightly more complicated, phase of activation (Olshausen & Field, 1996; Rao & Ballard, 1995).

In Hebbian models of activity-dependent development, a key role is played by lateral local intracortical connections (longer-range excitatory connections are also present but develop later). Lateral connections are not present in the linear Helmholtz machines we have so far described, but they could play a role in inducing correlations between the hidden factors in the generative model, in the recognition model, or in both, perhaps replacing the correlation-inducing connections shown in Figure 2.

Purely linear models, such as those presented here, will not suffice to explain fully the intricacies of information processing in the cortical hierarchy. However, understanding how a factor analysis model can be learned using simple and local operations is a first step to understanding how more complex statistical models can be learned using more complex architectures involving nonlinear elements and multiple layers.

Acknowledgments

We thank Geoffrey Hinton for many useful discussions. This research was supported by the Natural Sciences and Engineering Research Council of Canada and by grant R29 MH55541-01 from the National Institute of Mental Health of the United States. All opinions expressed are those of the authors.

References

Barlow, H. B. (1989). Unsupervised learning. *Neural Computation, 1*, 295–311.
Dayan, P., & Hinton, G. E. (1996). Varieties of Helmholtz machine. *Neural Networks, 9*, 1385–1403.

Dayan, P., Hinton, G. E., Neal, R. M., & Zemel, R. S. (1995). The Helmholtz machine. *Neural Computation, 7*, 889–904.

Dempster, A. P., Laird, N. M, & Rubin, D. B. (1977). Maximum likelihood from incomplete data via the EM algorithm. *Proceedings of the Royal Statistical Society, B39*, 1–38.

Everitt, B. S. (1984). *An introduction to latent variable models.* London: Chapman and Hall.

Felleman D. J., & Van Essen, D. C. (1991). Distributed hierarchical processing in the primate cerebral cortex. *Cerebral Cortex, 1*, 1–47.

Földiák, P. (1989). Adaptive network for optimal linear feature extraction. In *Proceedings of the International Joint Conference on Neural Networks, Washington, DC* (Vol. I, pp. 401–405).

Grenander, U. (1976–1981). *Lectures in pattern theory I, II and III: Pattern analysis, pattern synthesis and regular structures.* Berlin: Springer-Verlag.

Hasselmo, M. E., & Bower, J. M. (1993). Acetylcholine and memory. *Trends in Neurosciences, 16*, 218–222.

Hebb, D. O. (1949). *The organization of behavior: A neuropsychological theory.* New York: Wiley.

Hinton, G. E., Dayan, P., Frey, B., & Neal, R. M. (1995). The wake-sleep algorithm for self-organizing neural networks. *Science, 268*, 1158–1160.

Hinton, G. E., & Zemel, R. S. (1994). Autoencoders, minimum description length and Helmholtz free energy. In J. D. Cowan, G. Tesauro, & J. Alspector (Eds.), *Advances in neural information processing systems, 6* (pp. 3–10). San Mateo, CA: Morgan Kaufmann.

Jolliffe, I. T. (1986) *Principal component analysis,* New York: Springer-Verlag.

Jöreskog, K. G. (1967). Some contributions to maximum likelihood factor analysis, *Psychometrika, 32*, 443–482.

Jöreskog, K. G. (1969). A general approach to confirmatory maximum likelihood factor analysis, *Psychometrika, 34*, 183–202.

Jöreskog, K. G. (1977). Factor analysis by least-squares and maximum-likelihood methods. In K. Enslein, A. Ralston, & H. S. Wilf (Eds.), *Statistical methods for digital computers.* New York: Wiley.

Linsker, R. (1986). From basic network principles to neural architecture. *Proceedings of the National Academy of Sciences, 83*, 7508–7512, 8390–8394, 8779–9783.

Linsker, R. (1988). Self-organization in a perceptual network. *Computer, 21*, 105–128.

Miller, K. D. (1994). A model for the development of simple cell receptive fields and the ordered arrangement of orientation columns through activity-dependent competition between ON- and OFF-center inputs. *Journal of Neuroscience, 14*, 409–441.

Miller, K. D., Keller, J. B., & Stryker, M. P. (1989). Ocular dominance column development: Analysis and simulation. *Science, 245*, 605–615.

Miller, K. D., & MacKay, D. J. C. (1994). The role of constraints in Hebbian learning. *Neural Computation, 6*, 100–126.

Montague, P. R., & Sejnowski, T. J. (1994). The predictive brain: Temporal coincidence and temporal order in synaptic learning mechanisms. *Learning and Memory, 1*, 1–33.

Mumford, D. (1994). Neuronal architectures for pattern-theoretic problems. In C. Koch & J. Davis (Eds.), *Large-scale theories of the cortex* (pp. 125–152). Cambridge, MA: MIT Press.

Oja, E. (1989). Neural networks, principal components, and subspaces. *International Journal of Neural Systems, 1*, 61–68.

Olshausen, B. A., & Field, D. J. (1996). Emergence of simple-cell receptive field properties by learning a sparse code for natural images. *Nature, 381*, 607–609.

Plumbley, M. D. (1993). Efficient information transfer and anti-Hebbian neural networks. *Neural Networks, 6*, 823–833.

Rao, P. N. R., & Ballard, D. H. (1995). *Dynamic model of visual memory predicts neural response properties in the visual cortex* (Technical Rep. No. 95.4). Rochester, NY: Department of Computer Science, University of Rochester.

Rescorla, R. A., & Wagner, A. R. (1972). A theory of Pavlovian conditioning: The effectiveness of reinforcement and non-reinforcement. In A. H. Black & W. F. Prokasy (Eds.), *Classical conditioning II: Current research and theory* (pp. 64–69). New York: Appleton-Century-Crofts.

Rubin, D. B., & Thayer, D. T. (1982). EM algorithms for ML factor analysis. *Psychometrika, 47*, 69–76.

Sanger, T. D. (1989). Optimal unsupervised learning in a single-layer linear feedforward neural network. *Neural Networks, 2*, 459–473.

Sutton, R. S., & Barto, A. G. (1981). Toward a modern theory of adaptive networks: Expectation and prediction. *Psychological Review, 88*, 135–170.

von der Malsburg, C. (1973). Self-organization of orientation sensitive cells in the striate cortex. *Kybernetic, 14*, 85–100.

von der Malsburg, C., & Willshaw D. J. (1977). How to label nerve cells so that they can interconnect in an ordered fashion. *Proceedings of the National Academy of Sciences, 74*, 5176–5178.

Willshaw, D. J., & von der Malsburg, C. (1976). How patterned neural connections can be set up by self-organisation. *Proceedings of the Royal Society of London B, 194*, 431–445.

Willshaw, D. J., & von der Malsburg, C. (1979). A marker induction mechanism for the establishment of ordered neural mappings: Its application to the retinotectal problem. *Philosophical Transactions of the Royal Society B, 287*, 203–243.

18

Dimension Reduction by Local Principal Component Analysis

Nandakishore Kambhatla
Todd K. Leen
Department of Computer Science and Engineering, Oregon Graduate Institute of Science and Technology, Portland, Oregon 97291-1000, U.S.A.

Reducing or eliminating statistical redundancy between the components of high-dimensional vector data enables a lower-dimensional representation without significant loss of information. Recognizing the limitations of principal component analysis (PCA), researchers in the statistics and neural network communities have developed nonlinear extensions of PCA. This article develops a local linear approach to dimension reduction that provides accurate representations and is fast to compute. We exercise the algorithms on speech and image data, and compare performance with PCA and with neural network implementations of nonlinear PCA. We find that both nonlinear techniques can provide more accurate representations than PCA and show that the local linear techniques outperform neural network implementations.

1 Introduction

The objective of dimension reduction algorithms is to obtain a parsimonious description of multivariate data. The goal is to obtain a compact, accurate, representation of the data that reduces or eliminates statistically redundant components.

Dimension reduction is central to an array of data processing goals. Input selection for classification and regression problems is a task-specific form of dimension reduction. Visualization of high-dimensional data requires mapping to a lower dimension—usually three or fewer. Transform coding (Gersho & Gray, 1992) typically involves dimension reduction. The initial high-dimensional signal (e.g., image blocks) is first transformed in order to reduce statistical dependence, and hence redundancy, between the components. The transformed components are then scalar quantized. Dimension reduction can be imposed explicitly, by eliminating a subset of the transformed components. Alternatively, the allocation of quantization bits among the transformed components (e.g., in increasing measure according to their variance) can result in eliminating the low-variance components by assigning them zero bits.

Recently several authors have used neural network implementations of dimension reduction to signal equipment failures by novelty, or outlier, detection (Petsche et al., 1996; Japkowicz, Myers, & Gluck, 1995). In these schemes, high-dimensional sensor signals are projected onto a subspace that best describes the signals obtained during normal operation of the monitored system. New signals are categorized as normal or abnormal according to the distance between the signal and its projection[1].

The classic technique for linear dimension reduction is principal component analysis (PCA). In PCA, one performs an orthogonal transformation to the basis of correlation eigenvectors and projects onto the subspace spanned by those eigenvectors corresponding to the largest eigenvalues. This transformation decorrelates the signal components, and the projection along the high-variance directions maximizes variance and minimizes the average squared residual between the original signal and its dimension-reduced approximation.

A neural network implementation of one-dimensional PCA implemented by Hebb learning was introduced by Oja (1982) and expanded to hierarchical, multidimensional PCA by Sanger (1989), Kung and Diemantaras (1990), and Rubner and Tavan (1989). A fully parallel (nonhierarchical) design that extracts orthogonal vectors spanning an m-dimensional PCA subspace was given by Oja (1989). Concurrently, Baldi and Hornik (1989) showed that the error surface for linear, three-layer autoassociators with hidden layers of width m has global minima corresponding to input weights that span the m-dimensional PCA subspace.

Despite its widespread use, the PCA transformation is crippled by its reliance on second-order statistics. Though uncorrelated, the principal components can be highly statistically dependent. When this is the case, PCA fails to find the most compact description of the data. Geometrically, PCA models the data as a hyperplane embedded in the ambient space. If the data components have nonlinear dependencies, PCA will require a larger-dimensional representation than would be found by a nonlinear technique. This simple realization has prompted the development of nonlinear alternatives to PCA.

Hastie (1984) and Hastie and Stuetzle (1989) introduce their principal curves as a nonlinear alternative to one-dimensional PCA. Their parameterized curves $f(\lambda): R \to R^n$ are constructed to satisfy a self-consistency requirement. Each data point x is projected to the closest point on the curve $\lambda_f(x) = \text{argmin}_\mu \|x - f(\mu)\|$, and the expectation of all data points that project to the same parameter value λ is required to be on the curve. Thus $f(\Lambda) = E_x[x \mid \lambda_f(x) = \Lambda]$. This mathematical statement reflects the desire that the principal curves pass through the middle of the data.

---

[1] These schemes also use a sigmoidal contraction map following the projection so that new signals that are close to the subspace, yet far from the training data used to construct the subspace, can be properly tagged as outliers.

Hastie and Stuetzle (1989) prove that the curve $f(\lambda)$ is a principal curve iff it is a critical point (with respect to variations in $f(\lambda)$) of the mean squared distance between the data and their projection onto the curve. They also show that if the principal curves are lines, they correspond to PCA. Finally, they generalize their definitions from principal curves to principal surfaces.

Neural network approximators for principal surfaces are realized by five-layer, autoassociative networks. Independent of Hastie and Stuetzle's work, several researchers (Kramer, 1991; Oja, 1991; DeMers & Cottrell, 1993; Usui, Nakauchi, & Nakano, 1991) have suggested such networks for nonlinear dimension reduction. These networks have linear first (input) and fifth (output) layers, and sigmoidal nonlinearities on the second- and fourth-layer nodes. The input and output layers have width n. The third layer, which carries the dimension-reduced representation, has width $m < n$. We will refer to this layer as the *representation layer*. Researchers have used both linear and sigmoidal response functions for the representation layer. Here we consider only linear response in the representation layer.

The networks are trained to minimize the mean squared distance between the input and output and, because of the middle-layer bottleneck, build a dimension-reduced representation of the data. In view of Hastie and Stuetzle's critical point theorem, and the mean square error (MSE) training criteria for five-layer nets, these networks can be viewed as approximators of principal surfaces.[2]

Recently Hecht-Nielsen (1995) extended the application of five-layer autoassociators from dimension reduction to encoding. The third layer of his replicator networks has a staircase nonlinearity. In the limit of infinitely steep steps, one obtains a quantization of the middle-layer activity, and hence a discrete encoding of the input signal.[3]

In this article, we propose a locally linear approach to nonlinear dimension reduction that is much faster to train than five-layer autoassociators and, in our experience, provides superior solutions. Like five-layer autoassociators, the algorithm attempts to minimize the MSE between the original

---

[2] There is, as several researchers have pointed out, a fundamental difference between the representation constructed by Hastie's principal surfaces and the representation constructed by five-layer autoassociators. Specifically, autoassociators provide a continuous parameterization of the embedded manifold, whereas the principal surfaces algorithm does not constrain the parameterization to be continuous.

[3] Perfectly sharp staircase hidden-layer activations are, of course, not trainable by gradient methods, and the plateaus of a rounded staircase will diminish the gradient signal available for training. However, with parameterized hidden unit activations $h(x; a)$ with $h(x; 0) = x$ and $h(x; 1)$ a sigmoid staircase, one can envision starting training with linear activations and gradually shift toward a sharp (but finite sloped) staircase, thereby obtaining an approximation to Hecht-Nielsen's replicator networks. The changing activation function will induce both smooth changes and bifurcations in the set of cost function minima. Practical and theoretical issues in such homotopy methods are discussed in Yang and Yu (1993) and Coetzee and Stonick (1995).

data and its reconstruction from a low-dimensional representation—what we refer to as the *reconstruction error*. However, while five-layer networks attempt to find a global, smooth manifold that lies close to the data, our algorithm finds a set of hyperplanes that lie close to the data. In a loose sense, these hyperplanes locally approximate the manifold found by five-layer networks.

Our algorithm first partitions the data space into disjoint regions by vector quantization (VQ) and then performs local PCA about each cluster center. For brevity, we refer to the hybrid algorithms as VQPCA. We introduce a novel VQ distortion function that optimizes the clustering for the reconstruction error. After training, dimension reduction proceeds by first assigning a datum to a cluster and then projecting onto the m-dimensional principal subspace belonging to that cluster. The encoding thus consists of the index of the cluster and the local, dimension-reduced coordinates within the cluster.

The resulting algorithm directly minimizes (up to local optima) the reconstruction error. In this sense, it is optimal for dimension reduction. The computation of the partition is a generalized Lloyd algorithm (Gray, 1984) for a vector quantizer that uses the reconstruction error as the VQ distortion function. The Lloyd algorithm iteratively computes the partition based on two criteria that ensure minimum average distortion: (1) VQ centers lie at the generalized centroids of the quantizer regions and (2) the VQ region boundaries are surfaces that are equidistant (in terms of the distortion function) from adjacent VQ centers. The application of these criteria is considered in detail in section 3.2. The primary point is that constructing the partition according to these criteria provides a (local) minimum for the reconstruction error.

Training the local linear algorithm is far faster than training five-layer autoassociators. The clustering operation is the computational bottleneck, though it can be accelerated using the usual tree-structured or multistage VQ. When encoding new data, the clustering operation is again the main consumer of computation, and the local linear algorithm is somewhat slower for encoding than five-layer autoassociators. However, decoding is much faster than for the autoassociator and is comparable to PCA.

Local PCA has been previously used for exploratory data analysis (Fukunaga & Olsen, 1971) and to identify the intrinsic dimension of chaotic signals (Broomhead, 1991; Hediger, Passamante, & Farrell, 1990). Bregler and Omohundro (1995) use local PCA to find image features and interpolate image sequences. Hinton, Revow, and Dayan (1995) use an algorithm based on local PCA for handwritten character recognition. Independent of our work, Dony and Haykin (1995) explored a local linear approach to transform coding, though the distortion function used in their clustering is not optimized for the projection, as it is here. Finally, local linear methods for regression have been explored quite thoroughly. See, for example, the LOESS algorithm in Cleveland and Devlin (1988).

In the remainder of the article, we review the structure and function of autoassociators, introduce the local linear algorithm, and present experimental results applying the algorithms to speech and image data.

2 Dimension Reduction and Autoassociators

As considered here, dimension reduction algorithms consist of a pair of maps $g: R^n \rightarrow R^m$ with $m < n$ and $f: R^m \rightarrow R^n$. The function $g(x)$ maps the original n-dimensional vector x to the dimension-reduced vector $y \in R^m$. The function $f(y)$ maps back to the high-dimensional space. The two maps, g and f, correspond to the encoding and decoding operation, respectively. If these maps are smooth on open sets, then they are diffeomorphic to a canonical projection and immersion, respectively.

In general, the projection loses some of the information in the original representation, and $f(g(x)) \neq x$. The quality of the algorithm, and adequacy of the chosen target dimension m, are measured by the algorithm's ability to reconstruct the original data. A convenient measure, and the one we employ here, is the average squared residual, or reconstruction error:

$$\mathcal{E} = E_x[\, \|x - f(g(x))\|^2\,].$$

The variance in the original vectors provides a useful normalization scale for the squared residuals, so our experimental results are quoted as normalized reconstruction error:

$$\mathcal{E}_{\text{norm}} = \frac{E_x[\,\|x - f(g(x))\|^2\,]}{E_x[\,\|x - E_x x\|^2\,]}. \tag{2.1}$$

This may be regarded as the noise-to-signal ratio for the dimension reduction, with the signal strength defined as its variance.

Neural network implementations of these maps are provided by autoassociators, layered, feedforward networks with equal input and output dimension n. During training, the output targets are set to the inputs; thus, autoassociators are sometimes called self-supervised networks. When used to perform dimension reduction, the networks have a hidden layer of width $m < n$. This hidden, or representation, layer is where the low-dimensional representation is extracted. In terms of the maps defined above, processing from the input to the representation layer corresponds to the projection g, and processing from the representation to the output layer corresponds to the immersion f.

2.1 Three-Layer Autoassociators. Three-layer autoassociators with n input and output units and $m < n$ hidden units, trained to perform the identity transformation over the input data, were used for dimension reduction by several researchers (Cottrell, Munro, & Zipser, 1987; Cottrell &

Metcalfe, 1991; Golomb, Lawrence, & Sejnowski, 1991). In these networks, the first layer of weights performs the projection g and the second the immersion f. The output $f(g(x))$ is trained to match the input x in the mean square sense.

Since the transformation from the hidden to the output layer is linear, the network outputs lie in an m-dimensional linear subspace of R^n. The hidden unit activations define coordinates on this hyperplane. If the hidden unit activation functions are linear, it is obvious that the best one can do to minimize the reconstruction error is to have the hyperplane correspond to the m-dimensional principal subspace. Even if the hidden-layer activation functions are nonlinear, the output is still an embedded hyperplane. The nonlinearities introduce nonlinear scaling of the coordinate intervals on the hyperplane. Again, the solution that minimizes the reconstruction error is the m-dimensional principal subspace.

These observations were formalized in two early articles. Baldi and Hornik (1989) show that optimally trained three-layer linear autoassociators perform an orthogonal projection of the data onto the m-dimensional principal subspace. Bourlard and Kamp (1988) show that adding nonlinearities in the hidden layer cannot reduce the reconstruction error. The optimal solution remains the PCA projection.

2.2 Five-Layer Autoassociators.

To overcome the PCA limitation of three-layer autoassociators and provide the capability for genuine nonlinear dimension reduction, several authors have proposed five-layer autoassociators (e.g., Oja, 1991; Usui et al., 1991; Kramer, 1991; DeMers & Cottrell, 1993; Kambhatla & Leen, 1994; Hecht-Nielsen, 1995). These networks have sigmoidal second and fourth layers and linear first and fifth layers. The third (representation) layer may have linear or sigmoidal response. Here we use linear response functions. The first two layers of weights carry out a nonlinear projection $g: R^n \to R^m$, and the last two layers of weights carry out a nonlinear immersion $f: R^m \to R^n$ (see Figure 1). By the universal approximation theorem for single hidden-layer sigmoidal nets (Funahashi, 1989; Hornik, Stinchcombe, & White, 1989), any continuous composition of immersion and projection (on compact domain) can be approximated arbitrarily closely by the structure.

The activities of the nodes in the third, or representation layer form global curvilinear coordinates on a submanifold of the input space (see Figure 1b). We thus refer to five-layer autoassociative networks as a global, nonlinear dimension reduction technique.

Several authors report successful implementation of nonlinear PCA using these networks for image (DeMers & Cottrell, 1993; Hecht-Nielsen, 1995; Kambhatla & Leen, 1994) and speech dimension reduction, for characterizing chemical dynamics (Kramer, 1991), and for obtaining concise representations of color (Usui et al., 1991).

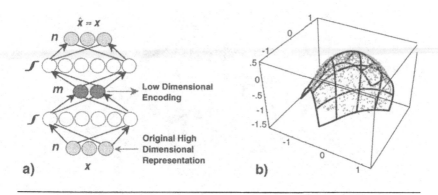

Figure 1: (a) Five-layer feedforward autoassociative network with inputs $x \in R^n$ and representation layer of dimension m. Outputs $x' \in R^n$ are trained to match the inputs, that is, to minimize $E[\, \|x - x'\|^2\,]$. (b) Global curvilinear coordinates built by a five-layer network for data distributed on the surface of a hemisphere. When the activations of the representation layer are swept, the outputs trace out the curvilinear coordinates shown by the solid lines.

3 Local Linear Transforms

Although five-layer autoassociators are convenient and elegant approxima-tors for principal surfaces, they suffer from practical drawbacks. Networks with multiple sigmoidal hidden layers tend to have poorly conditioned Hessians (see Rognvaldsson, 1994, for a nice exposition) and are therefore difficult to train. In our experience, the variance of the solution with respect to weight initialization can be quite large (see section 4), indicating that the networks are prone to trapping in poor local optimal. We propose an alternative that does not suffer from these problems.

Our proposal is to construct local models, each pertaining to a different disjoint region of the data space. Within each region, the model complexity is limited; we construct linear models by PCA. If the local regions are small enough, the data manifold will not curve much over the extent of the region, and the linear model will be a good fit (low bias).

Schematically, the training algorithm is as follows:

1. Partition the input space R^n into Q disjoint regions $\{R^{(1)}, \ldots, R^{(Q)}\}$.

2. Compute the local covariance matrices

$$\Sigma^{(i)} = E[\, (x - Ex)(x - Ex)^T \mid x \in R^{(i)}\,]; \quad i = 1, \ldots, Q$$

and their eigenvectors $e_j^{(i)}$, $j = 1, \ldots, n$. Relabel the eigenvectors so

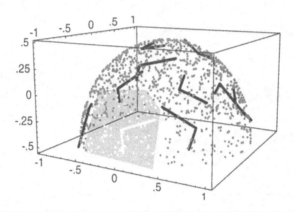

Figure 2: Coordinates built by local PCA for data distributed on the surface of a hemiphere. The solid lines are the two principal eigendirections for the data in each region. One of the regions is shown shaded for emphasis.

that the corresponding eigenvalues are in descending order $\lambda_1^{(i)} > \lambda_2^{(i)} > \cdots > \lambda_n^{(i)}$.

3. Choose a target dimension m and retain the leading m eigendirections for the encoding.

The partition is formed by VQ on the training data. The distortion measure for the VQ strongly affects the partition, and therefore the reconstruction error for the algorithm. We discuss two alternative distortion measures.

The local PCA defines local coordinate patches for the data, with the orientation of the local patches determined by the PCA within each region R_i. Figure 2 shows a set of local two-dimensional coordinate frames induced on the hemisphere data from figure 1, using the standard Euclidean distance as the VQ distortion measure.

3.1 Euclidean Partition. The simplest way to construct the partition is to build a VQ based on Euclidean distance. This can be accomplished by either an online competitive learning algorithm or by the generalized Lloyd algorithm (Gersho & Gray, 1992), which is the batch counterpart of competitive learning. In either case, the trained quantizer consists of a set of Q reference vectors $r^{(i)}$, $i = 1, \ldots, Q$ and corresponding regions $R^{(i)}$. The placement of the reference vectors and the definition of the regions satisfy Lloyd's optimality conditions:

1. Each region, $R^{(i)}$ corresponds to all $x \in R^n$ that lie closer to $r^{(i)}$ than to any other reference vector. Mathematically $R^{(i)} = \{x \mid d_E(x, r^{(i)}) <$

$d_E(x, r^{(j)})$, $\forall j \neq i$, where $d_E(a, b)$ is the Euclidean distance between a and b. Thus, a given x is assigned to its nearest neighbor r.

2. Each reference vector $r^{(i)}$ is placed at the centroid of the corresponding region $R^{(i)}$. For Euclidean distance, the centroid is the mean $r^{(i)} = E[x \mid x \in R^{(i)}]$.

For Euclidean distance, the regions are connected, convex sets called Voronoi cells.

As described in the introduction to section 3, one next computes the covariance matrices for the data in each region $R^{(i)}$ and performs a local PCA projection. The m-dimensional encoding of the original vector x is thus given in two parts: the index of the Voronoi region that the vector lies in and the local coordinates of the point with respect to the centroid, in the basis of the m leading eigenvectors of the corresponding covariance.[4] For example, if $x \in R^{(i)}$, the local coordinates are

$$z = \left(e_1^{(i)} \cdot (x - r^{(i)}), \ldots, e_m^{(i)} \cdot (x - r^{(i)}) \right). \tag{3.1}$$

The decoded vector is given by

$$\hat{x} = r^{(i)} + \sum_{j=1}^{m} z_j \, e_j^{(i)}. \tag{3.2}$$

The mean squared reconstruction error incurred is

$$\mathcal{E}_{\text{recon}} = E[\|x - \hat{x}\|^2]. \tag{3.3}$$

3.2 Projection Partition. The algorithm described above is not optimal because the partition is constructed independent of the projection that follows. To understand the proper distortion function from which to construct the partition, consider the reconstruction error for a vector x that lies in $R^{(i)}$,

$$d(x, r^{(i)}) \equiv \left\| x - r^{(i)} - \sum_{j=1}^{m} z_j \, e_j^{(i)} \right\|^2 = (x - r^{(i)})^T P^{(i)\,T} P^{(i)} (x - r^{(i)})$$

$$\equiv (x - r^{(i)})^T \Pi^{(i)} (x - r^{(i)}) , \tag{3.4}$$

where $P^{(i)}$ is the $m \times n$ matrix whose rows are the trailing eigenvectors of the covariance matrix $\Sigma^{(i)}$. The matrix $\Pi^{(i)}$ is the projection orthogonal to the local m-dimensional PCA subspace.

---

[4] The number of bits required to specify the region is small (between four and seven bits in all the experiments presented here) with respect to the number of bits used to express the double-precision coordinates within each region. In this respect, the specification of the region is nearly free.

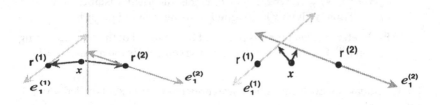

Figure 3: Assignment of the data point x to one of two regions based on (left) Euclidean distance and (right) the reconstruction distance. The reference vectors $r^{(i)}$ and leading eigenvector $e_1^{(i)}$ are shown for each of two regions ($i = 1, 2$). See text for explanation.

The reconstruction distance $d(x, r^{(i)})$ is the squared projection of the difference vector $x - r^{(i)}$ on the trailing eigenvectors of the covariance matrix for region $R^{(i)5}$. Equivalently, it is the squared Euclidean distance to the linear manifold that is defined by the local m-dimensional PCA in the ith local region. Clustering with respect to the reconstruction distance directly minimizes the expected reconstruction error $\mathcal{E}_{recon}$.

Figure 3 illustrates the difference between Euclidean distance and the reconstruction distance, with the latter intended for a one-dimensional local PCA. Suppose we want to determine to which of two regions the data point x belongs. For Euclidean clustering, the distance between the point x and the two centroids $r^{(1)}$ and $r^{(2)}$ is compared, and the data point is assigned to the cluster whose centroid is closest—in this case, region 1. For clustering by the reconstruction distance, the distance from the point to the two one-dimensional subspaces (corresponding to the principal subspace for the two regions) is compared, and the data point is assigned to the region whose principal subspace is closest—in this case, region 2. Data points that lie on the intersection of hyperplanes are assigned to the region with lower index.

Thus the membership in regions defined by the reconstruction distance can be different from that defined by Euclidean distance. This is because the reconstruction distance does not count the distance along the leading eigendirections. Neglecting the distance along the leading eigenvectors is exactly what is required, since we retain all the information in the leading directions during the PCA projection. Notice too that, unlike the Euclidean Voronoi regions, the regions arising from the reconstruction distance may not be connected sets.

Since the reconstruction distance (see equation 3.4) depends on the eigenvectors of $\Sigma^{(i)}$, an online algorithm for clustering would be prohibitively

---

[5] Note that when the target dimension m equals 0, the representation is reduced to the reference vector $r^{(i)}$ with no local coordinates. The distortion measure then reduces to the Euclidean distance.

expensive. Instead, we use the generalized Lloyd algorithm to compute the partition iteratively. The algorithm is:

1. Initialize the $r^{(i)}$ to randomly chosen inputs from the training data set. Initialize the $\Sigma^{(i)}$ to the identity matrix.

2. *Partition.* Partition the training data into Q regions $R^{(1)}, \ldots, R^{(Q)}$ where

$$R^{(i)} = \{x \mid d(x, r^{(i)}) \le d(x, r^{(j)}); \text{ all } j \ne i\} \tag{3.5}$$

with $d(x, r^{(i)})$ the reconstruction distance defined in (equation 3.4).

3. *Generalized centroid.* According to the Lloyd algorithm, the reference vectors $r^{(i)}$ are to be placed at the generalized centroid of the region $R^{(i)}$. The generalized centroid is defined by

$$r^{(i)} = \text{argmin}_r \, \frac{1}{N_i} \sum_{x \in R^{(i)}} (x - r)^T \, \Pi^{(i)} \, (x - r), \tag{3.6}$$

where N_i is the number of data points in $R^{(i)}$. Expanding the projection operator Π in terms of the eigenvectors $e_j^{(i)}$, $j = m + 1, \ldots, n$ and setting to zero the derivative of the argument of the right-hand side of equation 3.6 with respect to r, one finds a set of equations for the generalized centroid[6] (Kambhatla, 1995),

$$\Pi^{(i)} r = \Pi^{(i)} \bar{x} \tag{3.7}$$

where $\bar{x}$ is the mean of the data in $R^{(i)}$. Thus any vector r whose projection along the trailing eigenvectors equals the projection of $\bar{x}$ along the trailing eigenvectors is a generalized centroid of $R^{(i)}$. For convenience, we take $r = \bar{x}$. Next compute the covariance matrices

$$\Sigma^{(i)} = \frac{1}{N_i} \sum_{x \in R^{(i)}} (x - r^{(i)})(x - r^{(i)})^T$$

and their eigenvectors $e_j^{(i)}$.

4. Iterate steps 2 and 3 until the fractional change in the average reconstruction error is below some specified threshold.

Following training, vectors are encoded and decoded as follows. To encode a vector x, find the reference vector $r^{(i)}$ that minimizes the reconstruction distance $d(x, r)$, and project $x - r^{(i)}$ onto the leading m eigenvectors

---

[6] In deriving the centroid equations, care must be exercised to take into account the dependence of $e_j^{(i)}$ (and hence $\Pi^{(i)}$) on $r^{(i)}$.

of the corresponding covariance matrix $\Sigma^{(i)}$ to obtain the local principal components

$$z = \left(e_1^{(i)} \cdot (x - r^{(i)}), \ldots, e_m^{(i)} \cdot (x - r^{(i)}) \right). \tag{3.8}$$

The encoding of x consists of the index i and the m local principal components z. The decoding, or reconstruction, of the vector x is

$$\hat{x} = r^{(i)} + \sum_{j=1}^{m} z_j \, e_j^{(i)}. \tag{3.9}$$

The clustering in the algorithm directly minimizes the expected reconstruction distance since it is a generalized Lloyd algorithm with the reconstruction distance as the distortion measure. Training in batch mode avoids recomputing the eigenvectors after each input vector is presented.

3.3 Accelerated Clustering. Vector quantization partitions data by calculating the distance between each data point x and all of the reference vectors $r^{(i)}$. The search and storage requirements for computing the partition can be streamlined by constraining the structure of the VQ. These constraints can compromise performance relative to what could be achieved with a standard, or unconstrained, VQ with the same number of regions. However, the constrained architectures allow a given hardware configuration to support a quantizer with many more regions than practicable for the unconstrained architecture, and they can thus improve speed and accuracy relative to what one can achieve in practice using an unconstrained quantizer. The two most common structures are the tree-search VQ and the multistage VQ (Gersho & Gray, 1992).

Tree-search VQ was designed to alleviate the search bottleneck for encoding. At the root of the tree, a partition into b_0 regions is constructed. At the next level of the tree, each of these regions is further partitioned into b_1 regions (often $b_0 = b_1 = \ldots$), and so forth. After k levels, each with branching ratio b, there are b^k regions in the partition. Encoding new data requires at most kb distortion calculations. The unconstrained quantizer with the same number of regions requires up to b^k distortion calculations. Thus the search complexity grows only logarithmically with the number of regions for the tree-search VQ, whereas the search complexity grows linearly with the number of regions for the unconstrained quantizer. However, the number of reference vectors in the tree is

$$\frac{b}{b-1}(b^k - 1),$$

whereas the unconstrained quantizer requires only b^k reference vectors. Thus the tree typically requires more storage.

Multistage VQ is a form of product coding and as such is economical in both search and storage requirements. At the first stage, a partition into b_0 regions is constructed. Then all of the data are encoded using this partition, and the residuals from *all* b_0 regions $\epsilon = x - r^{(i)}$ are pooled. At the next stage, these residuals are quantized by a b_1 region quantizer, and so forth. The final k-stage quantizer (again assuming b regions at each level) has b^k effective regions. Encoding new data requires at most kb distortion calculations.

Although the search complexity is the same as the tree quantizer, the storage requirements are more favorable than for either the tree or the unconstrained quantizer. There are a total b^k regions generated by the multistage architecture, requiring only bk reference vectors. The unconstrained quantizer would require b^k reference vectors to generate the same number of regions, and the tree requires more. The drawback is that the shapes of the regions in a multistage quantizer are severely restricted. By sketching regions for a two-stage quantizer with two or three regions per stage, the reader can easily show that the final regions consist of two or three shapes that are copied and translated to tile the data space. In contrast, an unconstrained quantizer will construct as many different shapes as required to encode the data with minimal distortion.

4 Experimental Results

In this section we present the results of experiments comparing global PCA, five-layer autoassociators, and several variants of VQPCA applied to dimension reduction of speech and image data. We compare the algorithms' training time and distortion in the reconstructed signal. The distortion measure we use is the reconstruction error normalized by the data variance,

$$\mathcal{E}_{\text{norm}} \equiv \frac{E[\|x - \hat{x}\|^2]}{E[\|x - E[x]\|^2]}, \tag{4.1}$$

where the expectations are with respect to empirical data distribution.

We trained the autoassociators using three optimization techniques: conjugate gradient descent (CGD), stochastic gradient descent (SGD), and the Broyden-Fletcher-Goldfarb-Shanno (BFGS) quasi-Newton method (Press, Flannery, Teukolsky, & Vetterling, 1987). The gradient descent code has a momentum term, and learning rate annealing as in Darken and Moody (1991).

We give results for VQPCA using both Euclidean and reconstruction distance, with unconstrained, multistage, and tree-search VQ. For the Euclidean distortion measure with an unconstrained quantizer, we used online competitive learning with the annealed learning rate schedule in Darken and Moody (1991).

We computed the global PCA for the speech data by diagonalizing the covariance matrices using Householder reduction followed by QL.[7] The image training set has fewer data points than the input dimension. Thus the covariance matrix is singular, and we cannot use Householder reduction. Instead we computed the PCA using singular-value decomposition applied to the data matrix.

All of the architecture selection was carried out by monitoring performance on a validation (or holdout) set. To limit the space of architectures, the autoassociators have an equal number of nodes in the second and fourth (sigmoidal) layers. These were varied from 5 to 50 in increments of 5. The networks were regularized by early stopping on a validation data set.

For VQPCA, we varied the number of local regions for the unconstrained VQ from 5 to 50 in increments of 5. The multistage VQ examples used two levels, with the number of regions at each level varied from 5 to 50 in increments of 5. The branching factor of the tree-structured VQ was varied from 2 to 9.

For all experiments and all architectures, we report only the results on those architectures that obtained the lowest reconstruction error on the validation data set. In this sense, we report the best results we obtained.

4.1 Dimension Reduction of Speech.
We drew examples of the 12 monothongal vowels extracted from continuous speech in the TIMIT database (Fisher & Doddington, 1986). Each input vector consists of the lowest 32 discrete Fourier transform coefficients (spanning the frequency range 0–4 kHz), time-averaged over the central third of the vowel segment. The training set contains 1200 vectors, the validation set 408 vectors, and the test set 408 vectors. The test set utterances are from speakers not represented in the training or validation sets. Motivated by the desire to capture formant structure in the vowel encodings, we reduced the data from 32 to 2 dimensions.

The results of our experiments are shown in Table 1. Table 1 shows the mean and 2-σ error bars (computed over four random initializations) of the test set reconstruction error, and the Sparc 2 training times (in seconds). The numbers in parentheses are the values of architectural parameters. For example Autoassoc. (35) is a five-layer autoassociator with 35 nodes in each of the second and fourth layers. VQPCA-E-MS (40 × 40) is a Euclidean distortion, multistage VQPCA with 40 cells in each of two stages.

The VQPCA encodings have about half the reconstruction error of the global PCA or the five-layer networks. The latter failed to obtain significantly better results than the global PCA. The autoassociators show high variance in the reconstruction errors with respect to different random weight initializations. Several nets had higher error than PCA, indicating trapping

---

[7] The Householder algorithm reduces the covariance matrix to tridiagonal form, which is then diagonalized by the QL procedure (Press et al., 1987).

Table 1: Speech Dimension Reduction.

Algorithm	ε_{norm}	Training Time (seconds)
PCA	0.443	11
Autoassoc.-CGD (35)	0.496 ± .103	7784 ± 7442
Autoassoc.-BFGS (20)	0.439 ± .059	3284 ± 1206
Autoassoc.-SGD (35)	0.440 ± .016	35,502 ± 182
VQPCA-Eucl (50)	0.272 ± .010	1915 ± 780
VQPCA-E-MS (40 × 40)	0.244 ± .008	144 ± 41
VQPCA-E-T (15 × 15)	0.259 ± .002	195 ± 10
VQPCA-Recon (45)	0.230 ± .004	864 ± 102
VQPCA-R-MS (45 × 45)	0.208 ± .005	924 ± 50
VQPCA-R-T (9 × 9)	0.242 ± .005	484 ± 128

in particularly poor local optima. As expected, stochastic gradient descent showed less variance due to initialization. In contrast, the local linear algorithms are relatively insensitive to initialization.

Clustering with reconstruction distance produced somewhat lower error than clustering with Euclidean distance. For both distortion measures, the multistage architecture produced the lowest error.

The five-layer autoassociators are very slow to train. The Euclidean multistage and tree-structured local linear algorithms trained more than an order of magnitude faster than the autoassociators. For the unconstrained, Euclidean distortion VQPCA, the partition was determined by online competitive learning and could probably be speeded up a bit by using a batch algorithm.

In addition to training time, practicality depends on the time required to encode and decode new data. Table 2 shows the number of floating-point operations required to encode and decode the entire database for the different algorithms. The VQPCA algorithms, particularly those using the reconstruction distance, require many more floating-point operations to encode the data than the autoassociators. However, the decoding is much faster than that for autoassociators and is comparable to PCA. [8] The results indicate that VQPCA may not be suitable for real-time applications like videoconferencing where very fast encoding is desired. However, when only the decoding speed is of concern (e.g., for data retrieval), VQPCA algorithms are a good choice because of their accuracy and fast decoding.

---

[8] However, parallel implementation of the autoassociators could outperform the VQPCA decode in terms of clock time.

Table 2: Encoding and Decoding Times for the Speech Data.

Algorithm	Encode Time (FLOPs)	Decode Time (FLOPs)
PCA	158	128
Autoassoc.-CGD (35)	2380	2380
Autoassoc.-BFGS (20)	1360	1360
Autoassoc.-SGD (35)	2380	2380
VQPCA-Eucl (50)	4957	128
VQPCA-E-MS (40 × 40)	7836	192
VQPCA-E-T (15 × 15)	3036	128
VQPCA-Recon (45)	87,939	128
VQPCA-R-MS (45 × 45)	96,578	192
VQPCA-R-T (9 × 9)	35,320	128

In order to test variability of these results across different training and test sets, we reshuffled and repartitioned the data into new training, validation, and tests sets of the same size as those above. The new data sets gave results very close to those reported here (Kambhatla, 1995).

4.2 Dimension Reduction of Images. Our image database consists of 160 images of the faces of 20 people. Each image is a 64 × 64, 8-bit/pixel grayscale image. The database was originally generated by Cottrell and Metcalfe and used in their study of identity, gender, and emotion recognition (Cottrell & Metcalfe, 1991). We adopted the database, and the preparation used here, in order to compare our dimension reduction algorithms with the nonlinear autoassociators used by DeMers and Cottrell (1993).

As in DeMers and Cottrell (1993), each image is used complete, as a 4096-dimensional vector, and is preprocessed by extracting the leading 50 principal components computed from the ensemble of 160 images. Thus the base dimension is 50. As in DeMers and Cottrell (1993), we examined reduction to five dimensions.

We divided the data into a training set containing 120 images, a validation set of 20 images, and a test set of 20 images. We used PCA, five-layer autoassociators, and VQPCA for reduction to five dimensions. Due to memory constraints, the autoassociators were limited to 5 to 40 nodes in each of the second and fourth layers. The autoassociators and the VQPCA were trained with four different random initializations of the free parameters.

The experimental results are shown in Table 3. The five-layer networks attain about 30 percent lower error than global PCA. VQPCA with either Euclidean or reconstruction distance distortion measures attain about 40 per-

Table 3: Image Dimension Reduction.

Algorithm	$\mathcal{E}_{norm}$	Training Time (seconds)
PCA	0.463	5
Autoassoc.-CGD (35)	0.441 ± .090	698 ± 533
Autoassoc.-BFGS (35)	0.377 ± .127	18,905 ± 15,081
Autoassoc.-SGD (25)	0.327 ± .027	4171 ± 41
VQPCA-Eucl (20)	0.179 ± .048	202 ± 57
VQPCA-E-MS (5 × 5)	0.307 ± .031	14 ± 2
VQPCA-E-Tree (4 × 4)	0.211 ± .064	31 ± 9
VQPCA-Recon (20)	0.173 ± .050	62 ± 5
VQPCA-R-MS (20 × 20)	0.240 ± .042	78 ± 32
VQPCA-R-Tree (5 × 5)	0.218 ± .029	79 ± 15

Table 4: Encoding and Decoding Times (FLOPs) for the Image Data.

Algorithm	Encode Time (FLOPs)	Decode Time (FLOPs)
PCA	545	500
Autoassoc.-CGD (35)	3850	3850
Autoassoc.-BFGS (35)	3850	3850
Autoassoc.-SGD (25)	2750	2750
VQPCA-Eucl (20)	3544	500
VQPCA-E-MS (5 × 5)	2043	600
VQPCA-E-T (4 × 4)	1743	500
VQPCA-Recon (20)	91,494	500
VQPCA-R-MS (20 × 20)	97,493	600
VQPCA-R-T (5 × 5)	46,093	500

cent lower error than the best autoassociator. There is little distinction between the Euclidean and reconstruction distance clustering for these data.

The VQPCA trains significantly faster than the autoassociators. Although the conjugate gradient algorithm is relatively quick, it generates encodings inferior to those obtained with the stochastic gradient descent and BFGS simulators.

Table 4 shows the encode and decode times for the different algorithms. We again note that VQPCA algorithms using reconstruction distance clustering require many more floating-point operations (FLOPs) to encode an

Table 5: Image Dimension Reduction: Training on All Available Data.

Algorithm	$\mathcal{E}_{norm}$	Training Time (seconds)
PCA	0.405	7
Autoassoc.-SGD (30)	0.103	25,306
Autoassoc.-SGD (40)	0.073	31,980
VQPCA-Eucl (25)	0.026	251
VQPCA-Recon (30)	0.022	116

input vector than does the Euclidean distance algorithm or the five-layer networks. However, as before, the decode times are much less for VQPCA. As before, shuffling and repartitioning the data into training, validation, and test data sets and repeating the experiments returned results very close to those given here.

Finally, in order to compare directly with DeMers and Cottrell's (1993) results, we also conducted experiments training with all the data (no separation into validation and test sets). This is essentially a model fitting problem, with no influence from statistical sampling. We show results only for the autoassociators trained with SGD, since these returned lower error than the conjugate gradient simulators, and the memory requirements for BFGS were prohibitive. We report the results from those architectures that provided the lowest reconstruction error on the training data.

The results are shown in Table 5. Both nonlinear techniques produce encodings with lower error than PCA, indicating significant nonlinear structure in the data. For the same data and using a five-layer autoassociator with 30 nodes in each of the second and fourth layers, DeMers and Cottrell (1993) obtain a reconstruction error $\mathcal{E}_{norm} = 0.1317$.[9] This is comparable to our results. We note that the VQPCA algorithms train two orders of magnitude faster than the networks while obtaining encodings with about one-third the reconstruction error.

It is useful to examine the images obtained from the encodings for the various algorithms. Figure 4 shows two sample images from the data set along with their reconstructions from five-dimensional encodings. The algorithms correspond to those reported in Table 5. These two images were selected because their reconstruction error closely matched the average. The left-most column shows the images as reconstructed from the 50 principal components. The second column shows the reconstruction from 5 princi-

---

[9] DeMers and Cottrell report half the MSE per output node, $E = (1/2) * (1/50) * MSE = 0.001$. This corresponds to $\mathcal{E}_{norm} = 0.1317$.

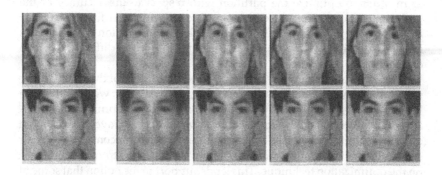

Figure 4: Two representative images: Left to right—Original 50 principal components reconstructed image, reconstruction from 5-D encodings: PCA, Autoassoc-SGD(40), VQPCAEucl(25), and VQPCA-Recon(30). The normalized reconstruction errors and training times for the whole data set (all the images) are given in Table 5.

pal components. The third column is the reconstruction from the five-layer autoassociator, and the last two columns are the reconstruction from the Euclidean and reconstruction distance VQPCA.

The five-dimensional PCA has grossly reduced resolution, and gray-scale distortion (e.g., the hair in the top image). All of the nonlinear algorithms produce superior results, as indicated by the reconstruction error. The lower image shows a subtle difference between the autoassociator and the two VQPCA reconstructions; the posture of the mouth is correctly recovered in the latter.

5 Discussion

We have applied locally linear models to the task of dimension reduction, finding superior results to both PCA and the global nonlinear model built by five-layer autoassociators. The local linear models train significantly faster than autoassociators, with their training time dominated by the partitioning step. Once the model is trained, encoding new data requires computing which region of the partition the new data fall in, and thus VQPCA requires more computation for encoding than does the autoassociator. However, decoding data with VQPCA is faster than decoding with the autoassociator and comparable to decoding with PCA. With these considerations, VQPCA is perhaps not optimal for real-time encoding, but its accuracy and computational speed for decoding make it superior for applications like image retrieval from databases.

In order to optimize the partition with respect to the accuracy of the projected data, we introduced a new distortion function for the VQ, the reconstruction distance. Clustering with the reconstruction distance does indeed provide lower reconstruction error, though the difference is data dependent.

We cannot offer a definitive reason for the superiority of the VQPCA representations over five-layer autoassociators. In particular, we are uncertain how much of the failure of autoassociators is due to optimization problems and how much to the representation capability. We have observed that changes in initialization result in large variability in the reconstruction error of solutions arrived at by autoassociators. We also see strong dependence on the optimization technique. This lends support to the notion that some of the failure is a training problem. It may be that the space of architectures we have explored does have better solutions but that the available optimizers fail to find them.

The optimization problem is a very real block to the effective use of five-layer autoassociators. Although the architecture is an elegant construction for nonlinear dimension reduction, realizing consistently good maps with standard optimization techniques has proved elusive on the examples we considered here.

Optimization may not be the only issue. Autoassociators constructed from neurons with smooth activation functions are constrained to generate smooth projections and immersions. The VQPCA algorithms have no inherent smoothness constraint. This will be an advantage when the data are not well described by a manifold.[10] Moreover, Malthouse (1996) gives a simple example of data for which continuous projections are *necessarily* suboptimal.

In fact, if the data are not well described by a manifold, it may be advantageous to choose the representation dimension locally, allowing a different dimension for each region of the partition. The target dimension could be chosen using a hold out data set, or more economically by a cost function that includes a penalty for model complexity. Minimum description length (MDL) criteria have been used for PCA (Hediger et al., 1990; Wax & Kailath, 1985) and presumably could be applied to VQPCA.

We have explored no such methods for estimating the appropriate target dimension. In contrast, the autoassociator algorithm given by DeMers and Cottrell (1993) includes a pruning strategy to reduce progressively the dimensionality of the representation layer, under the constraint that the reconstruction error not grow above a desired threshold.

Two applications deserve attention. The first is transform coding for which the algorithms discussed here are naturally suited. In transform coding, one transforms the data, such as image blocks, to a lower-redundancy

---

[10] A visualization of just such a case is given in Kambhatla (1995).

representation and then scalar quantizes the new representation. This produces a product code for the data. Standard approaches include preprocessing by PCA or discrete cosine transform, followed by scalar quantization (Wallace, 1991). As discussed in the introduction, the nonlinear transforms considered here provide more accurate representations than PCA and should provide for better transform coding.

This work suggests a full implementation of transform coding, with comparisons betweeen PCA, autoassociators, and VQPCA in terms of rate distortion curves. Transform coding using VQPCA with the reconstruction distance clustering requires additional algorithm development. The reconstruction distance distortion function depends explicitly on the target dimension, while the latter depends on the allocation of transform bits between the new coordinates. Consequently a proper transform coding scheme needs to couple the bit allocation to the clustering, an enhancement that we are developing.

The second potential application is in novelty detection. Recently several authors have used three-layer autoassociators to build models of normal equipment function (Petsche et al., 1996; Japkowicz et al., 1995). Equipment faults are then signaled by the failure of the model to reconstruct the new signal accurately. The nonlinear models provided by VQPCA should provide more accurate models of the normal data, and hence improve the sensitivity and specificity for fault detection.

Acknowledgments

This work was supported in part by grants from the Air Force Office of Scientific Research (F49620-93-1-0253) and the Electric Power Research Institute (RP8015-2). We thank Gary Cottrell and David DeMers for supplying image data and the Center for Spoken Language Understanding at the Oregon Graduate Institute of Science and Technology for speech data. We are grateful for the reviewer's careful reading and helpful comments.

References

Baldi, P., & Hornik, K. (1989). Neural networks and principal component analysis: Learning from examples without local minima. *Neural Networks, 2,* 53–58.

Bourlard, H., & Kamp, Y. (1988). Auto-association by multilayer perceptrons and singular value decomposition. *Biol. Cyb., 59,* 291–294.

Bregler, C., & Omohundro, S. M. (1995). Nonlinear image interpolation using manifold learning. In G. Tesauro, D. Touretzky, & T. Leen (Eds.), *Advances in neural information processing systems 7.* Cambridge, MA: MIT Press.

Broomhead, D. S. (1991, July). Signal processing for nonlinear systems. In S. Haykin (Ed.), *Adaptive Signal Processing, SPIE Proceedings* (pp. 228–243). Bellingham, WA: SPIE.

Cleveland, W. S., & Devlin, S. J. (1988). Locally weighted regression: An approach to regression analysis by local fitting. *J. Amer. Stat. Assoc.*, *83*, 596–610.

Coetzee, F. M., & Stonick, V. L. (1995). Topology and geometry of single hidden layer network, least squares weight solutions. *Neural Computation*, *7*, 672–705.

Cottrell, G. W., & Metcalfe, J. (1991). EMPATH: Face, emotion, and gender recognition using holons. In R. Lippmann, J. Moody, & D. Touretzky (Eds.), *Advances in neural information processing systems 3* (pp. 564–571). San Mateo, CA: Morgan Kaufmann.

Cottrell, G. W., Munro, P., & Zipser, D. (1987). Learning internal representations from gray-scale images: An example of extensional programming. In *Proceedings of the Ninth Annual Cognitive Science Society Conference* (pp. 461–473). Seattle, WA.

Darken, C., & Moody, J. (1991). Note on learning rate schedules for stochastic optimization. In R. Lippman, J. Moody, D. Touretzky, (Eds.), *Advances in neural information processing systems 3*. San Mateo, CA: Morgan Kaufmann.

DeMers, D., & Cottrell, G. (1993). Non-linear dimensionality reduction. In C. Giles, S. Hanson, & J. Cowan (Eds.), *Advances in neural information processing systems 5*. San Mateo, CA: Morgan Kaufmann.

Dony, R. D., & Haykin, S. (1995). Optimally adaptive transform coding. *IEEE Transactions on Image Processing* (pp. 1358–1370).

Fisher, W. M., & Doddington, G. R. (1986). The DARPA speech recognition research database: Specification and status. In *Proceedings of the DARPA Speech Recognition Workshop* (pp. 93–99). Palo Alto, CA.

Fukunaga, K., & Olsen, D. R. (1971). An algorithm for finding intrinsic dimensionality of data. *IEEE Transactions on Computers*, *C-20*, 176–183.

Funahashi, K. (1989). On the approximate realization of continuous mappings by neural networks. *Neural Networks*, *2*, 183–192.

Gersho, A., & Gray, R. M. (1992). *Vector quantization and signal compression*. Boston: Kluwer.

Golomb, B. A., Lawrence, D. T., & Sejnowski, T. J. (1991). Sexnet: A neural network identifies sex from human faces. In R. Lippmann, J. Moody, & D. Touretzky (Eds.), *Advances in neural information processing systems 3* (pp. 572–577). San Mateo, CA: Morgan Kauffmann.

Gray, R. M.(1984, April). Vector quantization. *IEEE ASSP Magazine*, pp. 4–29.

Hastie, T. (1984). *Principal curves and surfaces*. Unpublished dissertation, Stanford University.

Hastie, T., & Stuetzle, W. (1989). Principal curves. *Journal of the American Statistical Association*, *84*, 502–516.

Hecht-Nielsen, R. (1995). Replicator neural networks for universal optimal source coding. *Science*, *269*, 1860–1863.

Hediger, T., Passamante, A., & Farrell, M. E. (1990). Characterizing attractors using local intrinsic dimensions calculated by singular-value decomposition and information-theoretic criteria. *Physical Review*, *A41*, 5325–5332.

Hinton, G. E., Revow, M., & Dayan, P. (1995). Recognizing handwritten digits using mixtures of linear models. In G. Tesauro, D. Touretzky, & T. Leen (Eds.), *Advances in neural information processing systems 7*. Cambridge, MA: MIT Press.

Hornik, M., Stinchcombe, M., & White, H. (1989). Multilayer feedforward networks are universal approximators. *Neural Networks, 2*, 359–368.

Japkowicz, N., Myers, C., & Gluck, M. (1995). A novelty detection approach to classification. In *Proceedings of IJCAI*.

Kambhatla, N. (1995) *Local models and gaussian mixture models for statistical data processing*. Unpublished doctoral dissertation, Oregon Graduate Institute.

Kambhatla, N., & Leen, T. K. (1994). Fast non-linear dimension reduction. In J. D. Cowan, G. Tesauro, & J. Alspector (Eds.), *Advances in neural information processing systems 6*. San Mateo, CA: Morgan Kaufmann.

Kramer, M. A. (1991). Nonlinear principal component analysis using autoassociative neural networks. *AIChE Journal, 37*, 233–243.

Kung, S. Y., & Diamantaras, K. I. (1990). A neural network learning algorithm for adaptive principal component extraction (APEX). In *Proceedings of the IEEE International Conference on Acoustics Speech and Signal Processing* (pp. 861–864).

Malthouse, E. C. (1996). Some theoretical results on non-linear principal components analysis (Unpublished research report). Evanston, IL: Kellogg School of Management, Northwestern University.

Oja, E. (1982). A simplified neuron model as a principal component analyzer. *J. Math. Biology, 15*, 267–273.

Oja, E. (1989). Neural networks, principal components, and subspaces. *International Journal of Neural Systems, 1*, 61–68.

Oja, E. (1991). Data compression, feature extraction, and autoassociation in feedforward neural networks. In *Artificial neural networks* (pp. 737–745). Amsterdam: Elsevier Science Publishers.

Petsche, T., Marcantonio, A., Darken, C., Hanson, S. J., Kuhn, G. M., & Santoso, I. (1996) A neural network autoassociator for induction motor failure prediction. In D. S. Touretzky, M. C. Mozer, & M. E. Hasselmo (Eds.), *Advances in neural information processing systems 8*. Cambridge, MA: MIT Press.

Press, W. H., Flannery, B. P., Teukolsky, S. A., & Vetterling, W. T. (1987). *Numerical recipes—the art of scientific computing*. Cambridge: Cambridge University Press.

Rognvaldsson, T. (1994). On Langevin updating in multilayer perceptrons. *Neural Computation, 6*, 916–926.

Rubner, J., & Tavan, P. (1989). A self-organizing network for principal component analysis. *Europhysics Lett., 20*, 693–698.

Sanger, T. (1989). An optimality principle for unsupervised learning. In D. S. Touretzky (ed.), *Advances in neural information processing systems 1*. San Mateo, CA: Morgan Kaufmann.

Usui, S., Nakauchi, S., & Nakano, M. (1991). Internal color representation acquired by a five-layer neural network. In O. Simula, T. Kohonen, K. Makisara, & J. Kangas (Eds.), *Artificial neural networks*. Amsterdam: Elsevier Science Publishers, North-Holland.

Wallace, G. K. (1991). The JPEG still picture compression standard. *Communications off the ACM, 34*, 31–44.

Wax, M., & Kailath, T. (1985). Detection of signals by information theoretic criteria. *IEEE Transactions on Acoustics, Speech and Signal Processing, ASSP-33(2)*, 387–392.

Yang, L., & Yu, W. (1993). Backpropagation with homotopy. *Neural Computation,*
    5, 363–366.

19

A Resource-Allocating Network for Function Interpolation

John Platt
Synaptics, 2860 Zanker Road, Suite 206, San Jose, CA 95134 USA

We have created a network that allocates a new computational unit whenever an unusual pattern is presented to the network. This network forms compact representations, yet learns easily and rapidly. The network can be used at any time in the learning process and the learning patterns do not have to be repeated. The units in this network respond to only a local region of the space of input values.

The network learns by allocating new units and adjusting the parameters of existing units. If the network performs poorly on a presented pattern, then a new unit is allocated that corrects the response to the presented pattern. If the network performs well on a presented pattern, then the network parameters are updated using standard LMS gradient descent.

We have obtained good results with our resource-allocating network (RAN). For predicting the Mackey–Glass chaotic time series, RAN learns much faster than do those using backpropagation networks and uses a comparable number of synapses.

1 Introduction

Judd (1988) has shown that the problem of loading a multilayer perceptron with binary units is NP-complete. Loading sigmoidal multilayer networks is computationally expensive for large sets of real data, with unknown bounds on the amount of computation required.

Baum (1989) pointed out that the problem of NP-complete loading is associated only with a network of fixed resources. If a network can allocate new resources, then the problem of loading can be solved in polynomial time. Therefore, we are interested in creating a network that allocates new computational units as more patterns are learned.

Traditional pattern recognition algorithms, such as Parzen windows and k-nearest neighbors, allocate a new unit for every learned example. The number of examples in real problems forces us to use fewer than one unit for every learning example: we must create and store an abstraction of the data.

The network described here allocates far fewer units than the number of presented examples. The number of allocated units scales sublinearly with the number of presented inputs. The network can be used either for on-line or off-line learning.

Previous workers have used networks whose transfer function is a gaussian (Broomhead and Lowe 1988; Moody and Darken 1988, 1989; Poggio and Girosi 1990). The use of gaussian units was originally inspired by approximation theory, which describes algorithms that interpolate between irregularly spaced input–output pairs (Powell 1987). In fact, Lapedes discussed the hypothesis that multiple layers of sigmoidal units form gaussian-like transfer functions in order to perform interpolation (Lapedes 1987).

Gaussian units are well-suited for use in a resource-allocating network because they respond only to a local region of the space of input values. When a gaussian unit is allocated, it explicitly stores information from an input–output pair instead of merely using that information for gradient descent. The explicit storage of an input–output pair means that this pair can be used immediately to improve the performance of the system in a local region of the input space. A unit with a nonlocal response needs to undergo gradient descent, because it has a nonzero output for a large fraction of the training data.

The work of Moody and Darken (1988, 1989) is the closest to the work specified below. They use gaussian units, where the gaussians have variable height, variable centers, and fixed widths. The network learns the centers of the gaussians using the k-means algorithm (Lloyd 1957; Stark et al. 1962; MacQueen 1967), and learns the heights of the gaussians using the LMS gradient descent rule (Widrow 1960). The width of the gaussians is determined by the distance to the nearest gaussian center after the k-means learning.

Moody has further extended his work by incorporating a hash table lookup (Moody 1989). The hash table is a resource-allocating network where the values in the hash table become nonzero only if the entry in the hash table is activated by the corresponding presence of nonzero input probability.

Our work improves on previous work in several ways:

1. Although it has the same accuracy, our network requires fewer weights than do networks in either Moody and Darken (1989) or in Moody (1989).

2. Like the hashing approach in Moody (1989), our network automatically adjusts the number of units to reflect the complexity of the function that is being interpolated. Fixed-size networks either use too few units, in which case the network memorizes poorly, or too many, in which case the network generalizes poorly.

3. We use units that respond to only a local region of input space, similar to Moody and Darken (1988, 1989), but unlike backpropagation. The units respond to only a small region of the space of inputs so

that newly allocated units do not interfere with previously allocated units.

4. The RAN adjusts the centers of the gaussian units based on the error at the output, like Poggio and Girosi (1990). Networks with centers placed on a high-dimensional grid, such as Broomhead and Lowe (1988) and Moody (1989), or networks that use unsupervised clustering for center placement, such as Moody and Darken (1988, 1989), generate larger networks than RAN, because they cannot move the centers to increase the accuracy.

5. Parzen windows and k-nearest neighbors both require a number of stored patterns that grow linearly with the number of presented patterns. With our method, the number of stored patterns grows sublinearly, and eventually reaches a maximum.

2 The Algorithm

This section describes a resource-allocating network (RAN), which consists of a network, a strategy for allocating new units, and a learning rule for refining the network.

2.1 The Network. RAN is a two-layer network (Fig. 1). The first layer consists of units that respond to only a local region of the space of input values. The second layer aggregates outputs from these units and creates the function that approximates the input–output mapping over the entire space.

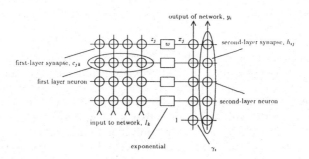

Figure 1: The architecture of the network. In parallel, the network computes the distances of the input vector $\mathbf{I}$ to the stored centers $\mathbf{c}_j$. The distance is then exponentiated to yield a weight x_j. The output $\mathbf{y}$ is a weighted sum of the heights $\mathbf{h}_j$ and an offset γ.

The units on the first layer store a particular region in the input space. When the input moves away from the stored region the response of the unit decreases. A simple function that implements a locally tuned unit is a gaussian:

$$z_j = \sum_k (c_{jk} - I_k)^2$$
$$x_j = \exp(-z_j/w_j^2) \tag{2.1}$$

We use a C^1 continuous polynomial approximation to speed up the algorithm, without loss of network accuracy:

$$x_j = \begin{cases} \left[1 - (z_j/qw_j^2)\right]^2, & \text{if } z_j < qw_j^2 \\ 0 & \text{otherwise} \end{cases} \tag{2.2}$$

where $q = 2.67$ is chosen empirically to make the best fit to a gaussian.

The inputs to the synapses of the second layer are the outputs of the units of the first layer. The purpose of each second-layer synapse is to define the contribution of each first-layer unit to a particular output y of the network. Each output of the network y is the sum of the first-layer outputs x_j, each weighted by the synaptic strength h_j plus a constant vector γ, which does not depend on the output of the first layer:

$$y = \sum_j h_j x_j + \gamma \tag{2.3}$$

The γ is the default output of the network when none of the first-layer units is active. The $h_j x_j$ term can be thought of as a bump that is added or subtracted to the constant term γ to yield the desired function.

2.2 The Learning Algorithm.

The network starts with a blank slate: no patterns are yet stored. As patterns are presented to it, the network chooses to store some of them. At any given point the network has a current state, which reflects the patterns that have been stored previously.

The allocator identifies a pattern that is not currently well represented by the network and allocates a new unit that memorizes the pattern. The output of the new unit extends to the second layer. After the new unit is allocated, the network output is equal to the desired output T. Let the index of this new unit be n.

The peak of the response of the newly allocated unit is set to the novel input,

$$c_n = I \tag{2.4}$$

The linear synapses on the second layer are set to the difference between the output of the network and the novel output,

$$h_n = T - y \tag{2.5}$$

The width of the response of the new unit is proportional to the distance from the nearest stored vector to the novel input vector,

$$w_n = \kappa \|I - c_{nearest}\| \tag{2.6}$$

where κ is an overlap factor. As κ grows larger, the responses of the units overlap more and more.

The RAN uses a two-part novelty condition. An input–output pair (I, T) is considered novel if the input is far away from existing centers,

$$\|I - c_{nearest}\| > \delta(t) \tag{2.7}$$

and if the difference between the desired output and the output of the network is large

$$\|T - y(I)\| > \epsilon \tag{2.8}$$

Typically, ϵ is a desired accuracy of output of the network. Errors larger than ϵ are immediately corrected by the allocation of a new unit, while errors smaller than ϵ are gradually repaired using gradient descent. The distance $\delta(t)$ is the scale of resolution that the network is fitting at the tth input presentation. The learning starts with $\delta(t) = \delta_{max}$, which is the largest length scale of interest, typically the size of the entire input space of nonzero probability density. The distance $\delta(t)$ shrinks until it reaches δ_{min}, which is the smallest length scale of interest. The network will average over features that are smaller than δ_{min}. We used a function

$$\delta(t) = \max[\delta_{max} \exp(-t/\tau), \delta_{min}] \tag{2.9}$$

where τ is a decay constant.

At first, the system creates a coarse representation of the function, then refines the representation by allocating units with smaller and smaller widths. Finally, when the system has learned the entire function to the desired accuracy and length scale, it stops allocating new units altogether.

The two-part novelty condition is necessary for creating a compact network. If only condition 2.7 is used, then the network will allocate units instead of using gradient descent to correct small errors. If only condition 2.8 is used, then fine-scale units may be allocated in order to represent coarse-scale features, which is wasteful.

By allocating new units, RAN eventually represents the desired function ever more closely as the network is trained. Fewer units are needed for a given accuracy if the first-layer synapses c_{jk}, the second-level synapses h_{ij}, and the thresholds γ_i are adjusted to decrease the error:

$$\mathcal{E} = ||\mathbf{y} - \mathbf{T}||^2 \tag{2.10}$$

We use the Widrow–Hoff LMS algorithm (Widrow and Hoff 1960) to decrease the error whenever a new unit is not allocated:

$$
\begin{aligned}
\Delta\mathbf{h}_j &= \alpha(\mathbf{T} - \mathbf{y})x_j \\
\Delta\gamma &= \alpha(\mathbf{T} - \mathbf{y})
\end{aligned}
\tag{2.11}
$$

In addition, we adjust the centers of the responses of units to decrease the error:

$$\Delta c_{jk} = 2\frac{\alpha}{w_j}(I_k - c_{jk})x_j\left[(\mathbf{T} - \mathbf{y})\mathbf{h}_j\right] \tag{2.12}$$

Equation 2.12 is derived from gradient descent and equation 2.1. Equation 2.12 also has an intuitive interpretation. Units whose outputs that would cancel the error have their centers pulled toward the input. Units whose outputs that would increase the error have their centers pushed away from the input. Empirically, equation 2.12 also works for the polynomial approximation 2.2.

The structure of the algorithm is shown below as pseudocode, including initialization code:

```
δ = δ_max
γ = T₀ (from the first input–output pair)
loop over presentations of input–output pairs (I, T)
    {
            evaluate output of network y = Σ_j h_j x_j(I) + γ
            compute error E = T − y
            find distance to nearest center d = min_j ||c_j − I||
            if ||E|| > ε and d > δ then
                {
                        allocate new unit, c_new = I, h_new = E
                        if this is the first unit to be allocated then
                                width of new unit = κδ
                        else
                                width of new unit = κd
                }
        else
                perform gradient descent on γ, h_j, c_jk
        if δ > δ_min
                δ = δ × exp(−1/τ)
    }
```

3 Results

One application of an interpolating RAN is to predict complex time series. As a test case, a chaotic time series can be generated with a nonlinear algebraic or differential equation. Such a series has some short-range time coherence, but long-term prediction is very difficult. The need to predict such a time series arises in such real-world problems as detecting arrhythmias in heartbeats.

The RAN was tested on a particular chaotic time series created by the Mackey–Glass delay-difference equation:

$$x(t+1) = (1-b)x(t) + a\frac{x(t-\tau)}{1+x(t-\tau)^{10}} \tag{3.1}$$

for $a = 0.2$, $b = 0.1$, and $\tau = 17$.

The network is given no information about the generator of the time series, and is asked to predict the future of the time series from a few samples of the history of the time series. In our example, we trained the network to predict the value at time $T + \Delta T$, from inputs at time T, $T - 6$, $T - 12$, and $T - 18$.

The network was tested using two different learning modes: off-line learning with a limited amount of data, and on-line learning with a large amount of data. The Mackey–Glass equation has been learned off-line, by other workers, using the backpropagation algorithm (Lapedes and Farber 1987), and radial basis functions (Moody and Darken 1989). We used RAN to predict the Mackey–Glass equations with the following parameters: $\alpha = 0.02$, 400 learning epochs, $\delta_{max} = 0.7$, $\kappa = 0.87$, and $\delta_{min} = 0.07$ reached after 100 epochs. RAN was simulated using $\epsilon = 0.02$ and $\epsilon = 0.05$. In all cases, $\Delta T = 85$.

Figures 2 and 3 compare the RAN to the other learning algorithms. Figure 2 shows the normalized error rate on a test set versus the size of the learning set for various algorithms. The test set is 500 points of the output of the Mackey–Glass equation at $T = 4000$. The normalized error is the rms error divided by the square root of the variance of the output of the Mackey–Glass equation.

When the RAN algorithm is optimized for accuracy ($\epsilon = 0.02$), then it attains accuracy comparable to hashing B-splines. Figure 3 shows the size of the network versus the size of the learning set. As the size of the learning set grows, the number of units allocated by RAN grows very slowly. The size of the network is measured via number of weights or parameters, which is an approximation to the complexity of the network. For backpropagation, the size is the number of synapses. For the RBF networks and for RAN, there are six parameters per unit: four to describe the location of the center, one for the width, and one for the height of the gaussian. For hashing B-splines, each unit has two parameters: the hash table index and its corresponding hash table value.

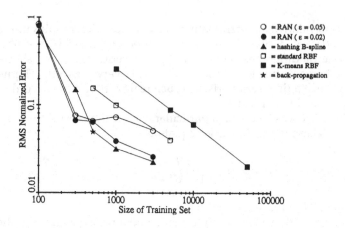

Figure 2: The normalized rms error on a test set for various off-line learning algorithms. Backpropagation, RAN, and hashing B-splines are all competitive in error rate. (Near the backpropagation symbol, the symbol for hashing B-splines is omitted for clarity.)

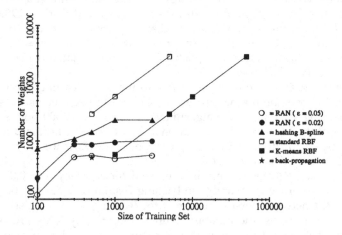

Figure 3: The number of weights in the network versus the size of the training set. RAN and backpropagation are competitive in the compactness of the network. Notice that as the training set size increases, the size of the RAN stays roughly constant.

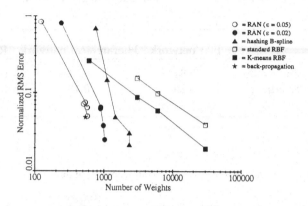

Figure 4: The error on a test set versus the size of the network. Backpropagation stores the prediction function very compactly and accurately, but takes a large amount of computation to form the compact representation. RAN is as compact and accurate as backpropagation, but uses much less computation to form its representation.

Figure 4 shows the efficiency of the various learning algorithms: the smallest, most accurate algorithms are toward the lower left. When optimized for size of network ($\epsilon = 0.05$), the RAN has about as many weights as backpropagation and is just as accurate. The efficiency of RAN is roughly the same as backpropagation, but requires much less computation: RAN takes approximately 8 min of SUN-4 CPU time to reach the accuracy listed in Figure 4, while backpropagation took approximately 30–60 minutes of Cray X-MP time.

The novelty criteria and the center adjustment are both important to the performance of the RAN algorithm. We tested off-line learning of Mackey–Glass predictions using three styles of network that share the same transfer function: a flat network whose centers are chosen with the k-means algorithm, a hierarchical network whose centers are chosen with the k-means algorithm, and a RAN. Each of these networks was tested with either center adjustment via gradient descent or no center adjustment at all. Table 1 shows the normalized rms error on a test set after training off-line on 500 examples. The nonhierarchical k-means network was formed with 100 units. The hierarchical k-means network was formed with three sets of centers: k-means was run separately for 75, 20, and 5 units. In both k-means networks, the widths of the units were chosen via equation 2.6, with a $\kappa = 0.87$. Using the same parameters as used above, and with $\epsilon = 0.05$, RAN allocated 100 units without center adjustment, and 95 units with center adjustment.

Table 1: Normalized rms error for various substrategies of RAN.

	Flat network	Hierarchical network	RAN
No center adjust	0.54	0.31	0.17
Center adjust	0.20	0.15	0.066

Table 2: Comparison between RAN and hashing B-splines.

Method	Number of units	Normalized rms error
RAN	143	0.054
Hashing B-spline 1 level of hierarchy	284	0.074
Hashing B-spline 2 levels of hierarchy	1166	0.044

Table 1 shows that the three substrategies of RAN are about equally important. Using hierarchy, adjusting the centers via gradient descent, and choosing units to allocate based on the novelty conditions all seem to improve the performance by roughly a factor of 1.5 to 2.

The Mackey–Glass equation has been learned using on-line techniques by hashing B-splines (Moody 1989). We used on-line RAN using the following parameters: $\alpha = 0.05$, $\epsilon = 0.02$, $\delta_{max} = 0.7$, $\delta_{min} = 0.07$, $\kappa = 0.87$, and δ_{min} reached after 5000 input presentations. Table 2 compares the on-line error versus the size of network for both RAN and the hashing B-spline (Moody, personal communication). In both cases, $\Delta T = 50$. The RAN algorithm has similar accuracy to the hashing B-splines, but the number of units allocated is between a factor of 2 and 8 smaller.

Table 3 shows the effectiveness of the ϵ novelty condition for on-line learning. When ϵ is set very low, the network performs very well, but is very large. Raising ϵ decreases the size of the network without substantially affecting the performance of the network. For $\epsilon > 0.05$, the network becomes very compact, but the accuracy becomes poor.

Figure 5 shows the output of the RAN after having learned the Mackey–Glass equation on-line. In the simulations, the network learns to roughly predict the time series quite rapidly. Notice in Figure 5a the

Table 3: Effectiveness of ϵ novelty condition.

ϵ	Number of units	Normalized rms error
0	189	0.055
0.01	174	0.050
0.02	143	0.054
0.05	50	0.071
0.10	26	0.102

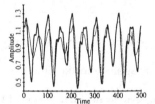 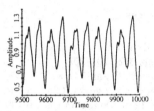

Figure 5: The output of the RAN as it learns on-line. The thick line is the output from the Mackey–Glass equation, the thin line is the prediction by the network. (a) The beginning of the learning. Very quickly, RAN picks up the basic oscillatory behavior of the Mackey–Glass equation. (b) The end of the on-line learning. At $T = 10,000$, the predictions match the actual output very well.

sudden jumps in the output of the network, which show that a new unit has been allocated. As more examples are shown, the network allocates more units and refines its predictions.

4 Conclusions

There are various desirable attributes for a network that learns: it should learn quickly, it should learn accurately, and it should form a compact representation. Formation of a compact representation is particularly important for networks that are implemented in hardware, because silicon area is at a premium. A compact representation is also important for statistical reasons: a network that has too many parameters can overfit data and generalize poorly.

Many previous network algorithms either learned quickly at the expense of a compact representation, or formed a compact representation only after laborious computation. The RAN is a network that can find a compact representation with a reasonable amount of computation.

Acknowledgments

Thanks to Carver Mead, Carl Ruoff, and Fernando Pineda for useful comments on the paper. Thanks to Glenn Gribble for helping to put the paper together. Special thanks to John Moody who not only provided useful comments on the paper, but also provided data on the hashing B-splines.

References

Baum, E. B. 1989. A proposal for more powerful learning algorithms. *Neural Comp.* **1**(2), 201–207.

Broomhead, D., and Lowe, D. 1988. Multivariable function interpolation and adaptive networks. *Complex Syst.* **2**, 321–355.

Judd, S. 1988. On the complexity of loading shallow neural networks. *J. Complex.* **4**, 177–192.

Lapedes, A., and Farber, R. 1987. *Nonlinear Signal Processing Using Neural Networks: Prediction and System Modeling.* Tech. Rep. LA-UR-87-2662, Los Alamos National Laboratory, Los Alamos, NM.

Lloyd, S. P. 1957. *Least Squares Quantization in PCM.* Bell Laboratories Internal Tech. Rep.

MacQueen, J. 1967. Some methods for classification and analysis of multivariate observations. In *Proceedings of the Fifth Berkeley Symposium on Mathematics, Statistics, and Probability*, L. M. LeCam and J. Neyman, eds., p. 281. University of California Press, Berkeley.

Moody, J., and Darken, C. 1988. Learning with localized receptive fields. In *Proceedings of the 1988 Connectionist Models Summer School*, D. Touretzky, G. Hinton, and T. Sejnowski, eds., pp. 133–143. Morgan-Kaufmann, San Mateo.

Moody, J., and Darken, C. 1989. Fast learning in networks of locally-tuned processing units. *Neural Comp.* **1**(2), 281–294.

Moody, J. 1989. Fast learning in multi-resolution hierarchies. In *Advances in Neural Information Processing Systems*, I, D. Touretzky, ed., pp. 29–39. Morgan-Kaufmann, San Mateo.

Poggio, T., and Girosi, F. 1990. Regularization algorithms for learning that are equivalent to multilayer networks. *Science* **247**, 978–982.

Powell, M. J. D. 1987. Radial basis functions for multivariable interpolation: A review. In *Algorithms for Approximation*, J. C. Mason and M. G. Cox, eds., pp. 143–167. Clarendon Press, Oxford.

Stark, L., Okajima, M., and Whipple, G. H. 1962. Computer pattern recognition techniques: Electrocardiographics diagnosis, *Commun. ACM* **5**, 527–532.

Widrow, B., and Hoff, M. 1960. Adaptive switching circuits. In *1960 IRE WESCON Convention Record*, pp. 96–104. IRE, New York.

20

Learning with Preknowledge:
Clustering with Point and Graph Matching Distance
Measures

Steven Gold
Department of Computer Science, Yale University,
New Haven, CT 06520-8285 USA

Anand Rangarajan
Department of Diagnostic Radiology, Yale University,
New Haven, CT 06520-8042 USA

Eric Mjolsness
Department of Computer Science and Engineering,
University of California at San Diego (UCSD),
La Jolla, CA 92093-0114 USA

Prior knowledge constraints are imposed upon a learning problem in
the form of distance measures. Prototypical 2D point sets and graphs
are learned by clustering with point-matching and graph-matching distance measures. The point-matching distance measure is approximately
invariant under affine transformations—translation, rotation, scale, and
shear—and permutations. It operates between noisy images with missing and spurious points. The graph-matching distance measure operates on weighted graphs and is invariant under permutations. Learning
is formulated as an optimization problem. Large objectives so formulated ($\sim$ million variables) are efficiently minimized using a combination of optimization techniques—softassign, algebraic transformations,
clocked objectives, and deterministic annealing.

1 Introduction

While few biologists today would subscribe to Locke's description of the
nascent mind as a tabula rasa, the nature of the inherent constraints—
Kant's preknowledge—that helps organize our perceptions remains much
in doubt. Recently, the importance of such preknowledge for learning
has been convincingly argued from a statistical framework (Geman *et al.*
1992). Several researchers have proposed that our minds may incorporate
preknowledge in the form of distance measures (Shepard 1989; Bienenstock and Doursat 1991). The neural network community has begun to

explore this idea via tangent distance (Simard *et al.* 1993) and model learning (Williams *et al.* 1993). However, neither of these distance measures has been invariant under permutation of the labeling of the feature points or nodes. Permutation-invariant distance measures must solve the correspondence problem, a computationally intractable problem fundamental to object recognition systems (Grimson 1990). Such distance measures may be better suited for the learning of the higher level, more complex representations needed for cognition. In this work, we introduce the use of more powerful, permutation-invariant distance measures in learning.

The unsupervised learning of object prototypes from collections of noisy 2D point-sets or noisy weighted graphs is achieved by clustering with point-matching and graph-matching distance measures. The point-matching measure is approximately invariant under permutations and affine transformations (separately decomposed into translation, rotation, scale, and shear) and operates on point-sets with missing or spurious points. The graph-matching measure is invariant under permutations. These distance measures and others like them may be constructed using Bayesian inference on a probabilistic model of the visual domain. Such models introduce a carefully designed bias into our learning, which reduces its generality outside the problem domain but increases its ability to generalize within the problem domain. From a statistical viewpoint, outside the problem domain it increases bias while within the problem domain it decreases variance. The resulting distance measures are similar to some of those hypothesized for cognition.

The distance measures and learning problem (clustering) are formulated as objective functions. Fast minimization of these objectives is achieved by a combination of optimization techniques—softassign, algebraic transformations, clocked objectives, and deterministic annealing. Combining these techniques significantly increases the size of problems that may be solved with recurrent network architectures (Rangarajan *et al.* 1996). Even on single-processor workstations, nonlinear objectives with a million variables can be minimized relatively quickly (a few hours). With these methods we learn prototypical examples of 2D point-sets and graphs from randomly generated experimental data.

2 Relationship to Previous Clustering Methods

Clustering algorithms may be classified as central or pairwise (Buhmann and Hofmann 1994). Central clustering algorithms generally use a distance measure, like Euclidean or Mahalonobis, that operates on feature vectors within a pattern matrix (Jain and Dubes 1988; Duda and Hart 1973). These algorithms calculate cluster centers (pattern prototypes) and compute the distances between patterns within a cluster and the cluster center (i.e., pattern–cluster center distances). Pairwise clustering algorithms, in contrast, may use only the distances between patterns and may operate on a proximity matrix (a precomputed matrix containing all the distances between every pair of patterns). Pairwise clustering algorithms need not produce a cluster center and do not have to recalculate distance measures during the algorithm.

We introduce central clustering algorithms that employ higher-level distance measures. In the few cases where higher-level distance measures have been used in clustering (Kurita *et al.* 1994) they have all, to our knowledge, been employed in pairwise clustering algorithms, which used precomputed proximity matrices and did not calculate prototypes. Consequently, while classification was learned the exemplars were not.

As is the case for central clustering algorithms, the algorithm employed here tries to minimize the cluster center–cluster member distances. However, because it uses complex distance measures it has an outer and inner loop. The outer loop uses the current values of the cluster center–cluster member distances to recompute assignments (reclassify). After reclassification, the inner loop recomputes the distance measures. The outer loop is similar to several other algorithms employing mean field approximations for clustering (Rose *et al.* 1990; Buhmann and Kuhnel 1993). It is also similar to fuzzy ISODATA clustering (Duda and Hart 1973), with annealing on the fuzziness parameter. The clustering algorithm used here is formulated as a combinatorial optimization problem, however, it may also be related to parameter estimation of mixture models using the maximum likelihood method (Duda and Hart 1973) and the expectation-maximization (EM) algorithm (Dempster *et al.* 1977; Hathaway 1986). The inner loop uses the newly discovered distance measures for point (Gold *et al.* 1995) and graph matching. In the following we will first describe these new distance measures and then show how they are incorporated in the rest of the algorithm.

3 Formulation of the Objective Functions

3.1 An Affine Invariant Point-Matching Distance Measure. The first distance measure quantifies the degree of dissimilarity between two unlabeled 2D point images, irrespective of bounded affine transformations, i.e., differences in position, orientation, scale, and shear. The two images may have a different number of points. The measure is calculated with an objective that can be used to find correspondence and pose for unlabeled feature matching in vision. Given two sets of points $\{X_j\}$ and $\{Y_k\}$, one can minimize the following objective to find the affine transformation and permutation that best maps some points of X onto some points of Y:

$$E_{pm}(m, t, A) = \sum_{j=1}^{J} \sum_{k=1}^{K} m_{jk} \|X_j - t - AY_k\|^2 + g(A) - \alpha \sum_{j=1}^{J} \sum_{k=1}^{K} m_{jk} \quad (3.1)$$

with constraints: $\forall j \sum_{k=1}^{K} m_{jk} \leq 1$, $\forall k \sum_{j=1}^{J} m_{jk} \leq 1$, $\forall jk \; m_{jk} \geq 0$ and

$$g(A) = \gamma a^2 + \kappa b^2 + \lambda c^2$$

A is the affine transformation, which is decomposed into scale, rotation, and two components of shear as follows:

$$A = s(a)R(\Theta)Sh_1(b)Sh_2(c)$$

where

$$s(a) \;\; = \;\; \begin{pmatrix} e^a & 0 \\ 0 & e^a \end{pmatrix} ,$$

$$Sh_1(b) \;\; = \;\; \begin{pmatrix} e^b & 0 \\ 0 & e^{-b} \end{pmatrix} ,$$

$$Sh_2(c) \;\; = \;\; \begin{pmatrix} \cosh(c) & \sinh(c) \\ \sinh(c) & \cosh(c) \end{pmatrix}$$

$R(\Theta)$ is the standard 2×2 rotation matrix. $g(A)$ serves to regularize the affine transformation by bounding the scale and shear components. m is a possibly fuzzy correspondence matrix that matches points in one image with corresponding points in the other image. The constraints on m ensure that each point in each image corresponds to at most one point in the other image. However, partial matches are allowed, in which case the sum of these partial matches may add up to no more than one. The inequality constraint on m permits a null match or multiple partial matches. [Note: simplex constraints on m, and its linear appearance in $E(m)$, imply that any local minimum of (m, A, t) occurs at a vertex in the m simplex. But m's trajectory can use the interior of the m simplex to avoid local minima in the optimization of A and t.]

The α term biases the objective toward matches. The decomposition of A in the above is not required, since A could be left as a 2×2 matrix and solved for directly in the algorithm that follows. The decomposition just provides for more precise regularization, i.e., specification of the likely kinds of transformations. Also $Sh_2(c)$ could be replaced by another rotation matrix, using the singular value decomposition of A.

Then given two sets of points $\{X_j\}$ and $\{Y_k\}$ the distance between them may be defined as

$$D(\{X_j\}, \{Y_k\}) = \min_{m,t,A}[E_{pm}(m, t, A) \mid \text{constraints on } m]$$

This measure is an example of a more general image distance measure derived from mean field theory assumptions in (Mjolsness 1993):

$$D(x, y) = - \log \frac{\Pr(x|y)}{\max_x \Pr(x|y)} \approx \min_T d[x, T(y)]$$

where

$$d(x,y) = -\log \frac{\hat{\mathrm{Pr}}(x|y)}{\max_x \hat{\mathrm{Pr}}(x,y)}$$

and T is a set of transformation parameters introduced by a visual grammar (Mjolsness 1994) and $\hat{\mathrm{Pr}}$ is the probability that x arises from y without transformations T.

We transform our inequality constraints into equality constraints by introducing slack variables, a standard technique from linear programming:

$$\forall j \sum_{k=1}^{K} m_{jk} \leq 1 \quad \rightarrow \quad \forall j \sum_{k=1}^{K+1} m_{jk} = 1$$

and likewise for our column constraints. An extra row and column is added to the permutation matrix m to hold our slack variables. These constraints are enforced by applying the Potts glass mean field theory approximations (Peterson and Soderberg 1989) and a Lagrange multiplier and then using an equivalent form of the resulting objective, which employs Lagrange multipliers and an $x \log x$ barrier function (Yuille and Kosowsky 1994; Rangarajan et al. 1996; Mjolsness and Garrett 1990):

$$
\begin{aligned}
E_{pm}(m,t,A) = & \sum_{j=1}^{J}\sum_{k=1}^{K} m_{jk}\|X_j - t - AY_k\|^2 + g(A) - \alpha \sum_{j=1}^{J}\sum_{k=1}^{K} m_{jk} \\
& + \frac{1}{\beta}\sum_{j=1}^{J+1}\sum_{k=1}^{K+1} m_{jk}(\log m_{jk} - 1) \\
& + \sum_{j=1}^{J}\mu_j\left(\sum_{k=1}^{K+1} m_{jk} - 1\right) + \sum_{k=1}^{K}\nu_k\left(\sum_{j=1}^{J+1} m_{jk} - 1\right) \quad (3.2)
\end{aligned}
$$

In this objective, we are looking for a saddle point. Equation 3.2 is minimized with respect to m, t, and A, that are the correspondence matrix, translation, and affine transform, and is maximized with respect to μ and ν, the Lagrange multipliers that enforce the row and column constraints for m. m is fuzzy, with the degree of fuzziness dependent on β.

The above defines a series of distance measures, since given the decomposition of A it is trivial to construct measures that are approximately invariant only under some subset of the transformations (such as rotation and translation). The regularization, $g(A)$, and α terms may also be individually adjusted in an appropriate fashion for a specific problem domain. For example, replacing A with $R(\Theta)$ in equation 3.1 and removing $g(A)$ would define a new distance measure, which is invariant only under rotation and translation.

3.2 Weighted Graph-Matching Distance Measures. The following distance measure quantifies the degree of dissimilarity between two unlabeled weighted graphs. Given two graphs, represented by adjacency matrices G_{jl} and g_{kp}, one can minimize the objective below to find the permutation which best maps G onto g (Rangarajan and Mjolsness 1994; von der Malsburg 1988; Hopfield and Tank 1986):

$$E_{gm}(m) = \sum_{j=1}^{J} \sum_{k=1}^{K} \left(\sum_{l=1}^{L} G_{jl}m_{lk} - \sum_{p=1}^{P} m_{jp}g_{pk} \right)^2$$

with constraints: $\forall j \; \sum_{k=1}^{K} m_{jk} = 1, \quad \forall k \; \sum_{j=1}^{J} m_{jk} = 1, \quad \forall jk \; m_{jk} \geq 0$. These constraints are enforced in the same fashion as in equation 3.2 with an $x \log x$ barrier function and Lagrange multipliers. The objective is simplified with a fixed point preserving transformation of the form $X^2 \rightarrow 2\sigma X - \sigma^2$. The additional variable (σ) introduced in such a transformation, described as a reversed neuron in Mjolsness and Garrett (1990), is similar to a Lagrange parameter. A self-amplification term is also added to push the match variables toward zero or one. This term (with the γ parameter below) is similarly transformed with a reversed neuron. The resulting objective is

$$\begin{aligned}
E_{gm}(m) = & \sum_{j=1}^{J} \sum_{k=1}^{K} \mu_{jk} \left(\sum_{l=1}^{L} G_{jl}m_{lk} - \sum_{p=1}^{P} m_{jp}g_{pk} \right) - \frac{1}{2} \sum_{j=1}^{J} \sum_{k=1}^{K} \mu_{jk}^2 \\
& -\gamma \sum_{j=1}^{J} \sum_{k=1}^{K} \sigma_{jk}m_{jk} + \frac{\gamma}{2} \sum_{j=1}^{J} \sum_{k=1}^{K} \sigma_{jk}^2 \\
& +\frac{1}{\beta} \sum_{j=1}^{J} \sum_{k=1}^{K} m_{jk}(\log m_{jk} - 1) \\
& +\sum_{j=1}^{J} \kappa_j \left(\sum_{k=1}^{K} m_{jk} - 1 \right) + \sum_{k=1}^{K} \lambda_k \left(\sum_{j=1}^{J} m_{jk} - 1 \right)
\end{aligned} \tag{3.3}$$

As in Section 2.1, we look for a saddle point. Equation 3.3 is minimized with respect to m and σ, which are the correspondence matrix and reversed neuron of the transform, and is maximized with respect to κ, λ, and μ, the Lagrange multipliers that enforce the row and column constraints for m and the reversed neuron parameter enforcing the first fixed point transformation. m may be fuzzy, so a given vertex in one graph may partially match several vertices in the other graph, with the degree of fuzziness dependent upon β; however, the self-amplification term dramatically reduces the fuzziness at high β.

A second, functionally equivalent, graph-matching objective is also used in the clustering problem (as explained in Section 3.3):

$$E_{gm'}(m) = \sum_{j=1}^{J} \sum_{l=1}^{L} \sum_{k=1}^{K} \sum_{p=1}^{P} m_{jk}m_{lp}(G_{jl} - g_{kp})^2 \tag{3.4}$$

with constraints: $\forall j \; \sum_{k=1}^{K} m_{jk} = 1, \quad \forall k \; \sum_{j=1}^{J} m_{jk} = 1, \quad \forall jk \; m_{jk} \geq 0$.

3.3 The Clustering Objective. The object learning problem is formulated as follows: Given a set of I noisy observations $\{X_i\}$ of some unknown objects, find a set of B cluster centers $\{Y_b\}$ and match variables $\{M_{ib}\}$ defined as

$$M_{ib} = \begin{cases} 1 & \text{if } X_i \text{ is in } Y_b\text{'s cluster} \\ 0 & \text{otherwise} \end{cases}$$

such that each observation is in only one cluster, and the total distance of all the observations from their respective cluster centers is minimized. The cluster centers are the learned approximations of the original objects. To find $\{Y_b\}$ and $\{M_{ib}\}$ minimize the cost function,

$$E_{\text{cluster}}(Y, M) = \sum_{i=1}^{I} \sum_{b=1}^{B} M_{ib} D(X_i, Y_b)$$

with constraints: $\forall i \sum_b M_{ib} = 1$, $\forall ib \; M_{ib} \geq 0$. $D(X_i, Y_b)$, the distance function, is a measure of dissimilarity between two objects. This problem formulation may be derived from Bayesian inference of a set of object models $\{Y\}$ from the data $\{X\}$ they explain (Mjolsness 1993). It is also a clustering objective with a domain-specific distance measure (Gold *et al.* 1994).

The constraints on M are enforced in a manner similar to that described for the distance measure, except that now only the rows of the matrix M need to add to one, instead of both the rows and the columns. The Potts glass mean field theory method is applied and an equivalent form of the resulting objective is used:

$$\begin{aligned} E_{\text{cluster}}(Y, M) &= \sum_{i=1}^{I} \sum_{b=1}^{B} M_{ib} D(X_i, Y_b) + \frac{1}{\beta_M} \sum_{i=1}^{I} \sum_{b=1}^{B} M_{ib}(\log M_{ib} - 1) \\ &+ \sum_{i=1}^{I} \lambda_i \left(\sum_{b=1}^{B} M_{ib} - 1 \right) \end{aligned} \tag{3.5}$$

Here, the objects are point-sets or weighted graphs. If point-sets are used, the distance measure $D(X_i, Y_b)$ is replaced by equation 3.1; if graphs are used it is replaced by equation 3.3, without the terms that enforce the constraints, or equation 3.4. For example, after replacing the distance measure by equation 3.1, we obtain

$$\begin{aligned} E_{\text{cluster}}(Y, M, t, A, m) &= \sum_{i=1}^{I} \sum_{b=1}^{B} M_{ib} \\ &\times \left[\sum_{j=1}^{J} \sum_{k=1}^{K} m_{ibjk}(\|X_{ij} - t_{ib} - A_{ib}Y_{bk}\|^2 - \alpha) + g(A_{ib}) \right] \\ &+ \sum_{i=1}^{I} \sum_{b=1}^{B} \left[\frac{1}{\beta_m} \sum_{j=1}^{J+1} \sum_{k=1}^{K+1} m_{ibjk}(\log m_{ibjk} - 1) \right] \end{aligned}$$

$$+ \sum_{j=1}^{J} \mu_{ibj} \left(\sum_{k=1}^{K+1} m_{ibjk} - 1 \right)$$

$$+ \sum_{k=1}^{K} \nu_{ibk} \left(\sum_{j=1}^{J+1} m_{ibjk} - 1 \right) \Bigg]$$

$$+ \frac{1}{\beta_M} \sum_{i=1}^{I} \sum_{b=1}^{B} M_{ib} (\log M_{ib} - 1)$$

$$+ \sum_{i=1}^{I} \lambda_i \left(\sum_{b=1}^{B} M_{ib} - 1 \right) \tag{3.6}$$

A saddle point is required. The objective is minimized with respect to Y, M, m, t, and A, which are, respectively, the cluster centers, the cluster membership matrix, the correspondence matrices, the translations, and other affine transformations. It is maximized with respect to λ, which enforces the row constraints for M, and μ and ν, which enforce the column and row constraints for m. M is a cluster membership matrix, indicating for each object i which cluster b it falls in, and m_{ib} is a permutation matrix that assigns to each point in cluster center Y_b a corresponding point in observation X_i. (A_{ib}, t_{ib}) gives the affine transform between object i and cluster center b. Both M and m are fuzzy, so a given object may partially fall in several clusters, with the degree of fuzziness depending on β_m and β_M.

Therefore, given a set of observations, X, we construct E_{cluster} and upon finding the appropriate saddle point of that objective, we will have Y, their cluster centers, and M, their cluster memberships.

An objective similar to equation 3.6 may be constructed using the graph-matching distance measure in equations 3.3 or 3.4 instead.

4 The Algorithm

4.1 Overview—Clocked Objective Functions.

The algorithm to minimize the clustering objectives consists of two loops—an inner loop to minimize the distance measure objective (either equation 3.2 or 3.3) and an outer loop to minimize the clustering objective (equation 3.5). Using coordinate descent in the outer loop results in dynamics similar to the EM algorithm for clustering (Hathaway 1986). The EM algorithm has been similarly used in supervised learning (Jordan and Jacobs 1994). All variables occurring in the distance measure objective are held fixed during this phase. The inner loop uses coordinate ascent/descent, which results in repeated row and column normalizations for m. This is described as a softassign (Gold et al. 1995; Gold and Rangarajan 1996; Rangarajan et al. 1996) (see Section 4.2). The minimization of m, and the distance measure variables (either t, A of equation 3.2 or μ, σ of equation 3.3), occurs in an incremental fashion—that is, their values are saved after each inner loop call from within the outer loop and are then used as initial values for the next call to the inner loop. This tracking of the values of the distance measure variables in the inner loop is essential to the efficiency of the algorithm since it greatly speeds up each inner loop optimization. Most coordinate ascent/descent phases are computed analytically, further speeding up the algorithm. Some poor local minima are avoided by deterministic annealing in both the outer and inner loops.

The resulting dynamics can be concisely expressed by formulating the objective as a clocked objective function (Mjolsness and Miranker 1993), which is optimized over distinct sets of variables in phases, as [letting $\mathcal{D}$ be the set of distance measure variables (e.g., $\{A,t\}$ for equation 3.2) excluding the match matrix],

$$E_{\text{clocked}} = E_{\text{cluster}} \left\langle \left\langle \left\langle (\mu, m)^A, (\nu, m)^A \right\rangle_\oplus, \mathcal{D} \right\rangle_\oplus, (\lambda, M)^A, Y^A \right\rangle_\oplus$$

with this special notation employed recursively: $E\langle x, y \rangle_\oplus$, coordinate descent on x, then y, iterated (if necessary); x^A, use analytic solution for x phase.

The algorithm can be expressed less concisely in English, as follows:

Initialize $\mathcal{D}$ to the equivalent of an identity transform, Y to random values
Begin Outer Loop
  Begin Inner Loop
  Initialize $\mathcal{D}$ with previous values
  Find m, $\mathcal{D}$ for each ib pair :
   Find m by softassign
   Find $\mathcal{D}$ by coordinate descent
  End Inner Loop
  If first time through outer loop increase β_m and repeat inner loop
  Find M,Y using fixed values of m, $\mathcal{D}$, determined in inner loop:
   Find M by softmax, across i
   Find Y by coordinate descent
  increase β_M, β_m
End Outer Loop

When the distances are calculated for all the X–Y pairs the first time through the outer loop, annealing is needed to minimize the objectives accurately. However, on each succeeding iteration, since good initial estimates are available for $\mathcal{D}$ (namely the values from the previous iteration of the outer loop), annealing is unnecessary and the minimization is much faster.

The speed of the above algorithm is increased by not recalculating the X–Y distance for a given ib pair when its M_{ib} membership variable drops below a threshold.

4.2 Inner Loop. The inner loop proceeds in two phases. In phase one, while $\mathcal{D}$ are held fixed, m is initialized with a coordinate descent

step, described below, and then iteratively normalized across its rows
and columns until the procedure converges (Kosowsky and Yuille 1994).
This phase is analogous to a softmax update, except that instead of enforcing a one-way, winner-take-all (maximum) constraint, a two-way, assignment constraint is being enforced. Therefore, we describe this phase
as a softassign (Gold *et al.* 1995; Gold and Rangarajan 1996; Rangarajan
et al. 1996). In phase two m is held fixed and $\mathcal{D}$ are updated using coordinate descent. Then β_m is increased and the loop repeats. Let E_{dmwc} be the
distance measure objective (equations 3.2 or 3.3) without the terms that
enforce the constraints (i.e., the $x \log x$ barrier function and the Lagrange
parameters).

In phase one m is updated with a softassign, which consists of a
coordinate descent update:

$$m_{ibjk} = \exp[-\beta_m \partial E_{dmwc}(X_i, Y_b)/\partial m_{ibjk}]$$

And then (also as part of the softassign) m is iteratively normalized across
j and k until $\sum_{j=1}^{J} \sum_{k=1}^{K} |\Delta m_{ibjk}| < \epsilon$:

$$m_{ibjk} = \frac{m_{ibjk}}{\sum_{j'=1}^{J+1} m_{ibj'k}} \; ; \qquad m_{ibjk} = \frac{m_{ibjk}}{\sum_{k'=1}^{K+1} m_{ibjk'}}$$

Using coordinate descent, the $\mathcal{D}$ are updated in phase two. If a member
of $\mathcal{D}$ cannot be computed analytically (such as the terms of A that are
regularized), Newton's method is used to compute the root of the func-
tion. So if d_n is the nth member of $\mathcal{D}$ then in phase two we update d_{ibn}
such that

$$\frac{\partial E_{dmwc}(X_i, Y_b)}{\partial d_{ibn}} \approx 0$$

Finally β_m is increased and the loop repeats.

By setting the partial derivatives of E_{dm} to zero and initializing the
Lagrange parameters to zero, the algorithm for phase one may be derived
(Rangarajan *et al.* 1996).

Beginning with a small β_m allows minimization over a fuzzy correspondence matrix m, for which a global minimum is easier to find.
Raising β_m drives the ms closer to 0 or 1, as the algorithm approaches a
saddle point.

4.3 Outer Loop. The outer loop proceeds in three phases: (1) distances are calculated by calling the inner loop, (2) M is projected across
b using the softmax function, (3) coordinate descent is used to update Y.
Therefore, using softmax, M is updated in phase two:

$$M_{ib} = \frac{\exp[-\beta_M D(X_i, Y_b)]}{\sum_{b'=1}^{B} \exp[-\beta_M D(X_i, Y_{b'})]} \tag{4.1}$$

Y, in phase three, is calculated using coordinate descent. Let y_n be the nth member of $\{Y\}$. y_n is updated such that

$$\frac{\partial E_{\text{cluster}}}{\partial y_{bn}} = 0 \tag{4.2}$$

Then β_M is increased and the loop repeats.

When learning prototypical point-sets, y_{bn} in equation 4.1 will be either the x or y coordinate of a point in the prototype (cluster center). If weighted graphs are being learned then y_{bn} will be a link in the cluster center graph. When clustering graphs, equation 3.3 is used for the distance in equation 4.1 while equation 3.4 is used to calculate y_{bn} in equation 4.2. This results in a faster calculation of equation 4.1, but for equation 4.2 results in an easy analytic solution.

5 Methods and Experimental Results

Five series of experiments were run to evaluate the learning algorithms. Point sets were clustered in four experiments and weighted graphs were clustered in the fifth. In each experiment, a set of object models was used. In one experiment handwritten character data were used for the object models and in the other experiments the object models were randomly generated. From each object model, a set of object observations was created by transforming the object model according to the problem domain assumed for that experiment. For example, an object represented by points in two-dimensional space was translated, rotated, scaled, sheared, and permuted to form a new point set. An object represented by a weighted graph was permuted. Independent noise of known variance was added to all real-valued parameters to further distort the object. Parts of the object were deleted and spurious features (points) were added. In this manner, from a set of object models, a larger number of object instances were created. Then, with no knowledge of the original object models or cluster memberships, we clustered the object instances using the algorithms described above.

The bulk of our experimental trials were on randomly generated patterns. However, to clearly demonstrate our methods and visually display our results, we will first report the results of the experiment in which we used handwritten character models.

5.1 Handwritten Character Models.
An X-windows tool was used to draw handwritten characters with a mouse on a writing pad. The contours of the images were discretized and expressed as a set of points in the plane. Twenty-five points for each character were used. The four characters used as models are displayed in row 1 of Figure 1. Each character model was transformed in the manner described above to create 32

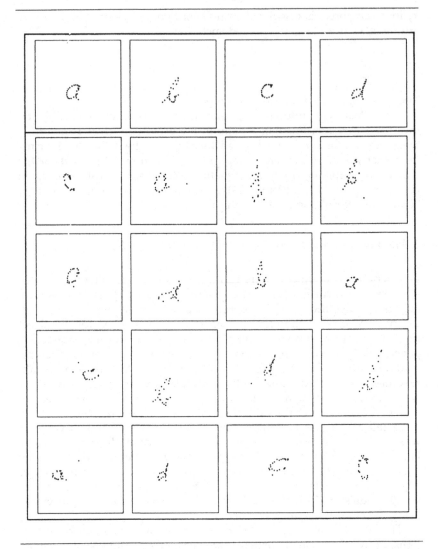

Figure 1: Row (1): Handwritten character models used to generate character instances. These models were not part of the input to the clustering algorithm. Rows (2–5): 16 character instances that (with 112 other characters) were clustered.

character instances (128 characters for all four). Specifically (in units normalized approximately to the height of b in Fig. 1): $\mathcal{N}(0, 0.02)$ of gaussian noise was added to each point. Each point had a 10% probability of being deleted and a 5% probability of generating a spurious point. The components of the affine transformation were selected from a uniform distribution within the following bounds; translation: ±0.5, rotation: $\pm27°$, $\log(scale)$: $\pm\log(0.7)$, $\log(vertical\ shear)$: $\pm\log(0.7)$, and $\log(oblique\ shear)$: $\pm\log(0.7)$. Note in equation 3.1, $a = \log(scale)$, $b = \log(vertical\ shear)$, and $c = \log(oblique\ shear)$. In rows 2–5 of Figure 1, 16 of the 128 characters generated are displayed. The clustering algorithm using the affine distance measure of Section 2.1 was run with the 128 characters as input and no knowledge of the cluster memberships. Figure 2 shows the results after 0, 4, 16, 64, 128, and 256 iterations of the algorithm. Note that the initial cluster center configurations (row 1 of Fig. 2) were selected at random from a uniform distribution over a unit square. The original models were reconstructed to high accuracy from the data, up to affine transformations within the allowed ranges.

5.2 Randomly Generated Models. In the next four experiments, the object models (corresponding to the models in Row 1 of Fig. 1) were generated at random. The results were evaluated by comparing the object prototypes (cluster centers) formed by each experimental run to the object models used to generate the object instances for that experiment. The distance measures used in the clustering were used for this comparison, i.e., to calculate the distance between the learned prototype and the original object. This distance measure also incorporates the transformations used to create the object instances. The mean and standard deviations of these distances were plotted (Fig. 3) over hundreds of trials, varying the object instance generation noise. The straight line appearing on each graph displays the effect of the gaussian noise only. It is the expected object model–object prototype distance if no transformations were applied, no features were deleted or added, and the cluster memberships of the object instances were known. It serves as an absolute lower bound on the accuracy of our learning algorithm. The variance of the real–valued parameter noise was increased in each series of trials until the curve flattened—that is, the object instances became so distorted by noise that no information about the original objects could be recovered by the algorithm.

In the first experiment (Fig. 3a), point set objects were translated, rotated, scaled, and permuted. Initial object models were created by selecting points with a uniform distribution within a unit square. The transformations to create the object instance were selected with a uniform distribution within the following bounds; translation: ±0.5, rotation: $\pm27°$, $\log(scale)$: $\pm\log(0.5)$. For example, within these bounds the largest object instances that are generated may be four times the size of the smallest. One hundred object instances were generated from 10 object models. All objects contained 20 points. The standard deviation of the gaussian noise was varied from 0.02 to 0.16 in steps of 0.02. At each noise level, there were 15 trials. The data point at each error bar represents 150 distances (15 trials times 10 model–prototype distances for each trial).

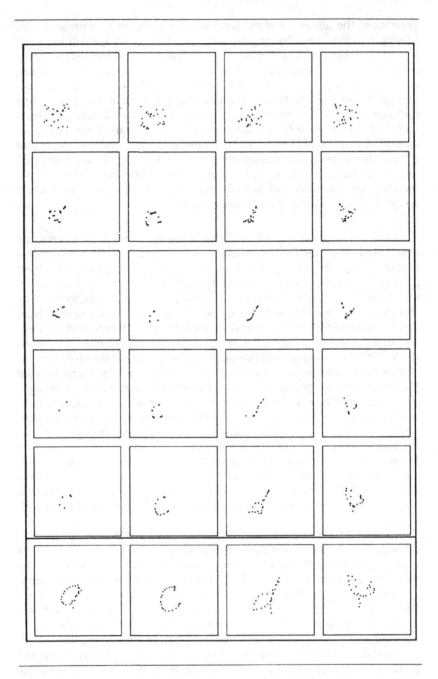

Figure 2: Row (1): initial cluster centers (randomly generated). Rows (2–6): character prototypes (cluster centers) after 4, 16, 64, 128, and 256 iterations.

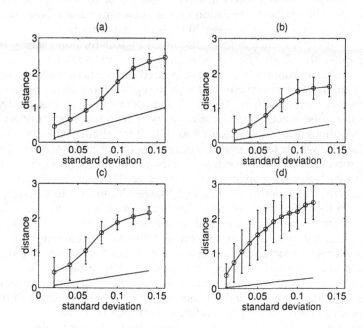

Figure 3: (a) Ten clusters, 100 point sets, 20 points each, scale, rotation, translation, 120 trials; (b) 4 clusters, 64 point sets, 15 points each, affine, 10% deleted,
5% spurious, 140 trials; (c) 8 clusters, 256 point sets, 20 points each, affine, 10%
deleted, 5% spurious, 70 trials; (d) 4 clusters, 64 graphs, 10 nodes each, 360
trials.

In the second and third experiments (Fig. 3b and c), point set objects
were translated, rotated, scaled, sheared (both components), and permuted. Each object point had a 10% probability of being deleted and a
5% probability of generating a spurious point. Object points and transformations were randomly generated as in the first experiment, except
for these bounds; $\log(scale)$: $\pm \log(0.7)$, $\log(vertical\ shear)$: $\pm \log(0.7)$, and
$\log(oblique\ shear)$: $\pm \log(0.7)$. In experiment 2, 64 object instances and 4
object models of 15 points each were used. In experiment 3, 256 object
instances and 8 object models of 20 points each were used. Noise levels
as in experiment 1 were used. Twenty trials were run at each noise level
in experiment 2 and 10 trials run at each noise level in experiment 3.

    In the fourth experiment (Fig. 3d), object models were represented by
fully connected weighted graphs. The link weights in the initial object
models were selected with a uniform distribution between 0 and 1. The
objects were then randomly permuted to form the object instance and
uniform noise was added to the link weights. Sixty-four object instances

were generated from 4 object models consisting of 10 node graphs with 100 links. The standard deviation of the noise was varied from 0.01 to 0.12 in steps of 0.01. There were 30 trials at each noise level.

In most experiments, at low noise levels ($\leq$ 0.06 for point sets, $\leq$ 0.03 for graphs), the object prototypes learned were very similar to the object models. As an example of what the plotted distances mean in terms of visual similarity, the average model–prototype distance in the handwritten character example (row 1 of Fig. 1 and row 6 of Fig. 2) was 0.5. Even at higher noise levels, object prototypes similar to the object models are formed, though less consistently. Results from about 700 experiments are plotted, which took several thousand hours of SGI R4400 workstation processor time. The objective for experiment 3 contained close to one million variables and converged in about 4 hr. The convergence times of the objectives of experiments 1, 2, and 4 were 120, 40, and 10 min, respectively. In these experiments the temperature parameter of the inner loop equaled the temperature parameter of the outer loop ($\beta_m = \beta_M$) and both were increased by a factor of 1.03 on each iteration of the outer loop. In the point set experiments, each trial was a best of four series. The object models and object instances were the same for each of the four executions within the trial, but the initial randomly selected starting cluster centers (Row 1 of Fig. 2) were varied for each execution and only the result from the execution with the lowest ending energy was reported.

The time for recognition, which simply involved running the distance measures alone, was at most a few seconds for the largest point-sets, which contained 25 points.

6 Conclusions

It has long been argued by many that learning in complex domains typically associated with human intelligence requires some type of prior structure or knowledge. We have begun to develop a set of tools that will allow the incorporation of prior structure within learning. Our models incorporate many features needed in complex domains like vision: parameter noise, missing and spurious features, nonrigid transformations. They can learn objects with inherent structure, like graphs. Many experiments have been run on experimentally generated data sets. Several directions for future research hold promise. One might be the learning of OCR data. Second, a supervised learning stage could be added to our algorithms, i.e., we may include some prior knowledge regarding the classification or labeling of our objects. While the experiments in this paper incorporated only a few missing points within the object sets, the point-matching distance measures are capable of matching objects arising from real image data with large amounts of occlusion and with feature points that do not necessarily lie in one-to-one correspondence with each other as did the artificially generated point sets of this paper (Gold *et al.*

1995). Supervised learning algorithms may be better able to exploit the power of these distance measures. Finally, more powerful, recently developed graph-matching distance measures (Gold and Rangarajan 1996) may be used that are able to operate on graphs with attributed nodes, multiple link types, and deleted or spurious nodes and links.

Acknowledgments

This work has been supported by AFOSR Grant F49620-92-J-0465 and ONR/DARPA Grant N00014-92-J-4048 and the Yale Neuroengineering and Neuroscience Center.

References

Bienenstock, E., and Doursat, R. 1991. Issues of representation in neural networks. In *Representations of Vision: Trends and Tacit Assumptions in Vision Research*, A. Gorea, ed. Cambridge University Press, Cambridge, England.

Buhmann, J., and Hofmann, T. 1994. Central and pairwise data clustering by competitive neural networks. In *Advances in Neural Information Processing Systems 6*, J. Cowan, G. Tesauro, and J. Alspector, eds., pp. 104–111. Morgan Kaufmann, San Mateo, CA.

Buhmann, J., and Kuhnel, H. 1993. Complexity optimized data clustering by competitive neural networks. *Neural Comp.* 5(1), 75–88.

Dempster, A. P., Laird, N. M., and Rubin, D. B. 1977. Maximum likelihood from incomplete data via the EM algorithm. *J. R. Statist. Soc. Ser. B* 39, 1–38.

Duda, R., and Hart, P. 1973. *Pattern Classification and Scene Analysis*. John Wiley, New York.

Geman, S., Bienenstock, E., and Doursat, R. 1992. Neural networks and the bias/variance dilemma. *Neural Comp.* 4(1), 1–58.

Gold, S., and Rangarajan, A. 1996. A Graduated Assignment Algorithm for Graph Matching. *IEEE Trans. Patt. Anal. Mach. Intell.* (In press.)

Gold, S., Mjolsness, E., and Rangarajan, A. 1994. Clustering with a domain specific distance measure. In *Advances in Neural Information Processing Systems 6*, J. Cowan, G. Tesauro, and J. Alspector, eds., pp. 96–103. Morgan Kaufmann, San Mateo, CA.

Gold, S., Lu, C. P., Rangarajan, A., Pappu, S., and Mjolsness, E. 1995. New algorithms for 2-D and 3-D point matching: Pose estimation and correspondence. In *Advances in Neural Information Processing Systems 7*, G. Tesauro, D. S. Touretzky, and T. K. Leen, eds., pp. 957–964. MIT Press, Cambridge, MA.

Grimson, E. 1990. *Object Recognition by Computer: The Role of Geometric Constraints*. MIT Press, Cambridge, MA.

Hathaway, R. 1986. Another interpretation of the EM algorithm for mixture distributions. *Statist. Probability Lett.* 4, 53–56.

Hopfield, J. J., and Tank, D. W. 1986. Collective computation with continuous variables. In *Disordered Systems and Biological Organization*, pp. 155–170. Springer-Verlag, Berlin.

Jain, A. K., and Dubes, R. C. 1988. *Algorithms for Clustering Data*. Prentice-Hall, Englewood Cliffs, NJ.

Jordan, M. I., and Jacobs, R. A. 1994. Hierarchical mixtures of experts and the EM algorithm. *Neural Comp.* 6(2), 181–214.

Kosowsky, J. J., and Yuille, A. L. 1994. The invisible hand algorithm: Solving the assignment problem with statistical physics. *Neural Networks* 7(3), 477–490.

Kurita, T., Sekita, I., and Otsu, N. 1994. Invariant distance measures for planar shapes based on complex autoregressive model. *Patt. Recogn.* 27(7), 903–911.

Mjolsness, E. 1993. Bayesian inference on visual grammars by relaxation nets. Unpublished manuscript.

Mjolsness, E. 1994. Connectionist grammars for high-level vision. In *Artificial Intelligence and Neural Networks: Steps Toward Principled Integration*, V. Honavar, and L. Uhr, eds., pp. 423–451. Academic Press, San Diego, CA.

Mjolsness, E., and Garrett, C. 1990. Algebraic transformations of objective functions. *Neural Networks* 3, 651–669.

Mjolsness, E., and Miranker, W. 1993. *Greedy Lagrangians for Neural Networks: Three Levels of Optimization in Relaxation Dynamics*. Tech. Rep. YALEU/DCS/TR-945, Department of Computer Science, Yale University.

Peterson, C., and Soderberg, B. 1989. A new method for mapping optimization problems onto neural networks. *Int. J. Neural Syst.* 1(1), 3–22.

Rangarajan, A., and Mjolsness, E. 1994. A Lagrangian relaxation network for graph matching. In *IEEE International Conference on Neural Networks (ICNN)*, Vol. 7, pp. 4629–4634. IEEE Press, New York.

Rangarajan, A., Gold, S., and Mjolsness, E. 1996. A novel optimizing network architecture with applications. *Neural Comp.* (in press).

Rose, K., Gurewitz, E., and Fox, G. 1990. Statistical mechanics and phase transitions in clustering. *Phys. Rev. Lett.* 65(8), 945–948.

Shepard, R. 1989. Internal representation of universal algorithms: A challenge for connectionism. In *Neural Connections, Mental Computation*, L. Nadel, L. Cooper, P. Culicover, and R. Harnish, eds., pp. 104–134. Bradford/MIT Press, Cambridge, MA.

Simard, P., le Cun, Y., and Denker, J. 1993. Efficient pattern recognition using a new transformation distance. In *Advances in Neural Information Processing Systems 5*, S. Hanson, J. Cowan, and C. Giles, eds., pp. 50–58. Morgan Kaufmann, San Mateo, CA.

von der Malsburg, C. 1988. Pattern recognition by labeled graph matching. *Neural Networks*, 1, 141–148.

Williams, C., Zemel, R., and Mozer, M. 1993. *Unsupervised Learning of Object Models*. Tech. Rep. AAAI Tech. Rep. FSS-93-04, Department of Computer Science, University of Toronto.

Yuille, A. L., and Kosowsky, J. J. 1994. Statistical physics algorithms that converge. *Neural Comp.* 6(3), 341–356.

21

Learning to Generalize from Single Examples in the Dynamic Link Architecture

Wolfgang Konen
Christoph von der Malsburg
Institut für Neuroinformatik, Ruhr-Universität Bochum, Germany

A large attraction of neural systems lies in their promise of replacing programming by learning. A problem with many current neural models is that with realistically large input patterns learning time explodes. This is a problem inherent in a notion of learning that is based almost entirely on statistical estimation. We propose here a different learning style where significant relations in the input pattern are recognized and expressed by the unsupervised self-organization of dynamic links. The power of this mechanism is due to the very general a priori principle of conservation of topological structure. We demonstrate that style with a system that learns to classify mirror symmetric pixel patterns from single examples.

1 Introduction

Learning is the ability of animals and humans to absorb structure from one scene and apply it to others. The literal storage of whole sensory input fields is of little value since scenes never recur in all detail within our lifetime. Essential for learning is therefore the ability to extract significant patterns from an input field containing mostly patterns with accidental feature constellations, and to apply those significant patterns to the interpretation of later scenes.

How can significant patterns be identified? Theories of learning based on layered neural networks [e.g., backpropagation of errors (Rosenblatt 1962, Rumelhart *et al.* 1986) or the Boltzmann Machine (Ackley *et al.* 1985)] are based on the notion that significant patterns are, above all, recurring patterns. Such systems have an input layer, an output layer, and hidden units. During a learning phase, many examples are presented to input layer and output layer, and the system is enabled by some plasticity mechanism to pick up and represent patterns that recur with statistical significance in the input training set. This method of identifying significant patterns may be the obvious one—going back to the original definition of significance based on recurrence—but with realistic inputs taken from natural environments it is far too costly, in terms of the number of inputs required to discriminate significant patterns from accidental

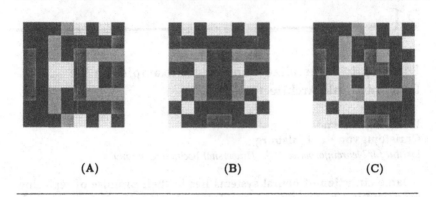

(A)　　　　　　　　　(B)　　　　　　　　　(C)

Figure 1: Symmetrical pixel patterns. Input patterns are arrays of $N \times N$ pixels, here $N = 8$. Pixel a has gray level feature value $F_a \in \{1, \ldots, F_{max}\}$. In most of our simulations, $F_{max} = 10$. In each input image, pixel values are random, but equal for points symmetrical with respect to one of three axes: (A) horizontal, (B) vertical, (C) diagonal. The system has to solve the task of assigning input patterns to classes according to these symmetries, and to learn this performance from examples.

patterns. The reason for this difficulty lies in the combinatorial explosion in the number of subsets that can be selected from large input fields (there are, for instance, 10^{3432} possible subsets of size 1000 in a set of 10^6). Among those subsets there are only relatively few of significant interest (in vision, for example, the criterion of spatial continuity alone singles out relatively very few subsets). There obviously are potent methods, presumably based on a priori knowledge built into the system, to extract significant patterns from a scene.

It is generally recognized that methods based purely on scene statistics must be complemented (if not supplanted) by more powerful ones based on a priori structure. One widespread piece of advice is to use input representations that are already adapted to the problem at hand. Down that alley there is, of course, the pitfall of hand-wiring instead of learning the essential structure. The real challenge is to find simple and general architectures that can handle large classes of problems and that can learn with a minimum of scene statistics.

The particular problem we are considering here has originally been proposed by Sejnowski *et al.* (1986). It consists in learning to classify mirror-symmetrical pixel patterns (see Fig. 1). The authors solved the problem with the help of scene statistics. Their system, consisting of a layer of 12 hidden units and 3 output units corresponding to the 3 symmetry classes, learned as a Boltzmann Machine, which is a variant of supervised learning. With input arrays of 10×10 pixels the system needed about 40,000 training examples in order to reach a success level of 85%.

The system (Sejnowski *et al.* 1986) demonstrates the strength and the weakness of statistical pattern classification. The strength is full generality with respect to possible patterns. This is best demonstrated with the thought experiment of applying a permutation to the pixels in the input field—the same permutation to all patterns presented. The system would now have the same learning performance, in spite of the complete destruction of topological structure. The weakness is an explosion in the number of examples required when scaling to larger input arrays. This weakness the system shares with a wide class of learning algorithms, which all are based on the statistical detection of classes as clusters in input space and their subsequent representation by single prototypes. Prominent examples are the k-nearest neighbor (kNN) algorithm (Fix and Hodges 1951; Cover and Hart 1967), the RCE algorithm (Reilly *et al.* 1982), which is a neural version of kNN, and adaptive vector quantization (LVQ, LVQ2) (Kohonen *et al.* 1988). None of those algorithms can easily deal with the symmetry classification problem. The reason is that already with modest problem size there are astronomically many patterns in a symmetry class (10^{32} for the 8×8 pixels of 10 features each in Fig. 1) and that these do not form clusters in input space and thus cannot be detected in a small training set. It is this that leads to the exploding thirst in learning time and number of prototypes.

Our treatment of the problem is based on the Dynamic Link Architecture (DLA) (von der Malsburg 1981). The strength of the DLA essential in the present context is its ability to detect pattern correspondences. An application of this ability to the problem of invariant pattern recognition has been reported previously (Bienenstock and von der Malsburg 1987; von der Malsburg 1988; Lades *et al.* 1993). Here we demonstrate that with it symmetry classes can be recorded from single examples for later recognition. Our treatment is based on the a priori restriction that significant relations within the input pattern are those which preserve topological structure. It is in this sense less general than the Boltzmann Machine, not being able to deal with the permutation symmetries mentioned above. On the other hand its extreme speed of adaptation to new symmetries makes it more potent than the Boltzmann Machine. Most of what is achieved in other neural systems with the help of statistical learning is performed here by the self-organization of an explicit representation of the symmetry in the input pattern.

2 Symmetry Detection by Dynamic Link Matching—Qualitative Model

Dynamic link matching is capable of finding and representing topological, feature-preserving mappings between parts of the input plane.

Such mappings are systems of pair-wise links that are neighborhood-preserving and that connect pairs of points with the same local properties in the input pattern. In this section we describe the network and its function qualitatively and establish its relationships to other, previously published models (von der Malsburg 1988; Bienenstock and von der Malsburg 1987; Buhmann et al. 1989; Lades et al. 1993; von der Malsburg and Buhmann 1992), and to the circuitry of cortical structures. In the next section we will describe an explicit quantitative, though somewhat simplified, model.

The network resembles primary visual cortex in representing visual images in a columnar fashion: Each resolution unit ("pixel") of the sensory surface is subserved by a collection ("column") of neurons, each neuron reacting to a different local feature. (In our concrete model, local features will simply be gray values. In a more realistic version, features would refer to texture, color, and the like.) There are intracolumnar connections, whose function will be explained below, and intercolumnar connections. The latter are what we will refer to as "dynamic links," are of rather large range in visual space, and are restricted to pairs of neurons with the same feature type. (In our explicit model the connections will run between cells responding to the same gray value in the image.) When a pattern is presented as visual input, those neurons in a column are selected that code for a feature that is present in the corresponding pixel. We refer to the selected cells as "preactivated" neurons. The set of all preactivated neurons represents the input image.

During the presentation of an image, the preactivated cells are actually not allowed to fire all at the same time. Rather, activity in the network takes the form of a sequence of "blob activations." During a blob activation, only those preactivated neurons are permitted to fire that lie in a group of neighboring columns. A blob activation corresponds to the "flash of the searchlight of focal attention" discussed, for instance, by Crick (Crick 1984). In the absence of any other control of attention, blob activations are created spontaneously in random positions in a rapid sequence of "cycles."

When a blob is active, its active cells send out signals that excite preactivated neurons of the same feature type in other locations. Thus, within the total network those preactivated neurons are excited whose type is represented in the active blob. Most of these cells form a diffuse spray over the image domain. If there is a symmetry in the image, however, there will be a location where all the feature types in the active blob are assembled locally again. With appropriate dynamics, those neurons are activated as well, forming a "shadow blob." The network thus has discovered the significant relationship between two symmetrical regions in the image, and with the help of rapid synaptic plasticity in the intercolumnar connections ("dynamic links") it is possible to record it, simply strengthening the synaptic connections between all pairs of neurons lying one in each blob. During a sequence of many blob pairs, a full consistent system of point-to-point connections will get established, forming a topological mapping between the symmetric parts of the image.

This sequence of events constitutes the dynamic link mapping mechanism. It is very robust. Occasional erroneous blob pairs are of little consequence whereas all correct blob pairs form a cooperative system of mutual reinforcement. Once the covering of the image with blobs is fairly complete the plexus of reinforced connections stabilizes signal correlations between symmetric points and, as our simulations show, false blob pairs do no longer occur. For each new image (or for each new fixation of an image, for that matter), a new mapping of dynamic links has to be built up.

A slow, and simpler, version of the dynamic link mapping mechanism was first described in Willshaw and von der Malsburg (1976) to account for the ontogenetic establishment of retinotopic mappings from retina to tectum. A dynamic link mapping system using feature labels has later been proposed as a solution to the problem of invariant object recognition (von der Malsburg 1988; Bienenstock and von der Malsburg 1987; Buhmann et al. 1989; Lades et al. 1993). As a mapping system, the present model goes beyond previous work in needing dramatically fewer activation cycles. The columnar connectivity pattern described here was introduced as part of a proposed solution to the figure ground segmentation problem (Schneider 1986; von der Malsburg and Buhmann 1992).

In the explicit model described below some network details are just necessary to realize the qualitative behavior described above. Others, however, we introduced to simplify the dynamics of our system. Prominent among these is the introduction of an "activator cell" (or X-cell) and a "collector cell" (or Y-cell) for each column (see Fig. 2A). The activator cells spontaneously create the active blob and activate all sensorily preactivated neurons in their column. The collector cells sum up all activity that arrives in the preactivated neurons of their column and that comes from the active blob, and they interact to form the shadow blob. Also, active collector cells gate the preactivated neurons in their columns into full activity. The presence of activator cells and collector cells ensures that all preactivated neurons in a column make their firing decision together. Global inhibition between all activator cells and between all collector cells ensures that there is exactly one active blob and exactly one shadow blob at any one time. An activator cell is kept by a compensating inhibitory connection from exciting the collector cell of its own column via its feature cells.

In our explicitly simulated network described below we make the simplifying assumption that during the presentation of an image exactly one of the feature cells in a column is active (corresponding to one of a number of possible gray values). As a consequence, at most one intercolumnar connection is active between two columns at any one time (exactly when the two columns are preactivated with the same gray value). This justifies our introduction of "compound connections" from the ac-

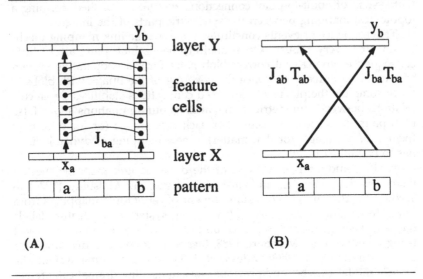

(A)   **(B)**

Figure 2: Architecture of the dynamic link network. (A) The complete architecture. The columns in two positions, a and b are shown. Feature cells
are preactivated by the pattern presented. Columns are connected with each
other by feature-preserving links. These links are rapidly modifiable ("dynamic
links"). Both the activator cells (layer X) and the collector cells (layer Y) have
short-range excitatory and long-range inhibitory connections (not shown) and
each have the tendency to form a local blob. Coupling from an X-cell a to a
Y-cell b is via the preactivated cells in column a, intercolumnar links, and the
preactivated cells in column b. (B) In our case, where only one feature is active
per column, a functionally equivalent description uses the effective connections
$J_{ba}T_{ba}$, where T_{ba} encodes the feature similarity between image positions a and
b (cf. equation 3.1), and J_{ba} is the rapidly modifiable strength of the dynamic
link.

tivator cells to the collector cells, treating all columnar quality cells and
their connections implicitly (see Fig. 2B).

3 Symmetry Detection by Dynamic Link Matching—Explicit Model

After these preparatory heuristic discussions we are ready to introduce
the explicit dynamic link mapping network that we have simulated. It
has the following parts (cf. Fig. 2B). Our image domain is formed by a
grid of 8×8 pixels. Positions in the image domain are designated by
letters $a, b, \ldots$. An input image is described by a distribution of features F_a
over the pixel positions a, where $F_a \in \{1, \ldots, F_{max}\}$ (see Fig. 1). The image
domain is covered by two layers of cells, the X-layer and the Y-layer. The

connection from cell a in the X-layer to cell b in the Y-layer is controlled by the dynamic link variable J_{ba}, which is subject to the dynamic described below. The constraint of feature specificity is formulated with the help of the similarity constraint matrix

$$T_{ba} = \begin{cases} 1 & \text{if } F_a = F_b \text{ and } b \neq a \\ 0 & \text{else} \end{cases} \tag{3.1}$$

The total connection from cell a in the X-layer to cell y in the Y-layer is described by the "effective coupling" $J_{ba}T_{ba}$.

The activities of cells are designated x_a or y_a. Both layers have homogeneous internal connections of the form

$$K_{aa'} = G_{aa'} - \beta \tag{3.2}$$

Here, $G_{aa'}$ is a short-range excitatory connection kernel, and β is the strength of a long-range (here: global) inhibitory connection. For both X and Y we assume wrap-around boundary conditions.

The dynamic of the X-layer is governed by the differential equations

$$\dot{x}_a = -\alpha x_a + \sum_{a'} K_{aa'} S(x_{a'}) + \rho \tag{3.3}$$

Here, $S(x)$ is a sigmoidal nonlinearity that saturates at $S(x) = 0$ for low x and at $S(x) = 1$ for high x, whereas ρ is a constant excitation.

The dynamic of the Y-layer is governed by the differential equations

$$\dot{y}_b = -\alpha y_b + \sum_{b'} K_{bb'} S(y_{b'}) + e \sum_a J_{ba} T_{ba} S(x_a) \tag{3.4}$$

With given effective connections and small noisy initial values (as a model for spontaneous activity) for the x_a, the activator and collector cell activities evolve on a fast time scale towards an equilibrium distribution in the form of local blobs of active cells ($S \approx 1$), with the rest of the cells in the layer X or Y inactive ($S \approx 0$). The size of the blob is controlled by the parameters α, β, and σ, whereas their position is determined by the noise input in the case of X and by the profile of the activation in the case of Y.

Once the activity in X and Y has settled, the dynamic link variables J_{ba} are modified by three consecutive substitutions:

$$\begin{aligned} J_{ba} &\rightarrow J_{ba} + \epsilon J_{ba} T_{ba} S(y_b) S(x_a) \\ &\rightarrow J_{ba} / \sum_{a'} J_{ba'} \\ &\rightarrow J_{ba} / \sum_{b'} J_{b'a} \end{aligned} \tag{3.5}$$

The first step encapsulates the general idea of Hebbian plasticity, though regulated here by the constant ϵ for the rapid time scale of a single image presentation. After the second and third steps the new connections conform to divergent and convergent sum rules.

When an image is presented, the full sequence of events is the following. First, the connections J_{ba} are initialized with a constant value conforming to the sum rules. Then a number of activity-and-modification cycles are carried through. For each of these, the X-activities are initialized with noise distribution, the Y-activities are reset to 0, and the dynamics of X and Y are run according to equations 3.3 and 3.4 to reach stationary values. Then the dynamic links are updated according to equation 3.5. After typically 50–80 such cycles the dynamic links J relax into a stable configuration displaying the underlying symmetry of the actual input image. For a typical result see Figure 4. The network is now ready for permanently recording the symmetry type if it is new, or for recognizing it according to a previously recorded type.

If a link J_{ba} is active, the activity dynamics of equations 3.3 and 3.4 produces correlated activity in the connected cells: In the stationary state towards the end of each cycle, cells a and b are always active or inactive together. In comparison to the dynamic links, activity correlations have the distinction of graceful degradation: Even if a single link is corrupted, the correlation between the corresponding x and y cells is high if there are strong links in the neighborhood (remember that an activity blob always covers a neighborhood along with a given cell).

4 Recording and Recognizing a Symmetry

The main task necessary for solving the symmetry recognition problem is solved for our model by the unsupervised process of dynamic link mapping described in the last section. For a given symmetric pattern it constructs a temporary representation in the form of a set of active links. This set is the same for all input patterns belonging to the same symmetry class. In order to record a symmetry type it is now simply necessary to create hidden units as permanent representatives for some of the active links (or rather the correlations created by them) and to connect them to appropriate output units. Once a symmetry type has been represented by such a network, its second occurrence can be detected and the system is ready to recognize all patterns of this symmetry type as such.

Our recognition network structure is similar to the one used in Sejnowski et al. (1986) and is shown in the upper panel of Figure 3. It consists of three output units C_k, $k = 1, 2, 3$ (sufficient for three symmetry types) and, connected to each output unit, 6 hidden units. Each hidden unit i has a randomly chosen fixed reference cell $a(i)$ in X and plastic synapses w_{ib} from all cells b in Y.[1] The output h_i of a hidden unit is driven by a

---

[1]In principle, the number of hidden units per output cell could be one. Recognition is more reliable and faster, however, if the density of reference cells $a(i)$ is large enough so that most of the active blobs in X hit at least one of them.

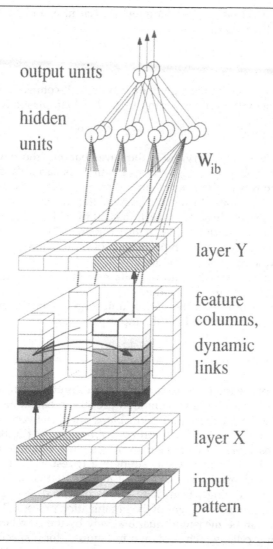

output units

hidden
units

W_{ib}

layer Y

feature
columns,

dynamic

links

layer X

input

pattern

Figure 3: The complete system. An input pattern (lowest layer) is represented by sets of preactivated neurons in the feature columns (marked here by
heavy outline, on the basis of gray levels). Columns are connected by feature-
preserving dynamic links (intercolumnar arrows). The dynamic link mechanism
creates simultaneous blobs in layers X ("active blob") and Y ("shadow blob")
in symmetrically corresponding positions (hatched areas). The symmetry type
is then recorded (when it is new) or recognized (when already known) in the
classification network (upper part). There are six hidden units per output unit
(only four of which are shown). Each hidden unit has one fixed connection to
its output unit, one connection from a randomly chosen X-cell, and has plastic
connections w_{ib} from all Y-cells. These latter connections record a symmetry
type permanently, by being concentrated into the Y-region lying symmetrically
to the location of the X-input of the hidden unit.

coincidence of activity $x_{a(i)}$ of its reference cell in X and activity within its receptive field w_{ib} in Y:

$$h_i = S(x_{a(i)}) \sum_b w_{ib} S(y_b) \tag{4.1}$$

In *recording mode*, hidden units modify their Y-connections w_{ib} at the end of each activity cycle according to the Hebbian plasticity rule:

$$\Delta w_{ib} = \eta S(y_b) \quad \text{if} \quad h_i > \theta \quad \text{and} \quad C_k > 0 \tag{4.2}$$

Synaptic plasticity is supervised in the sense that only those hidden units modify their connections whose output unit C_k is currently activated by a teacher (the role of the teacher simply being to fixate attention on one group of hidden units during the presentation of one pattern). In this way, a hidden unit whose X connection is hit by a blob learns to associate with it the corresponding blob in the Y plane. The whole process is completed for a symmetry type during one presentation (or in some cases two presentations, see below).

In *recognition mode*, the output units perform a leaky integration of the sum of the activities (equation 4.1) of their group of hidden units. After a number of cycles, the output unit with maximal signal is taken to indicate the class into which the input pattern falls.

5 Simulation Results

Simulations of the model were carried out for input patterns of size 8×8. The parameters for the blob formation process in equations 3.3 and 3.4 were adjusted to let the equilibrium blobs cover between 25 and 40% of the layer area; for example, with $\{\alpha, \beta, e, \eta, \epsilon, \rho, \theta\} = \{.3, .85, 1.8, .02, .8, .6, .125\}$ blobs cover 25% of their layer. As convolution kernel $G_{aa'}$ we used a gaussian of width 4 and strength 2.1, restricted, however, to a window of 5×5 pixels. For almost all input patterns, self-organization of the correct mapping J from X to Y was observed. Figure 4 shows a typical example in some stages of the organization process. The degree of organization can be measured quantitatively by the correlation between corresponding cells, which is shown in Figure 5 for a specific input example. During the first 40–50 activation cycles the correlation builds up and reaches almost the theoretical optimum 1. Thus, during all further cycles symmetrically corresponding points in X and Y are marked by strong correlations, whereas pairs of units in far-from-symmetrical positions would have correlation -1.

After learning the specific symmetries from either one or two training examples, the network can generalize almost perfectly to new input patterns of the same symmetry class. Figure 6A shows the classification performance on 200 new examples. There is a clear tradeoff between the reliability of recognition and the required time (in terms of activation

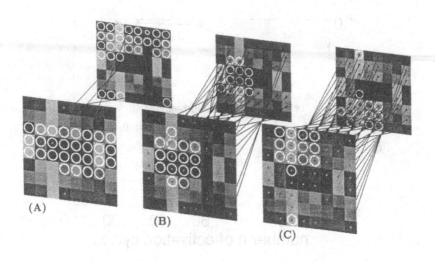

Figure 4: Dynamic link mapping. The network, with layers X (in front) and Y (in the rear) in different activation states, after 15 (A), 50 (B), and 80 (C) activity cycles, all generated for a fixed input pattern of symmetry class **A** (cf. Fig. 1). The dynamic link mapping process is based on a sequence of blob activations (white circles). Dynamic links $J_{ba} \in [0, 1]$ grow between temporally correlated cells. Only links with $J_{ba} \geq 0.4$ are shown in the figure.

cycles). In principle, one example can supply sufficient information for this performance. However, with our parameter settings two examples gave slightly more reliable results (see Fig. 6A).

Our network achieves a recognition reliability of 98%. Its level of reliability is only weakly affected by perturbations to the feature similarity matrix T up to $t = 40\%$ (Fig. 6B). This is due to the robustness of the dynamic link mapping mechanism (see Fig. 5), which creates near-to-perfect signal correlations between symmetric points. Since the hidden units are trained by these correlations, the presence of perturbations in the matrix T even during learning does not affect the performance of the system. We have verified numerically that after training the hidden units with $t = 40\%$ the performance is virtually the same as in Figure 6B, for example, 93% reliability if the recognition is forced after 100 cycles.

6 Discussion

We have presented here a network that is able to discover a system of relations in individual input patterns and to immediately generalize to

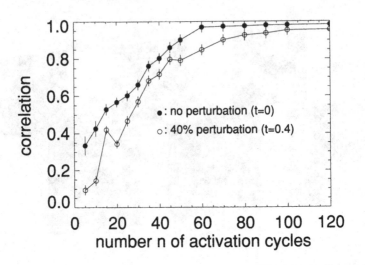

Figure 5: Mean correlation between pairs of corresponding cells in layer X and layer Y for a given state of the dynamic links J after n activation cycles (blob pairs). Correlation is computed as

$$C(x_a, y_{s(a)}) = \frac{\langle x_a y_{s(a)} \rangle - \langle x_a \rangle \langle y_{s(a)} \rangle}{\Delta x_a \, \Delta y_{s(a)}}$$

with $\Delta x = \sqrt{\langle (x - \langle x \rangle)^2 \rangle}$, and $s(a)$ denoting the the cell that lies symmetrically to a. To measure the correlation after n activation cycles, the link state $\{J_{ba}\}$ is frozen after n cycles (by setting $\epsilon = 0$), while the blob activation cycles continue. x_a and $y_{s(a)}$ are the equilibrium activities of cells a and $s(a)$, respectively, and $\langle \cdot \rangle$ denotes averaging over many cycles. Possible correlation values range from -1 for perfect anticorrelation to 1 for perfect correlation. What is displayed is the mean of $C(x_a, y_{s(a)})$ with respect to all possible positions a, and error bars denote the statistical errors when averaging over 900 cycles. Filled circles: Perfect feature similarity matrix $T_{ba} \in \{0, 1\}$. Open circles: All matches $T_{ba} = 1$ are replaced by random values $T_{ba} \in [1 - t, 1]$, all nonmatches $T_{ba} = 0$ by a random $T_{ba} \in [0, t]$, to mimic the effects of noisy feature information. The correlations are robust against this perturbation.

further examples of the same type. The network is based on dynamic link mapping. The self-organization of dynamic links in our model is extremely fast, requiring much less than 100 update cycles. This is due to the use of local feature information in conjunction with a topology constraint. For simplicity, we have used gray-values of single pixels as

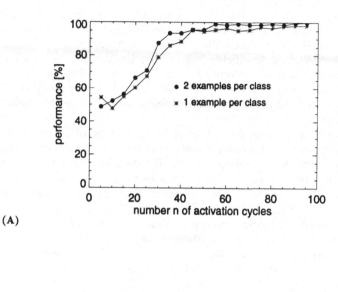

(A)

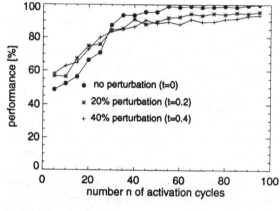

(B)

Figure 6: Symmetry recognition performance. A total of 200 input patterns are classified according to one of three possible symmetries (cf. Fig. 1). The symmetry types have been recorded previously. The percentage of correct decisions is displayed as a function of the number n of activation cycles until the decision is forced. (A) Unperturbed features, $T_{ba} \in \{0,1\}$, training with $k = 1$ or $k = 2$ examples per class, $120/k$ learning steps according to equation 4.2 for each example. (B) Influence on performance of perturbations in the feature similarity matrix T during recognition: The network can tolerate perturbations of $t = 20\%$ or even $t = 40\%$, where t is defined as in Figure 5.

our visual features. In applications to large pixel arrays this would be impractical. The number of dynamic links in the matrix J would have to grow with the fourth power of the linear extent of the input plane. However, if one replaced the gray-level sensitivity of our feature cells by extended receptive fields [e.g., of the Laplace type with a hierarchy of spatial scales, in analogy to the feature jets of (Buhmann et al. 1991)] one could cover the input plane with a fairly low-density set of sampling points and correspondingly operate with manageably small X and Y planes.

The main goal of our paper is to make a point about the learning issue, symmetry detection merely playing the role of an example. It may be interesting, though, to briefly discuss symmetry detection in humans and animals. Infants can detect symmetry at the age of four months (Bornstein et al. 1981). Pigeons learn to discriminate symmetry in very few trials (Delius and Nowak 1982), although one may suspect that they already come equipped with the ability of detecting symmetry and only have to be conditioned for the appropriate response. Our system may shed new light on the old discussion of nature vs. nurture with respect to the symmetry detection issue: Our demonstration that learning time could be extremely short makes it impossible to decide the issue by demonstrating the capability in naive or newborn subjects.

At first sight it is tempting to take our system directly as a model for symmetry detection in primary visual cortex, identifying all of our cell types (X and Y cells, feature cells and hidden units) with neurons found in cortical hypercolumns in area V1. This view would run, however, into a number of difficulties. One of them is the need, in our model, for long-range connections (intercolumnar links and the w_{ib} connections from Y cells to hidden units). With respect to area V1 this requirement creates a conflict, especially in view of the fact that humans are better at detecting symmetry around the vertical midline than around the horizontal (Barlow and Reeves 1979), and callosal connections are absent within V1 except for a narrow seam along the vertical meridian. [This difficulty is mitigated, though, by the fact that symmetry detection in humans relies mainly on a small strip along the symmetry axis of the input pattern, at least in random dot patterns (Julesz 1975).] The problem can be largely avoided by placing our model in a later area in which larger visual angles are spanned by horizontal fibers. Another hint to this effect is the observation that symmetry detection in humans may be based not on distributions of gray levels directly but rather on object shapes reconstructed from shading (Ramachandran 1988). Another difficulty for a direct biological application of our model [which it shares with the one of Sejnowski et al. (1986)] is its lack of invariance with respect to displacement of the symmetry axis, as for instance caused by eye movements during inspection of a pattern. All of these difficulties point to a slightly more complicated model, which would, however, obscure our main point.

Our system is not limited to mirror symmetry. It could equally record and recognize other pattern relations such as simple duplication with or without rotation (or, in a system of only slightly more general form, expansion). Humans, on the other hand, perform much worse on these (Corballis and Roldan 1974). The reason for such differences may be a rather superficial one. Even if the ontogeny of symmetry detection is of the nature we are putting forward here, the system will after some experience be dominated by the hidden units it has acquired. Once these have sufficient density, the dynamic link mechanism is no longer necessary for the recognition of familiar pattern relations [the same way the correct hidden units in Sejnowski *et al.* (1986) are activated directly by the known symmetries]. The relative performance on different problem types is then dominated by experience rather than by the nature of the ontogenetic mechanism. This would explain our bias toward vertical mirror symmetry. The heavy reliance of humans on a strip around the symmetry axis mentioned above may point to a mechanism relying on memorized symmetric shapes, such as butterfly patterns and the like, formed on the basis of a general learning mechanism but soon supplanting it by being more rapidly detected.

The structure of our model fits very well the general character of cortical columnar organization [as also employed in von der Malsburg and Buhmann (1992)]. Of central importance to our system is the encoding of significant relations with the help of temporal signal correlations. Candidate correlations of an appropriate nature have been observed in visual cortex (Gray *et al.* 1989; Eckhorn *et al.* 1988). The model may thus give support to the idea that correlations play an important functional role in cortical information processing.

The central point that we would like to make here refers to the general learning issue. The origin of knowledge in our mind has puzzled philosophers for centuries. Extreme empiricism is not tenable. Its most concrete formulation, nonparametric estimation, shows that it requires astronomical learning times. The opposite extreme, assuming all knowledge to be present in the brain at birth, is equally untenable, not doing justice to the flexibility of our mind, and just putting the burden of statistical estimation on evolution. The only possible way out of this dilemma is the existence of general principles simple enough to be discovered by evolution and powerful enough to make learning a very fast process. This can only be imagined in a universe with profound regularities. The one we are exploiting here is the wide-spread existence of similarities between simultaneously visible patterns. This regularity is captured in the rather simple structure of our network, enabling it to generalize from single examples of symmetrical patterns, in striking contrast to the system of Sejnowski *et al.* (1986), which is based on statistical estimation. With small modifications, dynamic link mapping can be used for the purpose of object recognition invariant with respect to translation, rotation and distortion, making the step from the correspondence of simultaneous patterns to those of consecutive patterns. Again, those transformations could be learned from few examples.

The very simple a priori principles incorporated in the learning system that we have presented are feature correspondence, topology, and rapid synaptic plasticity. We feel that it is structural principles of this general style that make natural brains so extremely efficient in extracting significant structure from complex scenes. Although statistical estimation certainly plays a role for animal learning, it can evidently not be its only basis—natural scenes are too complex, and it is impossible to keep track of the whole combina orics of subpatterns. Potent mechanisms are required to identify significant patterns already within single scenes. Ours may be a candidate.

Acknowledgments

Supported by a grant from the Bundesministerium für Forschung und Technologie (413-5839-01 IN 101 B/9), and a research grant from the Human Frontier Science Program.

References

Ackley, D. H., Hinton, G. E., and Sejnowski, T. S. 1985. A learning algorithm for Boltzmann machines. *Cogn. Sci.* **9**, 147–149.

Barlow, H. B., and Reeves, B. C. 1979. The versatility and absolute efficiency of detecting mirror symmetry in random dot displays. *Vision Res.* **19**, 783–793.

Bienenstock, E., and von der Malsburg, C. 1987. A neural network for invariant pattern recognition. *Europhys. Lett.* **4**, 121–126.

Bornstein, M. H., Ferdinandsen, K., and Gross, C. G. 1981. Perception of symmetry in infancy. *Dev. Psychol.* **17**, 82–86.

Buhmann, J., Lange, J., and von der Malsburg, C. 1989. Distortion invariant object recognition by matching hierarchically labeled graphs. In *IJCNN International Conference on Neural Networks, Washington*, pp. 155–159. IEEE, New York.

Buhmann, J., Lange, J., von der Malsburg, C., Vorbrüggen, J. C., and Würtz, R. P. 1991. Object recognition in the dynamic link architecture—parallel implementation on a transputer network. In *Neural Networks: A Dynamical Systems Approach to Machine Intelligence*, B. Kosko, ed., pp. 121–160. Prentice Hall, New York.

Coolen, A. C. C., and Kuijk, F. W. 1989. A learning mechanism for invariant pattern recognition in neural networks. *Neural Networks* **2**, 495.

Corballis, M. C., and Roldan, C. E. 1974. On the perception of symmetrical and repeated patterns. *Percept. Psychophys.* **16**, 136–142.

Cover, T. M., and Hart, P. E. 1967. Nearest neighbor pattern classification. *IEEE Transact. Inform. Theory* **IT-13**, 21–27.

Crick, F. 1984. Function of the thalamic reticular complex: The searchlight hypothesis. *Proc. Natl. Acad. Sci. U.S.A.* **81**, 4586–4590.

Delius, J. D., and Nowak, B. 1982. Visual symmetry recognition by pigeons. *Psychol. Res.* **44**, 199–212.

Eckhorn, R., Bauer, R., Jordan, W., Brosch, M., Kruse, W., Munk, M., and Reitboeck, H. 1988. Coherent oscillations: A mechanism of feature linking in the visual cortex? *Biol. Cybern.* **60**, 121.

Fix, E., and Hodges, J. L. 1951. *Discriminatory analysis, non-parametric discrimination.* Tech. Rep. USAF School of aviation medicine, Project 21-49-004. Rept. 4.

Gray, C. M., König, P., Engle, A. K., and Singer, W. 1989. Oscillatory responses in cat visual cortex exhibit inter-columnar synchronization which reflects global stimulus properties. *Nature (London)* **338**, 334–337.

Julesz, B. 1975. Experiments in the visual perception of texture. *Sci. Am.* **4**.

Kohonen, T., Barna, G., and Chrisely, R. 1988. Statistical pattern recognition with neural networks: benchmarking studies. *Proceedings of the IEEE ICNN,* San Diego.

Lades, M., Vorbrüggen, J. C., Buhmann, J., Lange, J., von der Malsburg, C., Würtz, R. P., and Konen, W. 1993. Distortion invariant object recognition in the dynamic link architecture. *IEEE Transact. Computers* **10**, 300.

Ramachandran, V. 1988. Perceiving shape from shading. *Sci. Am.* **10**, 76–83.

Reilly, D. L., Cooper, L. N., and Elbaum, C. 1982. A neural model for category learning. *Biol. Cybern.* **45**, 35–41.

Rosenblatt, F. 1962. *Principles of Neurodynamics: Perceptrons and the Theory of Brain Mechanisms.* Spartan Books, Washington, DC.

Rumelhart, D. E., Hinton, G. E., and Williams, R. J. 1986. Learning representations by backpropagating errors. *Nature (London)* **323**, 533–536.

Schneider, W. 1986. Anwendung der Korrelationstheorie der Hirnfunktion auf das akustische Figur-Hintergrund-Problem (Cocktailparty-Effekt). Ph.D. thesis, Universität Göttingen, 3400 Göttingen, Germany.

Sejnowski, T. J., Kienker, P. K., and Hinton, G. E. 1986. Learning symmetry groups with hidden units: Beyond the perceptron. *Physica* **22D**, 260–275.

von der Malsburg, C. 1981. The correlation theory of brain function. Internal report, 81-2, Max-Planck-Institut für Biophysikalische Chemie, Postfach 2841, 3400 Göttingen, Germany.

von der Malsburg, C. 1988. Pattern recognition by labeled graph matching. *Neural Networks* **1**, 141–148.

von der Malsburg, C., and Buhmann, J. 1992. Sensory segmentation with coupled neural oscillators. *Biol. Cybern.* **67**, 233–242.

Willshaw, D. J., and von der Malsburg, C. 1976. How patterned neural connections can be set up by self-organization. *Proc. R. Soc. London* **B194**, 431–445.

Index

Printed in the United States
By Bookmasters